OPTIMIZING COGNITIVE REHABILITATION

Optimizing
Cognitive Rehabilitation

EFFECTIVE INSTRUCTIONAL METHODS

McKay Moore Sohlberg
Lyn S. Turkstra

Foreword by Barbara A. Wilson

THE GUILFORD PRESS
New York   London

© 2011 The Guilford Press
A Division of Guilford Publications, Inc.
72 Spring Street, New York, NY 10012
www.guilford.com

Printed in the United States of America

This book is printed on acid-free paper.

Last digit is print number: 9 8 7 6 5 4 3 2

The authors have checked with sources believed to be reliable in their efforts to provide
information that is complete and generally in accord with the standards of practice that are
accepted at the time of publication. However, in view of the possibility of human error or
changes in behavioral, mental health, or medical sciences, neither the authors, nor the editor
and publisher, nor any other party who has been involved in the preparation or publication
of this work warrants that the information contained herein is in every respect accurate or
complete, and they are not responsible for any errors or omissions or the results obtained from
the use of such information. Readers are encouraged to confirm the information contained in
this book with other sources.

Library of Congress Cataloging-in-Publication Data

Sohlberg, McKay Moore.
   Optimizing cognitive rehabilitation : effective instructional methods / McKay Moore
Sohlberg and Lyn S. Turkstra.
      p. ; cm.
   Includes bibliographical references and index.
   ISBN 978-1-60918-200-7 (hardback: alk. paper)
   1. Brain—Diseases—Patients—Rehabilitation.   2. Cognition Disorders—Patients—
Rehabilitation.   I. Turkstra, Lyn.   II. Title.
   [DNLM: 1. Brain Diseases—rehabilitation.   2. Cognition Disorders—rehabilitation.
WL 348]
   RC386.S64 2011
   616.8′043—dc22
                                                          2011005900

To my parents,
Brian and Sue Moore
—M. M. S.

To my husband, Erwin Montgomery, Jr.
—L. S. T.

About the Authors

McKay Moore Sohlberg, PhD, CCC-SLP, is Full Professor at the University of Oregon, in Eugene, where she directs the master's and PhD training programs in Communication Disorders and Sciences. She is widely known for her pioneering work in the field of cognitive rehabilitation, having authored numerous journal articles, two leading texts in the field, and a number of widely used evidence-based clinical programs. Her research focuses on the development and evaluation of methods to manage acquired deficits in attention, memory, and executive functions. Dr. Sohlberg is supported by a number of federal grants to develop and evaluate assistive technology for individuals with cognitive impairment. She has been active at the national level in the development of evidence-based practice guidelines for cognitive rehabilitation.

Lyn S. Turkstra, PhD, CCC-SLP, is Associate Professor at the University of Wisconsin–Madison, where she directs the Communication and Cognition Laboratory. She is known internationally for her research on cognitive–communication disorders in adolescents and adults with traumatic brain injury (TBI) and has published numerous articles in this area. Her research aims to advance understanding of the cognitive basis of communication problems in individuals with brain injury, particularly in relation to social communication. Dr. Turkstra is board certified by the Academy of Neurologic Communication Disorders and Sciences. She is the lead author of national evidence-based practice guidelines for assessment of individuals with cognitive–communication disorders after TBI and has been active in the development of guidelines for cognitive rehabilitation and interdisciplinary collaboration.

Foreword

This is an exciting time to be involved in neurorehabilitation. Changes are occurring almost daily. Recent important developments include computational modeling to understand recovery from lesions to the brain; new assessment procedures to identify cognitive and emotional problems; new treatment strategies for cognitive, emotional, and psychosocial problems; new theoretical models to improve our understanding of the consequences of brain injury; new technology to help people to compensate for their difficulties; and an increasing recognition of the need to find new ways to evaluate the efficacy of rehabilitation. What has been missing until now, however, is detailed advice on *how* to provide instruction to survivors of brain injury to enable them to learn more efficiently and how to teach them effectively. McKay Moore Sohlberg and Lyn S. Turkstra, two of the most eminent practitioners in neurorehabilitation, have now filled this gap by providing an excellent book with comprehensive, practical, and meticulous advice on how to impart effective instruction to our brain-injured patients receiving rehabilitation.

The main structure or, as the authors say, the *scaffolding*, of the instructional method advocated, is the PIE method (Plan, Implement, and Evaluate). If rehabilitation is not *planned* properly, it is likely to fail. Correct *implementation* requires methods that ensure effective and long-lasting learning and *evaluation*, both within and outside treatment sessions, is essential for measuring success and for making decisions about future management. Quite rightly, the authors insist that we collect clinical data throughout our sessions because they provide essential information that enables us to make evidence-based decisions about the success and failure of our treatments. In addition to the PIE structure, we are encouraged to ask six basic questions for all of our interventions: "Who is the learner?", "What am I teaching?", "Where is the target environment?", "When will the learner implement the target?", "Why am I training this target?", and "How will I teach the target?" The PIE scaffolding and these basic questions are then used to illustrate the most practical part of the book, namely, chapters on training facts and concepts; training functional multistep routines; training the use of external cognitive aids; training the use of metacognitive strategies; and social skills training.

One of the main reasons why *Optimizing Cognitive Rehabilitation: Effective Instructional Methods* is so powerful is that the systematic instruction techniques described by the authors are derived from work in special education, neuropsychology, and cognitive psychology.

Rehabilitation needs a broad theoretical approach. To be constrained by one theory, model, or framework leads to poor clinical practice. The complexity of the process of rehabilitation and the heterogeneity of the people receiving rehabilitation, their many different needs, and the needs of their families means that we need to be guided by a number of different fields, theories, models, and approaches.

I am pleased that the contribution from special education is recognized because I began my professional career working with children who had severe developmental learning difficulties and severe behavior problems. The prevalent philosophy of the staff in the unit where I worked was that "if this child does not learn, it is because the therapists or psychologists have failed to find the right way to help him or her learn." In other words, it was the therapists' or psychologists' responsibility to find a solution or partial solution to any problems faced by these children. I then moved to neuropsychology and found that for many psychologists, the prevailing view was that if the patient failed to learn, it was because he or she had, for example, "frontal lobe damage" or "damage to the hippocampus." In other words, it was the patient's fault and the psychologist was exonerated. To be fair, therapists did not always follow this line of thinking, and many psychologists no longer think this way. I felt much more comfortable with the former theory and feel grateful to those colleagues who influenced me so many years ago. It is more than 30 years since I started working in brain injury rehabilitation, and I still maintain the belief that it is our responsibility to find a way to help our brain-injured patients to learn.

Now, thanks to McKay Moore Sohlberg and Lyn S. Turkstra, we have a book that will provide us with the guidance and structure to enable such learning to take place. I have no doubt that this important book will become essential reading for therapists, speech pathologists, and psychologists working in brain-injury rehabilitation.

BARBARA A. WILSON, PhD
Oliver Zangwill Centre
for Neuropsychological Rehabilitation
Ely, Cambridgeshire
United Kingdom

Acknowledgments

McKay Moore Sohlberg:

I gratefully acknowledge my research colleagues in the field of rehabilitation, education, and computer sciences. Some of you I have either never met or just enjoyed brief encounters at professional venues, but your writing and research have provided a foundation for clinical delivery and models for intervention research relevant to the populations I serve. Other colleagues have been ongoing beacons of research excellence helping our field to advance, notably Barbara A. Wilson and the late Mark Ylvisaker. Katy Mateer will forever be the most formative of mentors. In recent years, I also have been inspired by my computer science colleagues, principally Steve Fickas and Jason Prideaux, who are dedicated to using their trade to develop assistive tools and who are unparalleled in their commitment to people with cognitive impairments.

I thank my patients and their families who have participated in research projects or pursued therapy to improve cognitive functioning and increase independence. Ultimately, you have been my best clinical instructors and mentored me in the effective delivery of cognitive rehabilitation. I am most grateful, however, for your models of resilience, grace, and the power of human relationships to heal. You have helped me understand how meaning can indeed be gained from suffering.

I also thank my students. I am sure I learn more from you than I could ever impart. A special thanks to my doctoral students, whose energy, ideas, and able assistance have made my work possible. You know who you are. The best part is watching you graduate and take up the cognitive rehabilitation challenge in mind and heart.

Finally, I am especially grateful to my parents and siblings, who have shaped and encouraged me in all my endeavors, and to my extended family for being there. Most of all, I wish to acknowledge my husband and daughters. Olof, I must have done something very, very good in my past life to land you for my mate. The same goes for our miraculous girls, Ericka, Tatum, and Emma. You each provide me the inspiration, joy, and encouragement to pursue my interests. I love you so.

Lyn S. Turkstra:

Like McKay, I am sincerely grateful to rehabilitation pioneers like Barbara A. Wilson who have devoted their careers to advancing clinical practice for individuals with brain injury. I would like to give a special acknowledgment to my professional "parents," Audrey Holland and the late Mark Ylvisaker, who taught me what it means to be a lifelong learner, advocate, and multidisciplinary scholar and to take no prisoners when it comes to getting the best services for our clients. I have been privileged to train extraordinarily talented students who will carry these ideas forward and make their own unique contributions to this field.

I thank the many individuals with brain injury, and their families, whom I have come to know over the years. Our shared experiences were the basis for my contributions to this book. You have inspired me to always aim for the highest standard of clinical practice. To therapists who read this book, please tell your clients that the book was made possible by people like them who participated in research and student training.

To my large, creative, and complicated family, I am most indebted. You have participated in my research studies, let me practice nonstandardized tests on you, and contributed wonderful examples for my talks and publications (you probably did not know that last bit). I would particularly like to acknowledge my mother, an early childhood educator, who has been a good listener for so many years that she is now an expert on the differential diagnosis of aphasia versus right-hemisphere communication disorders. I truly could not have done any of this work without the support of all of you.

Both of us wish to acknowledge the staff at The Guilford Press, particularly Editor Rochelle Serwator for her gentle but steady pressure to write this book and for smoothing the way. We would like to thank Senior Production Editor Louise Farkas for her stellar production work and the production staff for their able assistance at every step. We are grateful to Dana Longstreth and an anonymous reviewer for their helpful comments on an earlier version of the book.

Contents

PART I

FOUNDATIONS

CHAPTER 1

Introduction and Overview

WHY A NEUROREHABILITATION BOOK ON INSTRUCTION?

The term *rehabilitation* stems from the latin roots *re-* (again) and *-habilitare* (make fit); the very definition incorporates the concept of teaching actions, behaviors, or information that will make the recipient "fit." *Instruction* is the process of teaching a fact, concept, set of skills, or strategies to another person—precisely the charge to rehabilitation professionals. Physical therapists teach motor sequences to improve patients' mobility, or they teach safety precautions to allow use of an adaptive device. Occupational therapists commonly instruct patients in efficient ways to complete multistep activities of daily living, such as grooming or cooking tasks. Speech–language pathologists frequently teach the use of memory compensation strategies or sequences for safe swallowing. Nurses instruct patients on medication management. Psychologists provide brain injury education or review stress management routines. Instructional targets are central to the rehabilitation process for all professionals.

Neurorehabilitation presents a specific challenge when patients have cognitive impairments that hamper their ability to learn. Myriad acquired neurological conditions can lead to temporary or chronic cognitive impairments, including conditions in which at least some recovery is expected (e.g., traumatic brain injury, stroke, anoxia) as well as progressive conditions in which continued decline is expected (e.g., dementia and other progressive diseases such as multiple sclerosis and Parkinson disease). Acquired neurological injury or disease may cause impairments in the cognitive processes of attention, memory, self-awareness, and executive functioning (Sohlberg & Mateer, 2001b). Each of these cognitive processes plays an important role in rehabilitation, which involves acquisition, mastery, maintenance, and generalization of new learning. Effective rehabilitation for people with acquired cognitive impairments requires professionals to use *specialized* instructional techniques.

Despite the centrality of instruction to the mission of the rehabilitation profession, many disciplines provide little training in the design and delivery of effective teaching methods. In a survey of medical speech–language pathologists working in clinical settings throughout the United States, only one third reported following a systematic

3

instructional approach, and nearly half reported making clinical decisions based on intuition and experience only (Lemoncello & Sohlberg, 2005). The goal of this manual is to fill this gap in professional training programs by providing evidence-based methods for the design, implementation, and evaluation of instructional techniques that are specialized for neurorehabilitation.

SYSTEMATIC INSTRUCTION: INSTRUCTIONAL THEORY IS CRITICAL TO THE DELIVERY OF EFFECTIVE REHABILITATION

Instruction involves both teaching and learning. Other terms for instruction are *training*, *coaching*, *mentoring*, *guiding*, and *co-learning*. In the rehabilitation context, the clinician is generally viewed as the instructor and the client as the learner. This book uses the terms *therapist* and *clinician* to refer to the professional who is planning and facilitating the structured learning. *Client*, *learner*, *patient*, and *individual* are used interchangeably to refer to the person seeking rehabilitation. Support people in the client's life also may be viewed as learners and are key for the success of the training. Depending on the nature of the instruction, these individuals may operate either as co-therapists or as clients receiving the instruction. Support people include *family*, *significant others*, *care providers*, and *community sources of support*. Delivering effective rehabilitation to the learner requires that clinicians understand the roles each of these different people play in the process.

When consulting a professional manual, readers should expect that recommended techniques are based on research evidence whenever it is available, or, at minimum, are grounded in a solid theoretical framework and follow principles of rational decision making (Ylvisaker, 2002). The techniques discussed in this manual can be classified as *systematic instruction* (Ehlhardt, Sohlberg, et al., 2008). The theory underlying systematic instruction is that persons with learning challenges benefit most from structured training that includes *explicit models*, *a minimization of errors* during initial acquisition (to prevent the learning of errors), *strategies to promote learner engagement*, and *carefully guided practice* to enhance mastery, maintenance, and generalization across contexts. The key to systematic instruction is the deliberate use of specific techniques designed to enhance the likelihood that information will be learned and stored in memory. In this book, we provide methods for applying these techniques to the rehabilitation of individuals with acquired cognitive impairments.

Systematic instruction contrasts with other instructional models that rely on the learner to experiment and draw conclusions from his or her performance. The latter models include *discovery learning* (i.e., exploratory learning) (Hammer, 1997) and *trial-and-error* learning (sometimes referred to as "learning through errors" or "learning from consequences"). In a trial-and-error model, the clinician sets up the environment to allow the client to explore and develop his or her own understanding of target concepts or strategies. The instructor's role is to observe errors and provide feedback. Readers may be familiar with this approach as the educational foundation of the Montessori method (Montessori & George, 1912). The assumption underlying this approach is that learners are capable of critically analyzing events and forming their own conclusions about their experiences; most important, it assumes that the learners are *able to learn from their mistakes*. Trial-and-error learning is the most common instructional method in rehabilitation; however, often it is not the most effective method for clients with significant cognitive impairments. Robust research supports the use of systematic instruction rather than trial-and-error learning for individuals with acquired cognitive impairments. This research is summarized in Chapter 2.

The systematic instruction techniques described in this manual were derived from work in special education, neuropsychology, and cognitive psychology. In the next section, we provide an overview of relevant foundational work from each of these disciplines.

Influences from Special Education

The field of special education has generated a substantial body of instructional research showing the efficacy of systematic instruction. The two research-based approaches within special education that have most influenced training practices in neurorehabilitation are *direct instruction* and *strategy instruction* (see detailed reviews in Ehlhardt et al., 2008, and Sohlberg & Ehlhardt, 2005).

Direct Instruction

The instructional model that has been subjected to the most experimental scrutiny is direct instruction (DI), pioneered by Engelmann and Carnine (1991). DI is a comprehensive, explicit instructional method shown to be effective in teaching a wide range of material across different populations with learning challenges, particularly individuals with learning disabilities (Engelmann & Carnine, 1991; Stein, Carnine, & Dixon, 1998). DI requires systematic design and delivery of instruction in order to facilitate efficient acquisition and generalization of a variety of targets, including facts, concepts, multistep procedures, skills, and strategies. The following key techniques are associated with the DI design–delivery process (Engelman & Carnine, 1991; Marchand-Martella & Slocum, 2004; Stein et al., 1998):

- Analyzing and sequencing instructional content (i.e., task analysis)
- Training in a broad range of examples
- Using simple, consistent instructional wording
- Establishing a high mastery criterion
- Providing models and carefully faded prompts
- Providing high amounts of correct massed practice following distributed practice
- Providing cumulative review

DI has been increasingly applied to the rehabilitation of individuals with acquired brain injury because of its effectiveness in teaching new facts and skills to people with profound anterograde memory impairments (Glang, Singer, Cooley, & Tish, 1992).

Strategy Instruction

Strategy-based instruction is another instructional approach that has been experimentally evaluated within special education (Englert, Raphael, Anderson, Anthony, &

Stevens, 1991; Graham, MacArthur, & Schwartz, 1995). This approach, which can be integrated with the previously described DI approach, teaches learners to monitor their own thinking. Different terms are sometimes used to describe strategy-based instruction, including *procedural facilitators*, *scaffolded instruction*, *cognitive strategies*, and *metacognitive strategy instruction* (Baker, Gersten, & Scanlon, 2002; Dunlosky, Hertzog, Kennedy, & Thiede, 2005; Englert et al., 1991; Harris & Pressley, 1991; Stein et al., 1998). Core strategy instructional techniques (Baker et al., 2002; Kim, Vaughn, Wanzek, & Wei, 2004; Swanson, 2001) include:

- Establishing the context for learning (i.e., helping learners see the "big picture") by using tools such as graphic organizers or simple outlines of important themes or concepts
- Using questions and/or prompts to encourage learner self-assessment
- Teaching the learner to use self-regulation scripts to summarize and elaborate on content (e.g., "Have I checked my work?")

Although the principles of strategy training are included in most types of rehabilitation, the most direct application occurs in *metacognitive strategy training* (Kennedy, Krause, & Turkstra, 2008), which is discussed in Chapter 8.

Several meta-analyses have attempted to parse out the most effective instructional practices and components within the special education literature (Adams & Engelmann, 2006; Kavale & Forness, 2000; Mastropieri, Scruggs, Bakken, & Whedon, 1996; Swanson, 1999, 2001; Swanson, Carson, & Sachse-Lee, 1996; Swanson & Hoskyn, 1998). Particularly pertinent is the series of meta-analyses by Swanson and colleagues (1996–2001). Following an extensive search yielding over 900 data-based articles, the authors selected 180 studies that met specific inclusion criteria (e.g., inclusion of a comparison/control group, sufficient data to calculate effect sizes). These studies were categorized into one of four groups based on the instructional techniques employed. The results indicated that a model using both DI and strategy instruction techniques *in concert* produced the largest effect size. Strategy instruction alone, DI alone, and nondirect or nonstrategy instruction showed respectively smaller effect sizes. A more recent meta-analysis by Graham and Harris (2003) also supported the effectiveness of self-regulation strategy development for a variety of students with and without disability. These meta-analyses are part of a rich experimental literature within the field of special education that supports the use of explicit, systematic instructional techniques to effectively teach individuals with learning disabilities (Sohlberg et al., 2005).

Influences from Neuropsychology

The field of neuropsychology has built upon the special education research and evaluated instructional design and teaching procedures for people with acquired neurogenic memory disorders. Chapter 2 examines the research literature on teaching procedures and information for individuals with acquired memory impairments due to brain injury or related conditions. The chapter restates and expands an evidence-based practice guideline paper for clinicians working in the field of cognitive rehabilitation (Ehlhardt et al., 2008). It is this body of research that led to the development of the current manual. Specific evidence-based methods discussed in that chapter include scaffolding instruction, errorless instruction, distribution of practice trials, and incorporation of metacognitive strategies.

Taken together, studies in educational psychology and neuropsychology have demonstrated the effectiveness of a combined approach that incorporates the principles of DI and strategy instruction. This approach has been specifically evaluated in students with learning disabilities and in adults with a variety of cognitive impairments.

Influences from Cognitive Psychology

Working effectively with clients who have cognitive impairments requires that clinicians have a basic understanding of memory processes, and it is in the discovery of these processes that cognitive psychology has made its greatest contribution to rehabilitation. In this section, we briefly review some key memory concepts from cognitive psychology that assist with understanding and implementing the techniques described in this manual. This information applies to any type of therapy: Whether training physical movements, daily activities, or behavioral routines, clinicians will want to exploit residual memory abilities and compensate for weaknesses in order to support their clients' learning.

Memory is not a unitary process, but a dynamic alliance of interrelated subsystems that rely on different brain structures and connections. We review two main constructs of memory that are critical for rehabilitation providers: (1) types of memory and (2) of key learning mechanisms.

Among memory types, a critical clinical distinction is between the two main time-dependent forms of memory—*long-term* versus *short-term memory*—which are primarily distinguished by (1) the duration of the memory store and (2) the capacity of the memory store. Long-term memory holds information in a permanent "store" and is thought to have unlimited capacity. Short-term memory is what is "on your mind" at any moment in time, your "mental workspace" (Baddely, Eysenck, & Anderson, 2009). It is what a person can hold in conscious thought (if he or she is not interrupted) and thus has a short duration and a limited capacity (about seven items or chunks of information). The original notion of short-term memory has been subsumed into the current term, *working memory*. The term *working memory* refers to both the short-term storage of information and also the active process of manipulating that information either for storage or retrieval (Baddely et al., 2009). Working memory allows us to temporarily hold information in mind while applying strategies such as elaboration during learning (Markowitsch, 1998), or while searching long-term memory for an idea or word we are trying to retrieve.

Working memory is important for rehabilitation specialists to understand because it is often disrupted following brain injury. It allows us to perform complex activities such as reasoning, learning, and comprehension. It also is the mental workspace for *executive functions*—the cognitive processes that underlie goal-directed behavior—and *metacognition*—the process of thinking about one's own thinking and making adjustments accordingly. A person with a working memory impairment might appear to have an executive function impairment, because he or she cannot hold information in mind long enough to plan, organize, or sequence it. What appears to be a deficit in metacognition (i.e., lack of awareness of one's deficits) also can be due to working memory impairments, because it is difficult to reflect on one's own performance when working memory resources are already consumed by task performance (Kennedy et al., 2008).

Long-term memory encompasses a number of different types of memory distinguished by the types of information stored and how that information is learned and retrieved. Table 1.1 provides definitions of key types of long-term memory. The most basic distinction is between *explicit* or *declarative* memory and *implicit* or *nondeclarative memory*. Declarative memory constitutes a knowledge base of information about which we have conscious awareness. Two distinct categories of declarative memory are semantic and episodic memory. *Semantic memory* is our mental encyclopedia and comprises our knowledge base. *Episodic memory* is memory for temporally related events and comprises our autobiographical memory. Although these represent different systems of learning, they are highly interdependent at both encoding and retrieval phases of learning. For example, existing knowledge (semantic knowledge) affects the learning of new episodic memories in both healthy and impaired learners (Greenberg & Verfaellie, 2010).

Declarative learning is enhanced by conscious strategies such as elaboration, trial-and-error, or discovery methods. It is not tied to the learning context, so it can be generalized to other situations. For example, you can probably recall a family holiday event from your childhood without physically being in the setting in which it occurred, although that setting might provide useful cues to help retrieve specific memories. Retrieval of long-term declarative memory is helped by meaning cues and prompts, as well as by an effortful search of long-term memory (e.g., thinking of relatives who might have been at that family event, or eliciting hints from family members). Because declarative memory is conscious, it is encoded and retrieved using working memory. This is another case in which a working memory impairment can masquerade as a long-term declarative memory impairment: If the client cannot hold information in mind long enough to use a strategy, he or she might appear to have a declarative memory impairment. If the information is divided into smaller chunks or made simpler, however, or if distractions are reduced, the client might perform normally.

Nondeclarative memory allows a person to learn without having conscious awareness of the learning. It is *probabilistic*: That is, what is learned is the information or skill that has the highest probability of being repeated, regardless of the importance of the stimulus. Stated another way, "Practice makes perfect." When nondeclarative memory

TABLE 1.1. Definitions of Content-Dependent Forms of Memory

Types of long-term memory	Description
Declarative memory	Explicit knowledge base; information held with conscious awareness
Episodic memory	Storage of events that are tagged in time and place
Semantic memory	Storage of facts and concepts
Metamemory	Awareness of one's own memory functioning
Prospective memory	Remembering to initiate future intentions
Nondeclarative memory	Implicit memory; doesn't require conscious awareness of learning
Procedural memory	Acquisition of rules, sequences, and perceptual motor skills
Emotional associations	Association of feelings with people and events
Priming	Increased probability of producing a response because of having previously produced it

fails, attempts to consciously retrieve it are unhelpful. For example, to remember the number of days in a month, many people have learned the "30 days has September ... " rhyme. To recall a particular month, it is often necessary to start at the beginning of the rhyme. Hints, cues, and encouragement to "try harder" (all of which rely on declarative memory processes) are likely to be less effective.

Unlike declarative memory, nondeclarative memory is highly context dependent. You might be able to recall a childhood family event by thinking consciously about it, but you are unlikely to remember procedural information such as how you learned the social skills you used on that day or how you learned to hold your fork at dinner. Because of this context dependence, nondeclarative memories do not automatically generalize except to situations with highly similar surface features. This *hyperspecificity* of learning is a challenge in rehabilitation and likely underlies much of the failure to generalize treatment gains outside of the clinic. Strategies to promote generalization of nondeclarative learning are discussed in subsequent chapters. As a resource for this manual and for clinicians working in the field of neurorehabilitation, Appendix 1.1 provides a list of terms relevant to learning and memory processes.

People with memory impairment may experience preservation of some types of memory and not others, which is why it is critical that rehabilitation professionals understand these distinctions. In general, the evidence suggests that the nondeclarative forms of memory that involve implicit learning and may allow learning without conscious awareness can be preserved in people with amnesia (Squire, 1992). Some of the techniques discussed in this book, such as spaced retrieval and errorless learning, take advantage of intact nondeclarative memory.

It can be helpful to understand disorders of memory and patterns of memory loss. *Anterograde memory loss* affects the ability to remember events occurring after the onset of a memory problem; most of the techniques described in this book address this type of memory loss. *Retrograde memory loss* refers to the inability to remember declarative information prior to a neurological insult. *Posttraumatic amnesia* involves the period of time, usually following decreased consciousness, when an individual is unable to consolidate or lay down new declarative memories.

THE NEUROREHABILITATION LANDSCAPE

The field of neurorehabilitation has traditionally classified treatment approaches as either those that attempt to decrease impairments in basic cognitive functions (i.e., "restorative approaches") or those that develop strategies to maximize function, with or without changes in underlying cognitive impairments (i.e., "compensatory approaches"). An example of a restorative, or impairment-based, cognitive intervention is direct attention training (Sohlberg, McLaughlin, Pavese, & Posner, 2005), a drill-oriented therapy with hierarchical exercises designed to increase attentional capacity. An example of a compensatory intervention might be teaching the use of external memory aids (e.g., Emslie, Wilson, Quirk, Evans, & Watson, 2007). This binary classification, however, quickly becomes muddy. Instructing individuals to use compensatory strategies may be associated with improved processing if their use of those strategies allows them to engage in thinking activities that improve cognitive functioning (e.g., there is some evidence that metacognitive strategy training improves other aspects of executive function;

Ylvisaker & Feeney, 2000). Conversely, improvements following restorative approaches may be due to a change in the individual's approach to a situation rather than a result of strengthening a cognitive ability. While we can categorize the *supposed target* of the treatment, it is not always possible to determine *which underlying mechanism was responsible* for changes.

In recent years, a third category has been added to the cognitive rehabilitation toolkit: therapies targeting metacognition (Kennedy et al., 2008), as noted above in the category of *strategy instruction. Metacognition* (literally, "knowing about knowing") refers to the processes involved in appraising one's own knowledge and skills and includes both the ability to monitor one's thinking and the ability to use that information to regulate one's behavior. Metacognitive deficits are the neuropsychological basis for *anosognosia*—the lack of awareness of deficits shown by individuals with certain types of brain injury—and often are seen in the early postinjury stage, regardless of lesion site. As common impediments to progress in rehabilitation and return to the community, metacognitive deficits are a logical target of intervention. An example of a metacognitive approach is training people in the use of a strategy that helps them monitor their own speed and accuracy during task completion (Levine et al., 2000).

Although the three approaches just discussed are based on different theoretical models and practice disciplines, all require some type of structured environmental experience in order for the client to learn, maintain, and transfer the skill to functional contexts. Structuring input in deliberate ways while providing multiple opportunities for repetition is at the heart of systematic instruction, whether repetitively stimulating an impaired cognitive process, training the steps of a specific functional activity, or practicing strategy use in a new context.

Exciting advances in the rehabilitation landscape are emerging from the field of neuroscience, including studies showing that brain structures and functions change in response to structured input and repetition (Kleim & Jones, 2008); such studies support the principles of systematic instruction. The umbrella term for the brain changes is *neuroplasticity*, and it encompasses the set of processes by which the healthy brain encodes experience and learns new behaviors and the damaged brain relearns lost behaviors or learns compensatory behaviors. Neurons have an extraordinary facility to modify their structure, connections, and function in response to differing internal and external forces across the lifespan (Turkstra, Holland, & Bays, 2003). A major focus of neuroscience research has been to explain the *underlying mechanisms* responsible for these changes, so that they can be applied to improve rehabilitation outcomes.

Kleim and Jones (2008) reviewed decades of basic neuroscience research and generated a list of neuroplasticity principles that they believe to be especially relevant to rehabilitation after brain damage. Whereas this research focused primarily on motor skills, a follow-up paper translated these findings into rehabilitation for aphasia (Raymer et al., 2008) and generated a road map for rehabilitation research in the future. Table 1.2 lists the principles outlined by Kleim and Jones (2008), and suggests implications for cognitive rehabilitation and instructional practices.

The principles in Table 1.2 suggest that a supportive rehabilitation environment will provide the opportunity for high-intensity, high-frequency repetition of meaningful and functional skills, in a context that is as similar as possible to the one in which those skills will be used, and extending into the chronic stage post-onset with the opportunity for maintenance of skills. This environment will consider the age of the learner (a

TABLE 1.2. Principles of Experience-Dependent Neural Plasticity

Principle	Description	Implication for instruction
Influences on design of instruction—planning matters		
Specificity	The nature of the training experience dictates the nature of the plasticity.	During initial acquisition training, strive to make stimuli and contexts as similar to target task as possible.
Interference	Plasticity in response to one experience can interfere with the acquisition of other behaviors.	During initial acquisition training, make sure that training does not address multiple salient targets simultaneously.
Salience matters	The training experience must be sufficiently salient to induce plasticity.	Target tasks and behaviors that are relevant and meaningful to the learner.
Time matters	Different forms of plasticity occur at different times during training: High-frequency intervention in the acute stage may be damaging to the brain but has been associated with significant benefits in the chronic stage.	Take careful data to evaluate response to intervention and do not assume that the opportunity for meaningful change ends after spontaneous recovery has peaked.
Age matters	The effects of intervention are different at different ages: Very young brains (<1 year) may have plasticity that is not adaptive; older brains (>65 years) are less plastic than younger brains (1–65 years).	Whereas younger brains may have a greater ability to substitute function, they have fewer established pathways to support learned behaviors. All ages can benefit from rehabilitation, but plasticity will operate differently at different ages.
Influences on implementation of instruction—practice matters		
Use it or lose it	Failure to use specific brain functions can lead to functional decline in those functions.	Gains require maintenance over time or they may reverse: Consider long-term maintenance schedules.
Use it and improve it	Training that drives a specific brain function can lead to an enhancement of that function.	Focus on specific, functional targets.
Repetition matters	Induction of plasticity requires sufficient repetition.	Provide high amounts of practice.
Intensity matters	Induction of plasticity requires sufficient training intensity.	Provide intensive practice (e.g., massed practice) during initial target acquisition.
Transference	Plasticity in response to one training experience can enhance the acquisition of similar behaviors.	Actively promote generalization to similar treatment targets.

Note. Adapted from Kleim and Jones (2008). Copyright 2008 by the American Speech–Language–Hearing Association. Adapted by permission.

growing concern with the aging population due to a lack of experimental literature on neurohabilitation in aging) and will capitalize on skills and knowledge that have developed over each individual's lifetime. It will provide opportunities for learning but not overwhelm the learner, and it will limit interference effects from competing simuli and goals.

Neuroplasticity research has shown that the brain changes in response to both internal input (e.g., medications that change neuronal responses) and external input (e.g., training and instruction). In this manual, we review the evidence-based practice techniques supporting effective *external input* to improve rehabilitation outcomes, with the understanding that effective instruction both promotes and exploits experience-dependent neuroplasticity. Many of the principles outlined in Table 1.2 match the instructional tenets articulated in this manual. For example, effective instructional planning requires careful consideration of generalizable features (i.e., specificity and interference), personal factors (i.e., age and time postonset), and environmental contextual factors (i.e., salience) that can enhance learning. Similarly, effective instruction can enhance neural plasticity by providing intensive practice (i.e., repetition and intensity) of functional rehabilitation targets (i.e., use it or lose it). In summary, there is a clear overlap between effective instructional practices and factors that enhance neuroplasticity.

Our understanding of neurological recovery mechanisms and response to stimulation is rapidly expanding, particularly with the advent of sophisticated functional imaging methods that permit the analysis of changes over time (Strangman et al., 2005). Practitioners should be aware of these studies, as they have direct implications for rehabilitation, and the results may influence not only the types and dosage schedules of treatment but also the measurement of outcomes.

TARGET AUDIENCE FOR THIS MANUAL

This instructional manual describes the research support for implementing systematic instructional practices, and it provides a framework for specifically planning, implementing, and evaluating such practices in a rehabilitation context. Here, we describe two facets of our target audience.

Practitioners

We hope that practitioners in a variety of rehabilitation disciplines will use this manual. We believe that all team members—including physicians, nurses, therapists, case managers, social workers, dieticians, and rehabilitation psychologists—can improve patient learning and ultimately patient outcomes by implementing aspects of systematic instruction.

Client Population

As discussed in Chapters 2 and 3, clients with a variety of cognitive impairments can benefit from the systematic instruction techniques we describe in this manual. The specific principles have been designed for learners with impairments in attention, memory, executive functions, or metacognition; for those with impairments that cross multiple cognitive domains; and for those with mild to severe impairments. The evidence to date and our own clinical experience also suggest that elements of systematic instruction can benefit individuals with progressive and nonprogressive conditions, during the acute, postacute, and chronic phases of recovery or disease.

ORGANIZATION OF THE BOOK

This instructional manual is divided into two parts. The first part—Chapters 1–4—provides the theoretical foundation. Chapter 2 presents a review of the literature regarding the use of specific instructional supports for individuals with acquired cognitive impairments. Chapter 3 provides a framework for considering additional contextual factors that affect learning and practice parameters that enhance neural plasticity. Chapter 4 outlines a framework for designing, delivering, and evaluating effective instruction, and it supports the organization of the second part of the book.

The second part—Chapters 5–9—provides specific guidelines for planning, implementing, and evaluating systematic instruction across specific domains. Application exercises are also provided to give clinicians practice opportunities with clinical concepts. The instructional targets include facts and concepts (Chapter 5), multistep procedures (Chapter 6), external aids (Chapter 7), strategies (Chapter 8), and social skills (Chapter 9). Each of these chapters contains clinical forms and examples to guide the design of instruction (i.e., planning), implementation (including scripts, steps, and procedures), data collection, and monitoring, and application exercises. To assist readers, relevant forms for clinicians to use in their clinical practice are provided in the Appendix and in .pdf format on the book's page on The Guilford Press website (*www.guilford.com*).

APPENDIX 1.1. Glossary of Key Memory and Learning Terms

anterograde amnesia: Impairment in ability to encode, store, or retrieve declarative information that is encountered after the neurological event that caused the amnesia occurred.

consolidation: The time-dependent processes that stabilize a memory trace in the neural connections after the initial acquisition.

declarative memory: The conscious, intentional recollection of experiences (episodic memory) and information (semantic memory); often used synonymously with *explicit memory*.

distributed practice: Breaking up practice into a series of shorter sessions; often conducted in an expanded rehearsal format where there is a gradual increase in the time interval between the practice trials.

elaboration: A process that encourages a deeper level of processing than simply rehearsing. Creating a visual image or trying to remember a special feature of target information are examples of elaboration.

episodic memory: Memory of autobiographical events (times, places, contextual knowledge) that can be explicitly stated. Together with semantic memory, it makes up the category of declarative memory.

errorless learning: The minimization of error responses during the presentation of target stimuli.

explicit memory: The conscious, intentional recollection of experiences (episodic memory) and information (semantic memory); often used synonymously with *declarative memory*.

implicit memory: Retrieval occurs from long-term memory through the repeated performance of tasks rather than conscious recall; often referred to as *nondeclarative memory*. Priming is an example of implicit memory, and procedural memory is a form of implicit memory. It uses a different memory system than explicit/declarative memory.

long-term memory: Memories that are a part of a durable store. Short-term memories become long-term memories through processes of repetition and association.

maintenance: Preservation of memories or skills over time.

metacognition: Knowledge about one's own thinking and an ability to regulate its functioning. The use of strategies to help remember information is an example of metacognitive ability.

nondeclarative memory: Retrieval occurs from long-term memory through the repeated performance of tasks rather than conscious recall; often referred to as *implicit memory*. It uses a different system than declarative/explicit memory.

posttraumatic amnesia (PTA): The state of confusion and inability to form new declarative memories after a traumatic brain injury; usually improves over time.

procedural memory: A form of implicit/nondeclarative memory that lets people perform actions, such as riding a bike or tying shoelaces, without conscious attempt at recall.

priming: The process whereby exposure to an item influences the processing of the subsequent item.

prospective memory: Remembering to initiate intended actions at a future time.

retrieval: The process of recovering an intended memory, usually through the use of cues that bring it into awareness.

retrograde amnesia: Impairment in declarative memory for information and events experienced prior to the event that caused the amnesia.

semantic memory: The storage of accumulated concept-based knowledge. Together with episodic memory, it makes up the category of declarative memory.

working memory: The processes responsible for holding information in short-term memory; often referred to as the "temporary scratch pad" for declarative memory and encompasses the processes necessary for holding on to and manipulating information.

CHAPTER 2

The Research Evidence

The purpose of this chapter is to review the research evidence supporting different instructional practices for people with acquired learning and memory problems. The chapter is divided into two sections. The initial section presents adapted portions of a published paper on clinical guidelines that analyzed two decades of neuropsychological intervention studies evaluating instructional practices for people with acquired brain injury (Ehlhardt et al., 2008).[1] The review of the guidelines paper is included in this book as a resource to those readers interested in an analysis of the instructional research literature. We recognize that it is more detailed than many clinicians will need or desire. However, we feel that it is important to have a place that consolidates and analyzes the research evidence supporting many of the techniques described in this book. Also, we want to support clinicians' use of prefiltered evidence, such as practice guidelines, to encourage engagement in evidence-based practice. The intervention practices described in Chapters 5–9 are based on the literature summarized here.

The second section reviews more recent articles published since the guidelines paper and compares them to the recommendations from that paper. Treatment implications of the research are discussed under the "Article Summary" and "Conclusion" subheadings for each section.

EVIDENCE-BASED PRACTICE GUIDELINES FOR INSTRUCTING INDIVIDUALS WITH ACQUIRED MEMORY IMPAIRMENTS: WHAT HAVE WE LEARNED IN THE PAST 20 YEARS?

The goal of this section is to identify effective instructional practices in cognitive rehabilitation that the research literature supports with a reasonable degree of certainty. The material in this section is part of a series of evidence-based practice guidelines for

---

[1] Adapted from Ehlhardt et al. (2008). Published by Psychology Press. Copyright 2008 by Taylor & Francis Group. Adapted by permission.

the treatment of individuals with traumatic brain injury (TBI), generated by the Academy of Neurologic Communication Disorders and Sciences (ANCDS; *www.ancds.org/ practice.html*). The literature search includes studies in which participants had acquired brain injury (ABI) of nontraumatic origin (e.g., via stroke, anoxia, tumors, infectious diseases), as well as individuals with progressive neurological disorders (e.g., dementia), to take advantage of research on other neurogenic populations in which learning and memory problems are a central deficit (Ylvisaker et al., 2002). Studies of individuals with schizophrenia also are reviewed, as there is increasing evidence that deficits in new learning and memory in this group are similar to those in people with ABI (McKenna, Clare, & Baddeley, 1995).

Identifying, Gathering, and Extracting Intervention Studies

The following data bases were searched for articles published between 1986 and 2006: Academic Search Premier, Education Research Complete, ERIC, Medline, Psychology and Behavioral Sciences Collection, and PsycINFO. The search methods initially yielded 2,155 records, which were narrowed to 857 records for review. The final evidence base included 51 studies. Readers are referred to the original article (Ehlhardt et al., 2008) for a detailed description of the search process, including key terms and inclusion criteria.

As part of the ANCDS practice guidelines for individuals with Alzheimer-type dementia, Hopper et al. (2005) conducted a systematic review of the literature on one specific memory technique, spaced retrieval training (SRT), so those studies were not included in this review. However, studies evaluating SRT in the TBI population were included in the review, as well as studies from the dementia literature that were not included in the review by Hopper and colleagues.

Reviewing and Coding Studies into Tables of Evidence

Tables of evidence were organized by identifying relevant parameters in four key domains: population sample, intervention, study design, and treatment outcomes. The full tables of evidence are presented in three appendices: Appendix 2.1 displays the coded population sample characteristics, Appendix 2.2 displays the coded intervention characteristics, and Appendix 2.3 displays the coded parameters related to study design and outcomes. There are three possible types of coding for each parameter: (1) a description of the relevant study content; (2) a mark of "1" or "0" indicating that the authors did or did not report that parameter; and (3) as described later, a mark of +, /, or – in relation to outcome of the treatment, indicating positive, qualified, or negative findings, respectively. There were 38 studies in ABI, 7 in dementia, and 6 in schizophrenia/ schizoaffective disorder, and these three separate groups are listed in each appendix to allow for population-specific analyses.

One author coded all 51 intervention studies, whereas another author conducted reliability coding for 26 out of the 51 (51%) for all coding parameters except for the type of instruction and four of the outcome components (immediate outcomes, ecological validity, generalization, and maintenance). A third author also coded these five parameters for all 51 studies. Interrater reliability was 90% or better for all coding parameters, and all disagreements were resolved by discussion.

Coding Results

This section summarizes relevant population sample characteristics across the three population groups (see Appendix 2.1 for details).

Number of Participants, Age, Gender, Etiology, Site of Injury, Time Postonset

ACQUIRED BRAIN INJURY

The 38 studies reviewed included 451 experimental participants with memory impairment, 42 control participants with acquired cognitive disabilities, and 163 nondisabled control participants. Ages ranged from 18 to 78 years, with two studies involving children ages 8–11 years. The experimental participants were predominantly adult males (>2:1). The etiology of memory impairment included a wide range of conditions: TBI, cerebral vascular accident (CVA; including anterior and posterior communicating artery hemorrhage), encephalitis, brain tumor, Korsakoff's syndrome, anoxia, brain abscess, Parkinson's disease, toxicity, encephalopathy, and cerebral infection. Site of injury and/or imaging findings were reported in 17/38 (45%) of the studies. Time postonset (TPO) was reported in 31/38 (82%) of the studies with the majority of participants between 1 year and several years postonset. Only three studies included participants with symptom onset of less than 1 year (Dou, Man, Ou, Sheng, & Tam, 2006; Glisky & Delaney, 1996; Wilson, Baddeley, Evans, & Shiel, 1994).

DEMENTIA

Across the seven studies, there were 55 experimental participants and 8 nondisabled control participants, ranging in age from 65 to 89 years. The participants were predominantly male, with Alzheimer's dementia as the most common etiology, followed by vascular dementia. Imaging findings were reported in 3/7 (43%) of the studies. Symptom onset date was reported in 2/7 (29%) of the studies and ranged from 18 months to 5 years prior to the study (Clare et al., 2000; Haslam, Gilroy, Black, & Beesley, 2006).

SCHIZOPHRENIA/SCHIZOAFFECTIVE DISORDER

Across the six studies in this group, there were 203 participants with schizophrenia/schizoaffective disorder and memory impairment, 21 control participants with schizophrenia/schizoaffective disorder without memory impairment, and 88 nondisabled control participants. The experimental participants were predominantly male, and ages ranged from 18 to 55 years, with the majority of participants in the 30- to 40-year age range. Site of injury/imaging findings were not reported. Symptom onset date was determined by the date of first hospitalization relative to the start of the study, and ranged from 1 month to 34.7 years.

Neuropsychological Testing, Premorbid IQ, Initial Severity, Memory Severity, Dual Diagnosis/Comorbidity, Selection Criteria

ACQUIRED BRAIN INJURY

Neuropsychological test data were included in all 38 studies; however, the type and number of measures used varied considerably across studies. Premorbid IQ was reported in 10/38 (26%) of the studies. Initial severity (length of coma and/or posttraumatic amnesia) was reported in 12/38 (32%) of the studies and was not relevant to participants in several studies because of the etiology (e.g., Korsakoff's syndrome). Severity of memory impairment was reported in 33/38 (87%) of the studies. Of these, 18/33 (55%) reported that the impairment was "severe," "profound," "marked," "significant," or "chronic, affecting everyday memory." Few studies described the specific type of memory impairment. Descriptors reported typically included "anterograde" or "episodic" memory impairments (e.g., Andrewes & Gielewski, 1999; Komatsu, Mimura, Kato, Wakamatsu, & Kashima, 2000).

Dual-diagnosis/comorbidity data were reported in 17/38 studies (45%). In addition to the memory impairments described above, other reported cognitive impairments included executive function and attention impairments, disorientation, anomia and other language impairments, visuoperceptual disorders, motor–speech impairments or motor slowing, diabetes, and seizures (e.g., Glang et al., 1992; Glisky, Schacter, & Tulving, 1986). Participants were excluded from several of the remaining studies on the basis of a dual diagnosis or comorbidity. (*Note*: Very few studies reported on vision, hearing, and motor status.) Selection criteria were reported in 16/38 (42%) studies.

DEMENTIA

Neuropsychological test data were available in all seven studies. Premorbid IQ was reported in 5/7 studies (71%). Two of the seven studies included participants with only minimal or mild dementia (Clare, Roth, Wilson, Carter, & Hodges, 2002; Clare et al., 2000), and the remaining studies included participants either from all severity groups or with moderate–severe dementia only (e.g., Metzler-Baddeley & Snowden, 2005; Ruis & Kessels, 2005). Six of the seven studies (86%) described participants as having "significant," "severe," or "profound" memory impairments. Dual-diagnosis/comorbidity data were provided in 3/7 (43%) studies. In addition to memory impairment, other cognitive impairments included general decline in intellectual ability, impaired concentration, disorientation, and word-finding difficulties (Haslam et al., 2006; Metzler-Baddeley, & Snowden, 2005; Winter & Hunkin, 1999). Selection criteria were reported in 6/7 (86%) studies.

SCHIZOPHRENIA/SCHIZOAFFECTIVE DISORDER

Neuropsychological testing was completed in all six studies; however, the number of measures used was often limited, thus precluding detailed descriptions of participant profiles. Premorbid IQ was not reported for participants. Severity of memory impairment was reported in only two (33%) studies and was determined via standardized test cutoff scores (Kern et al., 2005; O'Carroll, Russell, Lawrie, & Johnstone, 1999). Selection criteria were reported in 6/6 (100%) studies.

Treatment History, Medication Status, Education, Occupation, Living Situation

ACQUIRED BRAIN INJURY

Treatment history was reported in 9/38 (24%) of the studies. Medication status was reported in only 2/38 studies (1%) (Andrewes & Gielewski, 1999; Parkin, Hunkin, & Squires, 1998). Education levels were reported in 21/38 studies (55%), with the majority of the adult participants having completed high school, and many achieving some level of postsecondary education as well. Occupational history was stated in 13/38 studies (34%) and included reports of participant employment postintervention (e.g., Andrewes & Gielewski, 1999; Hillary et al., 2003). Postinjury living situation was reported in 18/38 (47%) and included home/community dwelling, assisted living centers, and long-term care residences.

DEMENTIA

Treatment history was not reported. Medication status was reported in 3/7 studies (43%) (Clare et al., 2002; Dunn & Clare, 2007; Metzler-Baddeley & Snowden, 2005). Education status was reported in 2/7 studies (29%) (Haslam et al., 2006; Ruis & Kessels, 2005), with participants having completed up to 10 years of education. Occupational history was reported in 4/7 studies (57%) (e.g., Clare et al., 2000, 2002; Metzler-Baddeley & Snowden, 2005), with participants having worked in a variety of jobs prior to their retirement (e.g., business owners, clerks, engineers). Living situation was reported in 6/7 studies (86%), with the majority of participants living with a family member.

SCHIZOPHRENIA/SCHIZOAFFECTIVE DISORDER

Treatment history was not reported. Medication status was reported in all six studies and included antipsychotic and neuroleptic medications. Education levels were reported in all six studies, with the majority of participants having completed at least high school. Occupational history was reported in only 1/6 studies (17%) (Kern et al., 2005). Living status was not consistently reported but was implied on the basis of the described treatment setting (e.g., inpatient hospital setting, outpatient clinic, community dwelling).

To summarize, the descriptions of population characteristics varied widely within and among the three population groups. Most studies provided sufficient information to develop a basic profile of study participants; however, there were notable gaps in the literature. For example, although most studies included neuropsychological test results, few provided clear links between test scores and the type and severity of memory impairment. This trend, in combination with the relative lack of information in domains such as treatment history and medication status, limited the studies' external validity—that is, the extent to which results can be generalized to individuals beyond those involved in the studies.

Intervention

This section summarizes the types of instructional methodologies and additional training components described in the 51 studies, as well as the treatment targets, dosage, treatment settings, providers, and outcome measurements (see Appendix 2.2 for details).

The reader will see the following abbreviations defined and used to describe treatment techniques: EL (errorless learning); EF (errorful learning), MVC (method of vanishing cues), and SR (spaced retrieval).

Instructional Methods

Two broad categories of instructional techniques emerged from the review: (1) systematic instructional methods and (2) conventional methods. Systematic instructional methods were originally developed in recognition of the need to control errors when training individuals with declarative learning impairments who learned primarily via classical conditioning. More broadly, *systematic* refers to educational approaches in which the instructional methods and sequence of learner steps are planned in advance, based on a careful analysis of learner characteristics, and build from simple to complex. This method contrasts with conventional approaches in which the materials and methods are adapted based on the learner's preferences or style or in response to the learner's errors. "Trial and error" or "test and correct" are common conventional instructional methods in which the learner is given feedback after an error is committed.

Error-control research in cognitive rehabilitation began in the 1980s with studies of patients with dense anterograde amnesia (e.g., Glisky et al., 1986a, 1986b). These individuals demonstrated the ability to learn new information and procedures if they rehearsed them enough, but had no conscious memory of either the learning event itself and would deny that they possessed the new knowledge and skills. In this category of techniques, errors are minimized during the acquisition phase by providing a model of the correct response *before* the client attempts to produce it (referred to as *most-to-least* cues), and guessing is discouraged (Baddeley & Wilson, 1994). This is in contrast to conventional, *least-to-most* cueing methods, in which the learner first attempts the target, then, if he or she fails, is provided with progressively more cues until he or she is able to produce the correct response. Systematic instruction was initially applied to the training of motor skills and later used to teach more complex behaviors and concepts such as metacognitive strategies.

Within the category of error-controlled instructional techniques, two specific methods have appeared in the ABI research literature: the method of vanishing cues (MVC) and spaced retrieval (SR) training. MVC is a form of error-controlled learning in which the client is given progressively stronger or weaker cues following recall attempts of the targeted information or skills (Glisky et al., 1986a, 1986b). In the initial versions of MVC, the patient was provided with the full target, then a single-letter cue with other letters added until he or she got the correct answer, then faded. For example, if the goal is learning to associate the name *Marilyn* with a photo of a woman, the client might be told the name initially, then given the cue *Mari* and asked to complete the name. If the client made an error, additional letters would be provided one at a time until the correct answer was produced (e.g., *Maril, Marily, Marilyn*). If the client answered correctly, the next presentation would have one less letter (i.e., *Mar*). As shown by this example, the original version of MVC was not an error-free technique, as the client could give the wrong answer four times before giving the correct answer. More recent versions of MVC use error control, typically by presenting the full stimulus then fading cues, rather than adding, guessing, then fading (Haslam, Moss, & Hodder, 2010).

SR, described in Chapter 5, is like MVC in that errors are minimized, but the focus is to manipulate the time intervals at which recall is elicited. SR is a form of *distributed practice*; that is, successful recall of information over expanded time intervals (McKitrick, Camp, & Black, 1992). In SR, the client is provided with the full correct response initially and asked to repeat it immediately, then to recall it at longer time intervals without cues (i.e., expanded rehearsal). If the client makes an error, he or she is immediately provided with the correct response and asked to repeat it, then the next recall interval is shortened to the last interval at which the client was successful. In the example above, the client would be told, "This person's name is Marilyn. So when I say 'What is her name?' you'll say her name, you'll say *Marilyn*. What is her name?" If the client responds correctly, he or she will be prompted again after 30 seconds. If that answer is correct, the recall interval will be doubled. If the client makes an error at 60 seconds, he or she will be immediately given the correct response, asked to repeat it, then asked again after a 30-second day (i.e., the last interval at which the client provided a correct response). SR is sometimes combined with MVC in the initial training phase if the person is unable to recall the target at the shortest time interval (Brush & Camp, 1998).

Although both MVC and SR training have been described as errorless learning techniques, they may be described more accurately as error-*control* methods. While MVC focuses more on the method of initial target acquisition and SR training focuses on long-term retention, both instructional methods emphasize explicit, carefully faded models/prompts. This approach contrasts with errorful or trial-and-error methods, which emphasize attempts by the individual to recall the target information or skill without prior models or prompts, with the trainer providing models only as feedback in response to errors. To continue with our example, the clinician would first ask, "What is the name of this person?" If the client made an error, he or she might be given an explicit hint (e.g., "It starts with the letter *M*" or "It's the first name of the shock-rock musician who was engaged to Evan Rachel Wood"), then ask the client to attempt recall again.

Another key component of systematic instruction is the provision of strategies or methods that encourage a deep level of processing to facilitate consolidation and retrieval of memories. We know that learning is facilitated when the learner is actively engaged and able to connect target content to existing information or elaborate incoming information and make it more salient, thereby increasing the likelihood that the memory will be durable. Examples of strategies include elaboration techniques such visualization and attention-enhancing strategies such as predicting performance. The potentially tricky part about systematic instruction is that these metacognitive strategies and the error minimization techniques discussed above can work against each other. Encouraging strategy use *may* allow more errors. There are some systematic instruction methods such as SR and MVC that focus on error control and do not provide for strategy instruction. Other instructional techniques are multidimensional and include both instructional approaches (e.g., using elaboration or visualization to generate the target, then SR to train it). The defining characteristic of systematic instruction is the deliberate and explicit delivery of information in a way designed to maximize retention.

The instructional literature reviewed in developing the practice guidelines contained examples of different types of systematic instructional techniques. Studies were grouped into the following six intervention categories:

1. *Errorless learning (EL).* The study evaluated errorless learning with no comparison condition or group.
2. *Errorless learning versus errorful learning (EL vs. EF).* The study compared EL versus EF, a comparison group, and/or an earlier EL training protocol.

3. *Method of vanishing cues (MVC)*. The study evaluated MVC with no comparison condition or group.
4. *Method of vanishing cues versus errorful or errorless learning (EF/EL)*. The study compared MVC with a comparison condition, such as errorful learning or errorless learning.
5. *Spaced retrieval/spaced presentations (SR)*. The study primarily evaluated spaced retrieval or spaced presentation of information.
6. *Systematic instructional packages*. The studies in this category evaluated a combination of systematic techniques (described on page 4) integrated into an instructional package and/or used a staged learning process (e.g., Phase 1 = acquisition, Phase 2 = application) with or without a comparison condition/group.

The target systematic instructional methodologies varied across the three etiology groups, as described in the following section.

ACQUIRED BRAIN INJURY

Most studies (11) in this group compared either EL versus EF or reported on the effects of systematic instructional packages (13). One study evaluated EL without a comparison condition/group (Parkin et al., 1998). Five studies evaluated MVC with no comparison group or condition, five evaluated MVC with a comparison, and three studies focused primarily on SR.

DEMENTIA

Three studies compared EL versus EF (Haslam et al., 2006; Metzler-Baddeley & Snowden, 2005; Ruis & Kessels, 2005), three evaluated systematic instructional packages (Clare et al., 2000, 2002; Dunn & Clare, 2007), and one study evaluated EL alone (Winter & Hunkin, 1999). Again, this overview does not include SR studies previously reviewed by Hopper, Drefs, Bayles, Tomoeda, & Dinu (2008), in their practice guidelines for intervention in dementia.

SCHIZOPHRENIA/SCHIZOAFFECTIVE DISORDER

Five studies compared EL versus EF methods, and one study evaluated two different systematic instructional packages with a control group. Across groups, documentation of specific training procedures for each instructional method varied. Several studies provided sufficient detail to allow for replication (e.g., Andrewes & Gielewski, 1999; Glisky & Schacter, 1989; Hunkin, Squires, Aldrich, & Parkin, 1998).

Additional Instructional Components

Several studies emphasized instructional components that researchers hypothesized would increase participants' active processing of the target information/procedures, while keeping errors to a minimum. These components took the form of either a strategy (e.g., verbal elaboration, imagery, prediction–reflection, evaluative questioning/self-generation of responses) or an emphasis on stimulus manipulation (e.g., using varied training examples for the targeted information/task step or stimulus preexposure that would increase client engagement).

ACQUIRED BRAIN INJURY

Eight studies included a strategy component (e.g., Evans et al., 2000; Tailby & Haslam, 2003), whereas 12 studies emphasized stimulus manipulation (e.g., Glisky & Schacter, 1987; Stark, Stark, & Gordon, 2005).

DEMENTIA

Almost half of the studies (3/7) included a strategy component (Clare et al., 2000, 2002; Metzler-Baddeley & Snowden, 2005), whereas none explicitly described stimulus manipulation.

SCHIZOPHRENIA/SCHIZOAFFECTIVE DISORDER

One out of the six studies (17%) emphasized strategy instruction (Young, Zakzanis, Campbell, Freyslinger, & Meichenbaum, 2002), and five described stimulus manipulation (e.g., Kern, Liberman, Kopelowicz, Mintz, & Green, 2002; Kern et al., 2005).

Instructional Targets

Instructional targets were grouped into two categories: information and procedures. *Information* targets included face–name associations, word lists, object names, facts, definitions, concepts, and curriculum content (e.g., math, reading). *Procedures* included a variety of multistep tasks, such as index card filing, word processing, data entry, programming electronic aids, external memory aid use, and route finding. Familiarity of the instructional targets varied, with both unfamiliar and familiar information and procedures trained across the three population groups.

ACQUIRED BRAIN INJURY

Most studies in this group (24/38) focused on training information, whereas 7/38 (18%) targeted procedures, and 7/38 targeted both.

DEMENTIA

Most of the studies (6/7) targeted information whereas one study (Clare et al., 2000) evaluated instruction that targeted both information and procedures.

SCHIZOPHRENIA/SCHIZOAFFECTIVE DISORDER

Three studies targeted information, and the other three taught procedures.

Treatment Dosage

Treatment dosage refers to the frequency of treatment sessions and the duration of treatment, both in terms of length of session and the total amount of time participants received treatment. It should be noted that treatment *dosage* and *intensity* are a function of treatment frequency (number of sessions per unit time) and duration (total number of minutes of therapy). The neuroplasticity literature reviewed in Chapter 1 suggests that high-intensity treatments, when delivered in the subacute or chronic stage postonset, are generally the most effective.

ACQUIRED BRAIN INJURY

Treatment frequency ranged from one session only to daily sessions. Treatment duration was also quite varied, with sessions lasting anywhere from 30 minutes to 2 hours, with total duration, when specified, from 1 week up to several months.

DEMENTIA

Treatment frequency ranged from a one session in each condition (two total) to 16 sessions. Total duration, when reported, ranged from 1 week up to 4 weeks.

SCHIZOPHRENIA/SCHIZOAFFECTIVE DISORDER

Treatment frequency ranged from one to six sessions, with durations up to 4 weeks.

Treatment Settings and Providers

ACQUIRED BRAIN INJURY

Half of the studies (19/38) reported treatment settings. These included laboratory or clinic settings, client job sites, and individuals' homes with treatment delivered via phone (Melton & Bourgeois, 2005). Treatment providers were reported in 20/38 studies (53%) and included experimenters and family members, as well as computer-delivered stimuli common to the studies by Glisky and colleagues (e.g., 1986, 1987, 1988, 1989, 1995).

DEMENTIA

Treatment settings and providers were reported in one study (14%) (Metzler-Baddeley & Snowden, 2005), which described a combination of clinic- and home-based therapy delivered by both the experimenter and the participants' spouses.

SCHIZOPHRENIA/SCHIZOAFFECTIVE DISORDER

Treatment settings and providers were reported in 5/6 studies (83%), with the majority conducted in hospital or clinic settings. Experimenters, supervisors, and assistants provided the treatment.

Measurement

Different types of outcome measures were used across the three population groups, with most studies incorporating more than one type. The most frequently used measure was the number, percentage, or proportion of targets correctly recalled, which was used in

77% of the studies overall: 74% in ABI, 100% in dementia, and 50% in schizophrenia/schizoaffective disorder.

Other outcome measures used across the three groups included documentation of error responses or intrusions (e.g., Glisky & Schacter, 1987; Komatsu et al., 2000; Leng, Copello, & Sayegh, 1991), task completion times (e.g., Glisky, 1995; Glisky & Schacter, 1987; Leng et al., 1991), levels of independence (Andrewes & Gielewski, 1999), number of trials/sessions to criterion (e.g., Ehlhardt, Sohlberg, Glang, & Albin, 2005; Glisky & Schacter, 1988; Turkstra & Bourgeois, 2005), scores on behavioral checklists/questionnaires (e.g., Hunkin, Squires, Aldrich, et al., 1998; Ownsworth & McFarland, 1999; Squires, Hunkin, & Parkin, 1996), and scores on standardized tests (e.g., Dou et al., 2006; Schmitter-Edgecombe, Fahy, Whelan, & Long, 1995; Winter & Hunkin, 1999). Qualifiers to these measures included whether the measure was implemented immediately following training or after a delay, whether recall was free or cued, and whether a recognition task was also included. These qualifiers were particularly relevant to studies in which a primary goal was to identify the memory system (e.g., implicit vs. explicit memory) that played the greatest role in successful performance (e.g., Hunkin, Squires, Parkin, & Tidy, 1998; Tailby & Haslam, 2003). In most studies it was unclear if evaluators were naïve to the training conditions when measuring outcomes; hence, for the majority of the studies, it was assumed that the trainer also served as the evaluator.

To summarize, the systematic instructional methods evaluated within and between etiology groups varied, although most used a form of EL or systematic instruction. The studies also varied in the extent to which the treatment procedures and dosages were sufficiently detailed to allow a naïve trainer to replicate the treatment; replicability is important for translating these findings into clinical practice. Treatment targets included a range of information and procedures. A number of studies evaluated word recall, whereas others selected targets such as face–name recall, computer-task completion, and external memory aid use. The most common outcome measure was correct versus incorrect target production, along with other measures specifically tailored to the treatment target (e.g., task completion time for multistep procedures). Lack of explicit information concerning the evaluators' knowledge of training conditions limited the assessment of internal validity. Design factors influencing internal validity are discussed in the next section.

Study Design

This section summarizes the classes of evidence, research designs, statistics, reliability, and validity of the reviewed studies (see Appendix 2.3 for details).

Design, Statistics, Reliability, and Validity

This section summarizes the methodological variables coded, including research design and experimental control conditions, statistics, reliability, and validity. These components are analyzed separately for each population group. Because ecological validity is a psychosocial rather than statistical construct, it is considered separately. For this review, the authors determined that ecological validity had been established when the intervention targets would be of direct benefit to the study participants in their daily lives (e.g., teaching the use of an external memory aid for use in the individual's workplace).

ACQUIRED BRAIN INJURY

Twenty-six of the 38 studies (68%) incorporated experimental control conditions. Of these, three were between-groups designs with random assignment. Experimental comparisons included comparison to pretreatment baseline data (Ownsworth & McFarland, 1999), a nontreatment condition (Schmitter-Edgecombe et al., 1995), or a different type of treatment (Dou et al., 2006). There were 12 within-subject experimental studies. In these, experimental comparisons were conducted between different treatment types, such as EL versus EF (e.g., Baddeley & Wilson, 1994; Evans et al., 2000), EL versus MVC, or different treatment or presentation conditions (e.g., Glisky et al., 1986a; Komatsu et al., 2000); or to pretreatment baseline data (Ehlhardt et al., 2005). Eight studies used combinations of between- and within-subject designs with comparison conditions similar to those listed above. Several studies reported counterbalanced treatment conditions and stimuli, as appropriate to the design. Three studies used combinations of between- or within-subject designs and case studies (Glang et al., 1992; Glisky & Delaney, 1996; Squires et al., 1996). Twelve studies did not use experimental control and were case studies with and without pre–posttreatment comparisons.

Levels of statistical significance were reported in 29/38 studies (76%) with analysis techniques such as t-tests, analysis of variance (ANOVA), and general linear model analysis, as well as nonparametric techniques. Statistics were not appropriate for selected within-subject studies that used visual inspection to determine effectiveness (e.g., Ehlhardt et al., 2005; Glang et al., 1992). Only four studies (11%) reported reliability or validity data related to measures (e.g., Ehlhardt et al., 2005; Melton & Bourgeois, 2005). Ecological validity was considered established in 12/38 (32%) of the studies.

DEMENTIA

Four of the seven studies used within-subject designs that included comparisons of EL versus EF (Clare et al., 2000; Metzler-Baddeley & Snowden, 2005; Ruis & Kessels, 2005) and use of a control set of stimulus items (Clare et al., 2002). Haslam and colleagues (2006) used both between- and within-subjects comparisons when evaluating EL vs. EF vs. a no-treatment control group. Clare and colleagues (2000) used a combination of experimental, within-subjects (stable baseline as control), and case study designs. Winter and Hunkin (1999) used a nonexperimental, pre–post comparison study of EL. Levels of statistical significance were reported in 5/6 studies (83%) and were calculated using t-tests, ANOVA, correlational analyses, and time series analyses. Reliability and validity were not reported in any of the studies. Ecological validity was established in one study (14%; Clare et al., 2000), in which participants demonstrated improved face–name recall and use of memory strategies in naturalistic settings.

SCHIZOPHRENIA/SCHIZOAFFECTIVE DISORDER

Four of the six studies (67%) used between-groups experimental designs comparing EL vs. EF, with and without a control group, and EL vs. symptom management (e.g., Kern et al., 2002, 2005). The two other studies used between- and within-subjects comparisons (Pope & Kern, 2006; Young et al., 2002). Young and colleagues (2002) compared two forms of systematic instruction—scaffolded instruction vs. direct instruction—and included a control group. Four of the six studies (67%) used randomized assignment (Kern, Wallace, Hellman, Womack, & Green, 1996; Kern et al., 2002, 2005; Young et al., 2002). Levels of statistical significance were reported in all of the studies and were calculated using t-tests, ANOVA, multivariate ANOVA (MANOVA), correlational tests and nonparametric tests. Reliability and validity were reported in 3/6 studies (50%) , with one study evaluating fidelity of treatment implementation (Kern et al., 2005). Ecological validity was addressed directly in one of the six studies (social problem solving; Kern et al., 2005).

To summarize, the research designs used across the three etiology groups included between-group and within-subject designs. These different study designs varied in the extent to which they established external and internal validity. Unfortunately, few studies documented reliability and validity of the procedures, limiting the extent to which changes in the dependent variables could be confidently linked to the targeted intervention.

Treatment Outcomes

This section summarizes immediate outcomes and generalization and maintenance of results (see Appendix 2.3 for details).

Three different types of immediate outcomes were described in the literature: *favorable* (designated by the "+" symbol in Appendix 2.3), assigned if the instructional method was reported to produce learning of the dependent variables or significantly stronger learning than a control instructional condition; *qualified* (designated by the "/" symbol), if the instructional method was associated with variable learning of the dependent measures; and *negative* (using the "–" symbol) if the method had limited or no advantage relative to the comparison condition.

Several studies, particularly those published in the 1980s and early 1990s, focused on the basic question of whether or not a specific systematic instructional method worked, or resulted in better performance than another method (e.g., MVC, Glisky et al., 1986a, 1986b; EL vs. EF, Baddeley & Wilson, 1994). As EL methods became accepted practice, later studies compared enhanced versions of these, such as EL with versus without preexposure to the targets (Kalla, Downes, & van den Broeck, 2001) or EL with versus without self-generated responses (Tailby & Haslam, 2003). Accordingly, the outcomes of these later studies were coded both according to the effectiveness of that established instructional method and according to the effectiveness of the hypothesized enhancement.

Immediate Outcomes

Outcomes were analyzed across the three population groups in order to evaluate global trends. A broad analysis of the aggregate immediate outcomes revealed strong evidence supporting the use of systematic instructional techniques. A total of 41 out of 51 studies (80%) reported favorable learning outcomes using EL (including MVC and SRT) or systematic instructional packages. Favorable outcomes occurred in each population group, with the least robust outcomes for the dementia population. In the ABI group, 34 out of 38 studies (89%) reported favorable immediate outcomes, four reported qualified outcomes, and one study that included children reported negative outcomes (Landis et al., 2006). Glang and colleagues (1992) also included children, but reported positive findings. The two studies differed considerably in terms of number of participants, severity levels, systematic instructional method, and study design. In the dementia group, two out of seven studies (29%) reported favorable immediate outcomes (Clare et al., 2000; Winter & Hunkin, 1999), four studies reported qualified outcomes, and one study reported a negative outcome (Dunn & Clare, 2007). With the exception of Kern et al. (2002), who reported qualified findings, five out of the six studies (83%) with participants who had schizophrenia reported favorable immediate outcomes (e.g., Kern et al., 2005; Pope & Kern, 2006).

Studies varied by type of instruction and outcome measures used to document treatment effects. The two studies evaluating EL reported only favorable outcomes (Parkin et al., 1998; Winter & Hunkin, 1999). In the 20 studies comparing EL with EF or a control group, 14 (56%) reported favorable outcomes (e.g., Squires, Hunkin, & Parkin, 1997; Van der Linden, Meulemans, & Lorrain, 1994; Young et al., 2002), with five studies reporting qualified findings (e.g., Evans et al., 2000; Metzler-Baddeley & Snowden, 2005; O'Carroll et al., 1999) and one study reporting negative outcomes (Landis et al., 2006). All five studies evaluating MVC reported favorable outcomes (e.g., Baddeley & Wilson, 1994; Glisky & Schacter, 1988; Glisky et al., 1986b). In the studies that compared MVC to another instructional condition, three out of five reported favorable findings (Glang et al., 1992; Glisky et al., 1986a; Riley, Sotirious, & Jaspal, 2004) and two reported qualified findings (Hunkin & Parkin, 1995; Thoene & Glisky, 1995). All three studies evaluating SR/spaced presentations reported favorable outcomes (Hillary et al., 2003; Melton & Bourgeois, 2005; Turkstra & Bourgeois, 2005). Most studies (16/17) evaluating systematic instructional packages reported favorable outcomes (e.g., Andrewes & Gielewski, 1999; Schmitter-Edgecombe et al., 1995; Winter & Hunkin, 1999).

Generalization

Generalization outcomes were coded for those studies that evaluated transfer of training to non-trained targets or natural settings. Studies were coded as positive (+) if any degree of generalization was reported and negative (−) if generalization was measured but not achieved.

ACQUIRED BRAIN INJURY

Generalization measures were taken in 19 out of 38 studies (50%). Of those studies, 15/19 (79%) reported partial or 100% generalization of treatment targets. For example, in the study by Ehlhardt and colleagues (2005), evidence for generalization of learning e-mail procedures was that all participants were able to use a slightly more complex e-mail interface. Other studies reported generalization from laboratory to naturalistic settings, and in some cases training in the natural environment also facilitated generalization (e.g., Andrewes & Gielewski, 1999; Glisky & Schacter, 1987).

DEMENTIA

Generalization was reported in one of the seven studies. Clare and colleagues (2000) reported generalization of face–name recall to a naturalistic setting for two of the six participants and use of memory strategies in new situations for one participant.

SCHIZOPHRENIA/SCHIZOAFFECTIVE DISORDER

Generalization measures were taken in two of the six studies (33%). Kern and colleagues (2005) reported that the experimental group generalized trained social problem-solving skills to novel problem-solving scenarios. Young and colleagues (2002) noted that a scaffolded instruction group demonstrated significant improvement on selected generalization assessment measures (e.g., object sorting task).

Maintenance

Maintenance outcomes were coded when reassessment of trained targets occurred more than 1 day following the cessation of training, as that was the minimum time described by authors as "maintenance."

ACQUIRED BRAIN INJURY

Maintenance checks were reported in 24 out of 38 studies (63%). All of these reported partial or 100% maintenance of treatment targets from a few days to 9 months postintervention (e.g., Andrewes & Gielewski, 1999; Thoene & Glisky, 1995).

DEMENTIA

Maintenance checks were reported in two of the seven studies (Clare et al., 2002, 2000) and revealed generally positive findings, with retention of therapy gains up to 6 months postintervention.

SCHIZOPHRENIA/SCHIZOAFFECTIVE DISORDER

Maintenance checks were reported in four out of six (67%) studies. Results were mixed. Kern and colleagues (2002) reported a decline in the performance of work-related tasks across both intervention groups at 3 months, whereas a later study by this group (Kern et al., 2005) reported maintenance of social problem-solving skills at 3 months after the end of treatment. One notable difference between the studies was that the first (Kern et al., 2002) included only two 45- to 60-minute sessions, with no opportunity to practice skills posttraining, whereas the second (Kern et al., 2005) included 6 hours of training over 2 days and an opportunity to practice skills posttraining.

To summarize, the results suggested that systematic instructional approaches can produce durable acquisition of skills and information. Further, the results of those studies measuring generalization underscored the importance of incorporating specific training components that would support "firm" skill and knowledge acquisition, maintenance, and generalization to "real-life," personally meaningful contexts.

Article Summary

Globally, the research evidence provided strong support for the effectiveness of systematic instruction. However, the literature lacked details that would make it possible to reproduce many of the treatments, and there was limited evidence that learning generalized to meaningful contexts; thus, much work remains to be done. The research did, however, suggest several general principles that may assist clinicians in designing, evaluating, and modifying instruction based on client performance.

Key Training Variables

SPECIFICITY OF TRAINING VERSUS GENERALIZATION

A dominant theme in the research was the need to reduce hyperspecificity of training conditions (e.g., by varying cues to the same target; Stark et al., 2005) and increase effortful processing in order to facilitate flexible learning and generalization. Most patients have some residual declarative memory ability and can benefit from explicit strategies like elaboration (e.g., "Spot is a dog" vs. "Spot is a dog who belongs to my neighbor, limps in cold weather, and ate my shoes last year") and self-generation (e.g., "What is it about Spot that's interesting to you and will help you remember his name?"). These strategies encourage effortful processing, which can lead to improved attention, encoding, and organization during acquisition as well as facilitate explicit retrieval (Riley & Heaton, 2000; Riley et al., 2004). However, these components also run the risk of increasing recall errors and may be less important when using training methods that rely on implicit or procedural learning. Maintaining a balance between constraining errors and encouraging effortful processing appears critical to careful treatment planning (e.g., Komatsu et al., 2000; Tailby & Haslam, 2003). The importance of errors versus effort is likely to vary as a function of the type and severity of the patient's memory impairment, as errors are more influential when learning primarily relies on implicit mechanisms; thus, patients with less severe impairments in declarative memory processes might be more likely to benefit from strategies that encourage conscious effort during encoding and retrieval, whereas patients with profound declarative memory impairments might benefit more from errorless procedures (Anderson & Craik, 2006). Also, patients with declarative memory impairments may benefit from conscious strategies during encoding, but still fail to generalize the information beyond the specific context in which it was taught (Oberg & Turkstra, 1998), perhaps because of impairments in executive function.

STRATEGIES

Studies were coded as having a "stimulus variation" component if there was an emphasis on training multiple exemplars (e.g., Glisky & Schacter, 1987; Stark et al., 2005) or the stimulus was enhanced in some other way (e.g., stimulus preexposure; Kalla et al., 2001). Studies were coded as having a "strategy component" if the intervention included techniques such as verbal elaboration, imagery, or self-generated responses (e.g., Clare et al., 2000; Tailby & Haslam, 2003). At least 16 of the 51 studies emphasized stimulus variability, with 15/16 (94%) of these reporting positive findings. Of the 51 total studies, 12 included a strategy component. Of these, 9/12 (75%) reported positive findings, and three reported qualified outcomes. Interestingly, in two of these latter studies (Evans et al., 2000; Thoene & Glisky, 1995), both cited the use of imagery or verbal elaboration as contributing to better recall. Both of these strategies were considered to contribute to more effortful processing compared to using EL or MVC alone.

PRACTICE

Another critical training variable was providing sufficient practice. There was a clear trend in this literature review suggesting that more practice leads to more durable learning. For example, 14 of the 16 studies targeting multistep procedures (e.g., for data entry or external memory aid use) reported favorable treatment outcomes, and all but one prescribed high treatment dosages, ranging from 6 to 30 sessions or more (e.g., Andrewes & Gielewski, 1999; Hunkin, Squires, Aldrich, & Parkin, 1998b). The two studies that did not report clear positive results held less than four total training sessions (Evans et al., 2000; Kern et al., 2002).

Spacing or distribution of practice trials (i.e., SR/expanded rehearsal) is another key training variable, a finding well supported in the literature for nondisabled individuals (Donovan & Radosevich, 1999) and for those with memory impairment due to dementia (Hopper et al., 2005). Hopper and colleagues reviewed 15 studies in which all participants learned some or all of the target information taught using SR. In the current review, three studies targeted SR or spaced presentations for individuals with TBI, all of which reported favorable outcomes (Hillary et al., 2003; Melton & Bourgeois, 2005; Turkstra & Bourgeois, 2005). Further, several other studies in this review that included SR/distributed practice as part of their EL or systematic instructional package also reported favorable outcomes (e.g., Clare et al., 2000; Ehlhardt et al., 2005). Of note, there is some suggestion that the type of task should influence practice distribution. Learning highly procedural, low-cognitive-demand tasks may be most responsive to distributed practice, whereas learning more complex tasks may require massed practice, at least initially (Donovan & Radosevich, 1999).

Both the frequency and distribution of practice trials contributed to mastering targeted skills and information; mastery is essential if one is to use the skills/information in daily life. A "criterion for mastery" is the a priori determination of the level of performance (e.g., accuracy, level of independence, time frame) indicative of such mastery. For example, a clinician and client might determine that mastery has been reached when a data entry task can be performed with 100% accuracy for three consecutive sessions, because only 100% is acceptable in that client's workplace. In this review, the majority of the studies did not establish a criterion for mastery since the primary research questions were concerned with whether a particular instructional method worked or if it was significantly better than another method. In other words, information/skill mastery was not always the primary goal. That said, there were 13 studies (25%) that included a criterion for mastery. Eleven of these (85%) reported positive outcomes, and several of these studies included high treatment dosages and distribution of practice trials, as described above (e.g., Ehlhardt et al., 2005; Glisky & Schacter, 1989).

TASK CHARACTERISTICS

A number of studies reminded readers of the importance of considering task characteristics when designing intervention. For example, several MVC studies by Glisky and colleagues (1986–1989) showed that complex procedures can be learned if they are broken into simple components and each component is specifically trained. Evans and colleagues (2000) showed that tasks and recall conditions that facilitated retrieval of *implicit* memory for learned material (e.g., learning names given a first-letter cue) benefited from EL methods, whereas those that required *explicit* recall of novel associations (e.g., programming a device) did not benefit from errorless learning.[2] There also is evidence that training of face–name association might be a special case (Thoene & Glisky, 1995; see discussion in Chapter 5). In a study of 12 patients with moderate-to-severe declarative memory impairments, Thoene and Glisky (1995) found that MVC was less effective than elaboration for learning face–name associations: Participants required significantly more trials to reach criterion than when they were given supplementary biographical information about the targets. This advantage was much smaller for delayed recall: Although items trained using elaboration were significantly more likely to be recalled after 3 or 4 days, this difference was small. The elaboration method was more effective across all levels of severity of memory impairment. This finding was surprising given that elaboration is thought to rely on declarative memory, which clearly was impaired in these participants. Two features of this study are important to note, however, when considering the generalization of the results to other learning targets. First, as the authors noted, face–name associations are particularly difficult to learn because they are completely arbitrary. Consistent with this point, in the MVC condition participants made many within-set errors—that is, they learned the names but associated them with the wrong faces. Second, the stimuli were created by the experimenters. It is not clear that results would generalize to everyday face–name associations, which are likely to carry semantic information that already has been associated with that target.

ECOLOGICAL VALIDITY

Of most interest to clinicians is the evidence that learning was useful beyond the clinic. As previously stated, instructional targets were defined as ecologically valid if the target constituted information or skills that the study participants would use in their own daily lives. Of the 51 studies, 14 (27%) used ecologically valid tasks. Targets included face–name associations, training the use of external memory aids, learning computer tasks, and academic skills. Of these studies, 100% reported positive findings. This high percentage of positive outcomes supports Bradely, Kapur, and Evan's (2003) assertion that task variables, such as motivational and emotional significance, help memories last. Specifically, the evidence suggested that learning may be facilitated when tasks or information are inherently functional to an individual. This is consistent with animal studies showing that learning is more rapid and enduring if the to-be-learned information has biological relevance to the organism (Kilgard & Merzenich, 1998). Another interesting trend noted in this subset of ecologically valid studies was that all reported high treatment dosages (with a minimum of six treatment sessions) and all incorporated task analyses to train procedures were explicit in identifying the target learning objective for the participant.

---

[2]Other authors would argue that such procedural tasks rely on implicit rather than explicit memory (e.g., Baddeley & Wilson, 1994; Page et al., 2006; Wilson et al., 1994).

Key Participant Variables

This analysis revealed no clear relationships between etiology of memory impairment and responsiveness to instructional methods. Individuals with memory impairment from a variety of causes were shown to benefit from systematic instruction, suggesting that it may be fruitful to look across neurogenic populations to evaluate instructional practices. One possible exception is the dementia population, where the outcomes were less clear and many studies reported qualified treatment effects. Of the studies reporting qualified findings across etiology groups, most reported differential outcomes for different memory severity levels. Riley and Heaton's (2000) study provides a clear example. These authors found that participants with poorer declarative learning ability benefited from a more gradual fading of cues, whereas those with better declarative learning showed positive results with more rapid fading. By contrast, other studies (e.g., Page, Wilson, Shiel, Carter, & Norris, 2006; Tailby & Haslam, 2003) have shown benefits of EL across memory severity levels. The influence of severity on candidacy for specific instructional practices was not clear from the articles reviewed.

The role played by an individual's cognitive profile in domains other than memory (e.g., attention, executive functions, awareness) was equally unclear. There was some evidence that clients with frontal lobe damage and concomitant impairments in awareness and executive functions might benefit less from MVC and EL techniques than patients with less frontal lobe dysfunction (e.g., Clare et al., 2002; Leng et al., 1991). Andrewes and Gielewski (1999) addressed this issue in their detailed report of positive outcomes following the training of vocational skills in a person with dense amnesia resulting from herpes encephalitis. They qualified their findings, noting that the participant's spared executive functions, high premorbid intelligence, and intact semantic memory may have allowed her to benefit from the training and achieve successful return to work. What was evident across studies was the need for therapists to match instructional techniques to specific client cognitive profiles and measure ongoing effects of learning in order to adjust instructional practices as necessary. The best procedures for matching clients to methods have not yet been established and constitute an important goal for future clinical research.

UPDATES: WHAT DOES THE NEWER RESEARCH SAY?

A growing body of research is devoted to evaluating the effectiveness of different types of instructional practices for people with cognitive impairments. In this section we review key studies published after the previously reviewed 2008 ANCDS guidelines paper (Ehlhardt et al., 2008) in addition to several studies that were omitted from that paper. Studies reviewed here were selected based on a hand search of key authors and journals identified from the 2008 review. The goal of this section is to evaluate whether the original conclusions and clinical recommendations continue to be supported, and to identify new findings in instructional practices for individuals with acquired cognitive impairments.

Recent studies confirm the tenet that structuring the manner in which target information or procedures are introduced to people with cognitive impairments can significantly enhance rate and quality of learning. The results also reinforce the need for clinicians to carefully plan training procedures, particularly in the areas discussed next.

Key Training Variables

Errorless Training

There is mounting evidence in the literature supporting the utility of constraining errors in the initial acquisition phase, particularly for highly proceduralized tasks and for individuals with moderate-to-severe declarative memory impairments. Todd and Barrow (2008) tested the acquisition of touch typing using a conventional computer software training package, supplemented by individual coaching, with two participants who had severely impaired memory functioning due to brain injury. Using EL with short sessions of distributed practice, both participants met criterion in speed and accuracy, and their performance was roughly comparable to that of two comparison participants without memory impairment. Another study of 20 patients with ABI compared route recall under conditions of EL versus trial-and-error learning and reported that route recall was significantly more accurate using errorless training methods (Lloyd, Riley, & Powell, 2009). Similarly, EL was evaluated using an experimental design of multiple baselines across interventions to determine if a patient with severe memory impairment due to TBI would experience less everyday memory impairments (Campbell, Wilson, McCann, Kernahan, & Rogers, 2007). The results were positive and again supported the use of EL.

EL techniques were evaluated to train the use of electronic aids to increase independence in apartment living for people with memory impairments due to ABI (Bowman, Linberg, Hemmingsson, & Barfai, 2010). Patients were showed sequences of steps, provided with clear instructions, and prevented from making errors. Reminders and learning support were adjusted according to the patients' learning performance. After 5 days in the training apartment, 3 of the 14 patients learned the use of the aids independently and 8 improved but required some ongoing support. Three were not able to learn to use the aids, suggesting that some individuals need more intensive, individualized training. The authors interpreted their findings as showing support for the systematic error-control instructional methods.

Bourgeois, Lenius, Turkstra, and Camp (2007) conducted a single-blind randomized controlled trial of EL techniques to train everyday memory goals in 38 adults with TBI. Goals were identified collaboratively with each participant and his or her caregiver, and participants were randomized to receive either SR training or training in the use of conventional instructional strategies (e.g., elaboration, association) for the same amount of treatment time. Participants in the SR group recalled twice as many of their goals than those in the instructional strategy group at the conclusion of therapy, and three times more after 1 month. Several findings from this study are of particular relevance to this manual: (1) the dropout rate was higher in the control group, and many participants stated that the techniques were unhelpful; (2) the average time required to achieve goal mastery in the SR group was eleven 30-minute sessions including six (one participant who had required 6 months to learn a single fact using traditional cueing hierarchies needed only six sessions); and (3) consistent with the hyperspecificity of EL techniques and despite the success of SR training, caregivers in the EL group reported no overall change in everyday life participation or generalization to other contexts in this group. These results suggest that if a patient is more successful with a given training approach, it might improve adherence. They also suggest that EL techniques can be significant time-savers with amnesic patients but it is important to address hyperspecificity.

The updated literature review yielded three articles (Bier et al., 2008; Dunn & Clare, 2007; Simard et al., 2009) that did not support superior effects of error reduction during learning. The first two evaluated face–name association learning in patients with early-stage dementia. These results suggested that this population could learn associations given systematic training, but error reduction might not facilitate greater improvement. The third study (Simard et al., 2009) evaluated the efficacy of cognitive training in a 10-week randomized controlled study involving 22 individuals presenting with mild cognitive impairment of the amnesic type (aMCI). A syndrome characterized by cognitive decline that is greater than expected for an individual's age and education level, aMCI does not interfere significantly with activities of daily life (Gauthier, 2006). When the cognitive decline is predominantly in the area of memory function—specifically, declarative learning and memory—the syndrome is referred to as *aMCI* (Gauthier, 2006). For this reason the literature on aMCI is relevant to the study of intervention for other memory-impaired groups as well.

In the study by Simard et al. (2009) participants in the experimental group (*n* = 11) learned face–name associations using a paradigm combining EL and SR, whereas participants in the control group (*n* = 11) were trained using an EF learning paradigm. Educational sessions on memory were also provided to all participants. After neuropsychological screening and baseline evaluations, the cognitive training took place in six sessions over a 3-week period. The posttraining and follow-up evaluations, at 1 and 4 weeks, respectively, were performed by research assistants blind to participants' study group. Results showed that regardless of training condition, all participants improved their capacity to learn face–name associations. There also was a significant increase in participant-reported satisfaction with everyday memory functioning and self-reported frequency of using strategies to support memory functions in daily life. The absence of differences between groups on all variables might be partly explained by the high variability of scores within the experimental group. As noted below, other studies are needed in order to verify the efficacy of EL learning and SR over EF in aMCI.

Promotion of Strategy Use and Engagement

Several recent studies show that simply encouraging active processing during training increases learning. A study compared the effectiveness of two instructional techniques for teaching people with brain injury a motor sequence: modeling (an active technique requiring the patient to imitate the clinician) and molding (a passive technique wherein the instructor shapes the patient's hand into the correct movements) (Zlotwitz et al., 2010). Results showed that the active technique was more effective for promoting long-term learning. The authors suggested that active response during learning engages implicit memory mechanisms more efficiently for people with severe brain injury. Similar findings were suggested by a study evaluating whether patients with memory impairments due to brain injury could learn to use a set of electronic memory aids in a training apartment (Bowman et al., 2010). Results suggested that learning was superior when individuals were actively trained on their use (e.g., use of a control panel to make sure the door was locked at night) versus those aids that were activated only if there was an error (e.g., kitchen alarm signaling that the stove was left on).

A number of studies has shown a benefit from instructional techniques in which the learner is not only active in the learning but generative. A laboratory study of word-list learning comparing EL versus elaborative, self-generated learning was conducted in individuals with aMCI (Lubinsky, Rich, & Anderson, 2009). Results showed that cued recall and recognition were best when EL and self-generated learning techniques were combined, but EL alone yielded the best results for free recall. Dunn and Clare (2007) compared the effects of four different learning techniques varying in level of effort required and number of errors on free recall, cued recall, and recognition of novel and previously known associations. Participants were adults with early-stage dementia. All conditions produced significant learning for both novel and familiar associations. Enhancing level of effort had no significant effects for familiar associations, but *high-effort* conditions were significantly more effective than low-effort conditions in facilitating cued recall of novel associations. The authors concluded that effort enhancement may be more important than EL in some conditions, such as the learning of novel associations in early-stage dementia.

The findings of both of the above studies are consistent with the results of a study comparing two learning conditions in a group of participants with Alzheimer's disease: SR alone versus SR plus elaborative encoding (Kinsella, Ong, Storey, Wallace, & Hester, 2007). In that study, the majority of participants exhibited superior free recall in the combined condition. Consistent with studies described earlier in this chapter (Andrewes & Gielewski, 1999; Clare et al., 2002; Leng et al., 1991), elaboration was more beneficial for individuals with stronger executive functions and attention. It should be emphasized that participants in both of these studies had relatively mild memory impairments; there are likely to be fewer benefits of elaboration and active engagement (i.e., conscious, declarative approaches) for individuals with more severe declarative memory problems. These authors subsequently conducted a randomized controlled trial investigating the efficacy of therapy supporting the use of compensatory strategies in 52 patients with aMCI (Kinsella et al., 2009). Their results showed that training patients in the use of memory strategies minimized everyday memory failures.

Distributed Practice

Not surprisingly, the results of current research support the importance of practicing target skills or material. Distributed practice, in particular, continues to be supported as an effective training technique. A randomized control trial was conducted with participants who had aMCI, to evaluate the effectiveness of a multidisciplinary group-based intervention (Troyer, Murphy, Anderson, Moscovitch, & Craik, 2008). The treatment participants showed an increase in memory strategy knowledge and use that was maintained for 3 months. It should be noted that maintenance of performance levels is considered a significant benefit in this group, given the expectation of decline. The intervention also successfully taught participants to use SR independently when learning new names. The benefit of distributed practice is consistent with the results of a study of skill acquisition for touch typing, in which patients with memory impairment received short sessions of distributed practice (Todd & Barrow, 2008).

Hawley, Cherry, Boudreaux, and Jackson (2008) compared the efficacy of two memory training schedules for adults with Alzheimer-type dementia: a conventional SR schedule versus a uniform expanded retrieval schedule, in which intervals between recall attempts were fixed for each session (e.g., 10 seconds for Session 1; 25 seconds for Session 2). The task was to learn name–face associations. Results showed a positive effect of conventional SR on the proportion of correct recall trials and greater success in transferring the learned information to the live target compared to the uniform expanded retrieval schedule. This study was interesting because all previous studies of SR in dementia had used an adjusted SR schedule, but it was not clear that this was a requirement, and there are practical advantages to having a fixed-interval schedule. A follow-up study (Cherry, Hawley, Jackson, & Boudreaux, 2009) showed that booster SR sessions provided at 6, 12, and 18 weeks after the original training yielded a positive effect, as participants were able to retain the name–face associations. Results of these studies suggest that it is not simply spacing that underlies the SR benefit, but rather spacing at progressively longer intervals.

Key Task Variables

Ecological Validity

The importance of training tasks that are meaningful to participants is obvious and continues to be underscored in the literature. A review of the training tasks in recent studies illustrates the range of ecologically valid targets that have been evaluated and shown to be successfully trained. Recent targets have included calendar use and leisure activities (listening to music on a radio, saying the rosary in a church group; Bier et al., 2008), training people to use electronic aids to increase their independence while living in an apartment (Bowman et al., 2010), using a mobile phone to prompt task completion (Stapleton, Adams, & Atterton, 2007), using a memory notebook entry and walking the dog (Campbell et al., 2007), learning touch typing (Todd & Barrow, 2008), and learning metamemory strategies (Troyer et al., 2008). In their randomized controlled trial of SR training for adults with TBI, Bourgeois et al. (2007) trained goals that were selected by each participant to meet his or her daily needs. These included face–names associations, appointment times, locations of personal items, and procedures related to the use of memory aids, completing chores, paying bills, returning phone calls, and taking medications. These functional tasks involved fact retrieval, learning multistep procedures, and applying internal strategies.

Three of the studies evaluated the learning of targets that had no apparent ecological validity for participants. Two of these trained face–name associations using black-and-white photographs unfamiliar to participants in a laboratory setting (Bier et al., 2008; Dunn & Clare, 2007), and one evaluated word-list learning (Lubinsky et al., 2009). These studies aimed to understand specific learning mechanisms, which then would be tested in clinical intervention trials.

Key Participant Variables

Etiology

As indicated by the studies just discussed, recent results continue to be mixed in regard to the benefit of certain types of structured training practices for people with mild memory impairments, particularly in the early stages of dementia or in aMCI. Some studies show benefits for EL for this population, whereas others indicate EF may be as or more important (Dunn & Clare, 2007). Even when findings are positive using instructional methods such as SR to teach this population new procedures and information (e.g., Hawley et al., 2008), the positive effects may not transfer to real-life contexts (Bier et al., 2008). Careful evaluation of training techniques and continued research are needed to understand variables affecting the learning process as individuals with dementing conditions progress from milder to more severe memory impairments.

Comorbid Cognitive Conditions

Another candidacy issue that remains largely unknown is the effect of other cognitive impairments on the learning process. The literature continues to hint that clients with concomitant executive function impairments or certain types of attention impairments may not respond as well to instructional methods as do participants who do not have these impairments (Kinsella et al., 2007; Stapleton et al., 2007), but this requires more formal study, and the appropriate test criteria have not yet been identified.

Delivery Models

Given restrictions in health care dollars, there is a welcome surge in evaluation of intervention models that are less time and resource intensive than previous practices. These include (1) the use of care providers as trainers, (2) group intervention, and (3) "telehealth" via the phone or internet. Campbell and colleagues (2007) examined whether EL applied by care providers in an everyday setting could reduce the frequency of everyday memory problems in an adult with severe memory impairment after TBI. The care providers were able to implement the EL techniques taught to them by an occupational therapist, and there was a resulting decrease in the frequency of memory lapses by the participant. Benefits were maintained at 3 months posttreatment. This study was also interesting in that it used self-generated cues whereby the care provider helped the participant develop his or her own wording for prompts.

Efficiency can also be gained by conducting therapy in groups. As reviewed, a group intervention using a systematic curriculum resulted in the successful use of memory strategies (Troyer et al., 2008). Another option to increase efficiency is to decrease office visits and provide support via telehealth, or distance therapies. A study evaluating the use of personal digital assistants (PDAs) for participants with memory and other cognitive impairments included a small number of introductory and training visits, followed by 8 weeks during which the participants were allowed to contact the therapists via telephone or e-mail (Gentry, Wallace, Kvarfordt, & Lynch, 2008). Results suggested that the brief training with distant support was successful in increasing use of the devices and improving the self-rating of memory performance. The study by Bourgeois and colleagues (2007), described above, was delivered entirely via telephone, with only one in-person visit for assessment.

The use of the Internet to deliver therapy is yet another option to increase efficiency. Participants receiving support to use a compensatory calendar system using an Internet-based messaging system showed superior use of the compensatory strategies compared to when they were trained using an online control condition that reviewed contents of the calendar but did not instruct the participants in how to use the tool (Bergquist et al., 2009). Of note, the Internet-based therapy was more effective for individuals who were already using some compensatory strategies at baseline.

Health care systems such as the Veterans Health Administration have made a significant investment in delivering care via telehealth, including mental health care, medical interventions, and rehabilitation. Telehealth has a significant benefit for rural health care delivery, and for individuals—like those with TBI or dementia—who are unable to drive to therapy. It also may have significant advantages for EL and SR training of personally relevant goals, because training conducted in this format can include the context in which the information will be used. We can expect to see a significant expansion of "telerehabilitation" services in the near future.

Conclusions

Findings from the newer research largely support the 2008 guidelines paper. Specifically, experimental work encourages the use of EL, the promotion of active learner engagement, and the selection of ecologically valid tasks; however, differential responses for different patient profiles and task conditions have been noted. For example, initial studies suggest that people with dementia or aMCI may respond less robustly to these instructional methods. Further studies are clearly needed. Overall, there is strong research support for the systematic techniques reviewed here, not only for individual treatment but also for group therapy and telerehabilitation.

SUMMARY

This chapter provides a broad literature review examining the evidence for implementing a variety of instructional methods. Although many questions remain about specific instructional practices that are effective for different patient profiles and goals, there is mounting evidence supporting the use of structured, systematic instruction with a thoughtful selection of targets that are meaningful to clients, with careful planning of the training regimen. Procedures and protocols described throughout the remainder of this manual rest on this literature base. It is hoped that these materials will facilitate evidence-based practice by clinicians charged with instructing patients who have cognitive impairments.

APPENDIX 2.1. Population Characteristics

ABI

Names and Dates	No.	Age	M:F	Etiology	Site of Injury	TPO	Neuropsych Tests	Pre-morbid IQ	Initial Severity	Memory Severity	Dual dx/Co-morbidity	Selection Criteria	Tx History	Medication	Education	Occupation	Living Situation
Glisky et al. (1986a)	Exp=4 / CG=4*	Exp M = 27.8 (24-32) / CG M = 32 (24-47)	1;3	Ss 1, 2, & 4 CHI / Ss 3 VE	0	2 yrs post injury	1	0		Ss 1: sev amnesia; Ss 2: mild amnesia; Ss 3 & 4: mod-sev amnesia; Ss #1: sev amnesia; Ss #2: mild-mod amnesia; Ss#3: mild-mod amnesia; Ss #4: mod-sev	naming pxs; attentional imp; extensive motor slowing	1	0	0	1	1	1
Glisky et al. (1986b)	Exp=4 / CG=4*	Exp M= 26 / CG = 35.3		CHI	1	2-5 yrs	1	0		sev amnesia	attention & visuoperceptual imp; extensive motor slowing	1	0	0	1	0	0
Glisky & Schacter (1987)	1	32 yrs	F	HSE	0	Dx 1980	1	0		sev amnesia	dysnomia	0	1	0	1	1	1
Glisky & Schacter (1988)	Exp = 8 / CG= 6*	Exp: M=33.6 / CG: M=30.8		Exp: CHI=4 with 1 each enceph, hypoxia, TIA, aneurysm / CG: 3 of 6 with CHI but no MI	0	2-5 yrs for Ss with CHI	1	0		mild-sev MI	attention, visuoperceptual imp; dysnomia, depressed IQ; extensive motor slowing	1	0	0	1	1	0
Leng et al. (1991)	1	18 yrs	M	severe TBI	1	Injury occurred in 1988	1	0	LOC not recorded; PTA at least 3 days	"impaired memory" (WMS quotient = 81)		0	1	0	1	0	0
Glang et al. (1992)	3	Ss 1: 8 yrs; Ss 2: 6 yrs; Ss 3: 10yrs	Ss 1: M; Ss 2: F; Ss 3: M	sev TBI	1	Ss 1: 15 mos.; Ss 2: 12 mos.; Ss 3: 19 mos	1	0	Ss 1: LOC 3 wks; Ss 2: LOC several mos.; Ss 3: LOC 3 mos.		attention imp, language imp, dysarthria, visuo-motor imp, behavior pxs; low avg IQ; r-sided weakness; motor imp; frontal lobe damage	0	1	0	1	0	0
Glisky (1992)	Exp=10 CG=5	Exp=36.8 CG=31.2		CHI, ACA, enceph, anoxia	1	M=5.9 yrs	1	0		mild-sev MI		0	0	0	1	0	0
Butters, Glisky & Schacter (1993)	Exp=6 CG=6	Exp=40 CG=42		CHI, enceph, aneurism	0		1	0		mild-sev MI		0	0	0	1	0	0
Baddeley & Wilson (1994)	ABI=16 / YCG=16 / OCG=16	M=44.18 (20-69) (ABI); M=35.56 (20-58) (YCG); M=67 (61-79) (OCG)	11;5, 10;6, 8;8	Enceph, TBI, ACA, PCA, CVA (thalamic), KS, toxicity, HSE	0		1	0		sev MI		0	0	0	1	0	0
Van der Linden et al. (1994)	Exp=2 / CG=2	Exp=49 yrs (both Ss)	F	KS	0	Ss 1: Dx 1986 / Ss 2: Dx 1988	1	0		Ss 1: profound amnesia / Ss 2: sev amnesia		0	0	0	1	1	1
Wilson et al. (1994)	5	31-68 yrs	M=5	HE; KS; CVA (thalamic); HI: ACA (right)	0	Ss 1: 11 yrs. post / Ss 4-several mos post	1	0	Ss 4: LOC 86 days; PTA = 251 days	sev MI	visual agnosia, dyslexia; exec func imp; confabulation; sev dysarthria, spastic quadriplegia	0	1	0	0	0	0
Glisky & Schacter (1989)	1	32 yrs	F	HSE	0	Dx 1980	1	0		prof MI	exec func imp; aphasia; motor imp	0	1	1	0	1	1
Glisky (1995)	1	29 yrs	M	ACA	1		1			sev MI		0	1	1	0	1	1
Hunkin & Parkin (1995)	Study 1=8, CG=8 / Study 2=16 (no CG)	Study 1: Ss with MI—M=53 / CG Ss—M=41.9 / Study 2: M=34.4	Study 1: 6:2 / 4:4 (CG group) / Study 2: 13:3	Study 1: CHI=6, VE=2 / Study 2: CHI=13, VE=3	1	Study 1: 10 mos-11 yrs / Study 2: 1 mo-1 yr	1	0		mod-sev MI	mild dyslexia, quadriplegia, visual field deficit	1	0	0	0	0	0
Schmitter-Edgecombe et al 1995	Exp=4 / CG=4*	Exp: M=29.9 / CG: M=26.8	6:2	CHI	0	Exp: M=77.7 mos / CG: M=86.6 mos	1	0	LOC Exp: M=39.7 days / CG:M=37.5 days	"everyday memory failures"		1	0	0	0	0	0
Theone & Glisky (1995)	12	M=45.6	6:6	CHI; CHI=3; AD=1; ACA=2; HE=1; A/H (left) =2; toxicity =1; tumor=2	0	M = 7.38 yrs (6 mos – 18 yrs)	1	0		MI primary deficit		1	0	0	0	0	0
Glisky & Delaney (1996)	Study 1: 8 with PTA; CG=8 / Study 2: 4 with PTA; CG=4	Study #1: M=30.9/29.1 / Study 2: M=31.5/30		CHI	0			0	Study 1: LOC M=10 days / PTA M= 53 days / Study 2: LOC M=7 days / PTA M=70 days	sev episodic MI	mod-sev generalized cortical atrophy	1	0	0	0	0	0
Squires et al. (1996)	1	70 yrs	M	CVA	1	At least 1 yr	1	0		sev, ant amnesia		0	1	0	0	1	1
Squires et al. (1997)	Study 1=16 / Study 2=16	Study 1 M=44.5 / Study 2 M=46.1	Study 1: 15:1 / Study 2: 14:2	CHI=11/10 / CVA=5/4 / Enceph=3/2	1		1	0				1	0	0	0	0	0
Hunkin et al. (1998a)	8	M=34.75 yrs (25-70)	6:2	CHI=5, VE=1, CVA=1, Anoxia=1	1	M=6,13 yrs (1-12 yrs)	1	0		mod-sev MI		0	0	0	0	0	0
Hunkin et al. (1998b)	1	33 yrs	M	VE	1	8 yrs	1	1		sev MI	seizures	0	0	0	0	1	0
Parkin et al. (1998)	1	63 yrs	M	HSE	0		1	1		marked MI	anomia	0	0	0	0	1	0
Andrewes & Gielewski (1999)	1	28	F	HSE	1	1 yr	1	0	Estimated length of PTA provided (0 days to over 8 weeks).	amnesia	Seizures, insulin dependent diabetes, depression	0	0	0	0	0	0
Ownsworth & McFarland (1999)	Exp=20 CG=31	Exp M=43.1 (23-65) / CG: 28.1 (20-40)	Exp: 19:1 / CG: 13:19	TBI=15, tumour, CVA, infection= 5	1	M=15 yrs (4-37 yrs)	1	0		poor memory (RBMT)		0	0	0	0	0	0

APPENDIX 2.1. (cont.)

Names and Dates	#	Age	M:F	Etiology	Site of Injury	TPO	Neuropsych Tests	Pre-morbid IQ	Initial Severity	Memory Severity	Dual dx/Co-morbidity	Selection Criteria	Tx History	Medication	Education	Occupation	Living Situation
Evans et al. (2000)	Study 1: 18 Study 2: 16 Study 3: 34	Study 1: M=43.3 Study 2: M=41.4 Study 3: M=36.4		Study 1: CVA=6; anoxia=5; HI=3; enceph=2; ETOH=2 Study 2: CVA=4; anoxia=4; HI=5; enceph=1; ETOH=2 Study 3: CVA=7; anoxia=11; HI=11; enceph=3; tumor=3; tumor=1.MD+CA=1	0	Study 1: M=22 mos* Study 2: M=66.45 mos* Study 3: M=21.2–67.7 mos (*excluding patients with alcoholism)	1	0		severity of MI determined by RBMT screening	unilateral neglect; language imp; attention + executive function imp	1	0	0	0	0	0
Komatsu et al. (2000)	Study 1 M=8 Study 2 M=4	Study 1 M=61 Study 2 M=58		KS	0	More than 1 yr.	1	0		sev ant. amnesia; varying degrees of ret. amnesia		0	0	0	0	0	0
Riley & Heaton (2000)	12	M=44 (19-61)	9:3	HI	0	M=11 yr.	1	1		varied severity MI	disorientation; exec func imp	1	0	0	1	1	1
Kalla et al. (2001)	12	M = 41	10:2	sev TBI = 11 CVA = 1	1	At least 12 mos post	1	1				1	0	0	0	0	1
Hillary et al. (2003)	20	M=41.5 (18-55)	16:4	mod-sev TBI	1	At least 1 yr (M=4.1 yrs)	1	0	Based on LOC over 24 hrs or positive neuroimaging findings			1	0	0	0	1	1
Tailby & Haslam (2003)	24	Group 1 (sev MI): M=43 Group 2 (mod MI): M=43.8 Group 3 (mild MI): M=37.5	Group 1 1:1 Group 2 3:1 Group 3 7:1	HI=12; CVA=6; hypoxia=3; dementia=1, HSE=1; Parkinson's=1 Study 1: CHI	0		1			mild, mod, sev MI		1	1	0	0	0	0
Riley et al. (2004)	Study 1=12 Study 2=12 Studies 3 & 4CG =20/24	Study 1: M=34 (19-54) Study 2: M=56 (38-66) Studies 3 & 4: NP		Study 2: CHI=4; CVA=8 (no participant overlap between Studies 1 & 2) Study 3: NA Study 4: NA	0	Study 1: M=3.8 yrs Study 2: M=2.6 yrs Study 3: NA Study 4: NA	1		Studies 1 & 2: GCS 8 or less and/or PTA in excess of 24 hours	mod MI			1	·	0	0	0
Ehlhardt et al. (2005)	4	M=47.25 (36-58)	2:2	TBI	0	M=23.25	1	0	LOC reported	significant MI	motor & visual imp	1	1	0	0	0	0
Melton & Bourgeois (2005)	7	35-56 yrs	3:4	TBI	0	2-30 yrs	1	0	LOC: 0-10 wks	chronic, "everyday" MI		0	1	0	0	1	1
Stark et al. (2005)	1: CG=3	Exp: 68 yrs CG: M=67 (63-72)	Exp: M CG: M	Anoxia	1	2 yrs	1	0	Comatose on admit to hospital	Profound ant amnesia; Ret amnesia		0	1	0	0	0	1
Turkstra & Bourgeois (2005)	1	M	M	TBI	1	7 yrs	0	0		sev ant amnesia, mild ret amnesia	mild speech ataxia	0	1	1	1	0	1
Dou et al. (2006)	CAMG =13 TAMG=11 CG=13*	M=38.067 (21-55)	27:10	TBI	1	In days CAMG M=270.15; TAMG M=161.27; CG M=226.77	1	0				1	0	0	1	1	0
Landis et al. (2006)	33 total Mild TBI=8 Mod TBI=9 Sev TBI=16	Mild: M=10.4 mod: M=11.5 sev: M=11.3	% male Mild: 87.5% mod: 77.8% sev: 93.8%	mild-severe TBI	0	yrs since injury: Mild: M=2.9 yrs mod: M=2.6 yrs sev: M=3 yrs	1	0	Mild, mod, or sev	Met criteria for MI		1	0	0	1	0	0
Page et al. (2006)	Study 1=23: CG=20 Study 2=20	Study 1: M=46 (26-69) Study 2: M=43 (21-80)	Study 1: 16:7 Study 2: 18:2	Study 1: TBI=9; CVA=4; enceph=4; hypoxia=2; KS=1; E=1; CR=1; CH=1 Study 2: TBI=8; CVA=5; KS=2; anoxia=2; enceph=1; SAH=2	0	Study 1 & 2: at least 1 yr post	1	0	TBI (GCS)	mod-sev MI		1	0	0	0	0	0

DEMENTIA

Names and Dates	#	Age	M:F	Etiology	Site of Injury	TPO	Neuropsych Tests	Pre-morbid IQ	Initial Severity	Memory Severity	Dual dx/Co-morbidity	Selection Criteria	Tx History	Medication	Education	Occupation	Living Situation
Winter & Hunkin (1999)	1	66	F	AD	1		1	1		sev MI, impaired new learning		0	0	0	0	0	1
Clare et al. (2000)	6	M=69.33 (69-75)	3:3	minimal-mild AD	0	MI noted 18 mos to 5 yrs prior to the study	1	1		sev MI	imp verbal fluency	0	0	0	0	1	1
Clare et al. (2002)	12	M=71 (57-83)	9:3	minimal-mild AD	1		1	1		significant MI		1	1	1	0	1	1
Metzler-Baddeley & Snowden (2005)	4	65-72 yrs	3:1	mixed sev AD	0		1	1		All participants MI; 2 with profound amnesia & sev impaired remote memory		1	0	1	0	0	1
Ruis & Kessels (2005)	10	Range: 73-89 yrs	5:5	mod-sev AD	0		1	1			mild anomia	1	1	1	1	1	1
Haslam et al. (2006)	Study 1: Exp=3; OCG=8 Study 2: Exp=2 Study 3: Exp=7	Study 1: Exp=81-89 yrs OCGs M=77.5 Study 2: 84 & 78 yrs Study 3: 67-87 yrs	Study 1: Exp=3 F; OCG=1:7 Study 2: 1:1 Study 3: NP	Study 1 & 2 AD Study 3: AD=2, VD=5	1		1	1		Study 1 & 2: general cognitive decline with MI primary deficit. Study 3: sev MI	deterioration in general intellectual ability; word finding difficulties, disorientation, imp concentration	1	0	0	1	0	0
Dunn & Clare (2007)	Exp=10	M=80.9 (76-86)	5:5	early AD, VD, mixed (AD + VD)	0		1	0		MI predominant		1	0	0	0	0	1

SCHIZOPHRENIA

APPENDIX 2.1. (cont.)

Names and Dates	#	Age	M:F	Etiology	Site of Injury	TPO	Neuropsych Tests	Pre-morbid IQ	Initial Severity	Memory Severity	Dual dx/Co-morbidity	Selection Criteria	Tx History	Medication	Education	Occupation	Living Situation
Kern et al. (1996)	23 (IE group=11; No IE group=12)	IE M=33.2; NIE M=30.1		schizophrenia/SD=IE 9; NIE 7. Remaining 7 participants: BD=1, depression=1, OPD=2, unspecified=3	0	Age at first hospitalization: IE group M=17.6 yrs; No IE group M=21.2 yrs	1	0				1	0	1	1	0	1
O'Carroll et al. (1999)	Group 1=20 schizophrenia w/MI; Group 2=21 schizophrenia wo MI; Group 3=20 (9CG)	Group 1 M=35.6; Group 2 M=36; Group 3 M=33	Group 1 M=11:9; Group 2 M=15:6; Group 3 M=12:8	schizophrenia	0	Chronicity (date of first hospitalization to testing): M=10 yrs (range 1 month-34.7 yrs)	1	0		MI group (score of less than 8 out of 10 on RBMT)		1	0	1	1	0	1
Kern et al. (2002)	65	EL M=32; CG M=33	26:6; 22:11	schizophrenia, SD	0	yrs since 1st hospitalization: Exp M=15.3; CG M=17.5	1	0				1	0	1	1	1	0
Young et al. (2002)	SI=15; DI=15; CG=15	Overall M=40-41 yrs; SI M=40.6; DI M=40.1; CG M=41.2	32:13	schizophrenia	0	Age of initial onset: SI M=19.9 yrs; DI M=18.9 yrs; CG M=23.1 yrs	1	0		MI severity levels based on 1st 3 trials of the CVLT		1	0	1	1	0	1
Kern et al. (2005)	Exp=29; CG=31	Exp. M=44.6; CG: M=42.6	Exp: 20.9; CG: 23.8	schizophrenia,SD	0	yrs since 1st hospitalization: Exp:17.9 yrs, CG: 15.7 yrs	1	0				1	0	1	1	0	1
Pope & Kern (2006)	Exp=36; CG=22	Exp M=42.4 CG=40.6	Exp group: 63.9% M; CG group: 68.2% M	schizophrenia, SD	0	Exp group: yrs since first hospitalization M = 17.4 yrs	1	0				1	0	1	1	0	0

Explanation of abbreviations in Appendices 2.1–2.3: − = negative outcome; / = qualified outcome; + = positive outcome; ABI = acquired brain injury; ACA = anterior communicating artery aneurysm rupture; AD = Alzheimer's dementia; AH = amygdala hippocampectomy; CA = cerebral atrophy; CAMG = computer-assisted memory training group; CG = control group; CG* (cognitive disabilities); CH = chronic hydrocephalus; CHI = closed head injury; CR = cyst removal; CVA = stroke; CVLT = California Verbal Learning Test; DAT = Alzheimer's type dementia; DI = direct instruction; DO = diary only; DSIT = diary and self-instructional training; EF = errorful learning; EL = errorless learning; ELWF = errorless learning without fading; EMQ = Everyday Memory Questionnaire; Enceph = encephalitis; ETOH = chronic alcoholism; Exp = experimental; f/u = follow-up; HE = herpes encephalitis; HI = head injury; HSE = herpes simplex encephalitis; I = information; IE = idiopathic epilepsy (disability); IE = initial errors; JOL = judgments of learning; KS = Korsakoff's syndrome; LOC = loss of consciousness; MCI = mild cognitive impairment; MD = mytonic dystrophy; MI = memory impairment; MOV = method of vanishing cues; MTL = medial temporal lobe; MVC = method of vanishing cues; OCG = older controls; OPD = organic personality disorder; P = Procedures; PCA = posterior cerebral anterior aneurysm rupture; PTA = posttraumatic amnesia; Pxs = pictures; RBMT = Rivermead Behavioral Memory Test; SA = standard anticipation; SAH = subarachnoid hemorrhage; SD = schizoaffective disorder; SI = scaffolded instruction; SP = spaced presentations; SIP = systematic instructional packages; SR = spaced retrieval; SRT = spaced retrieval training; Ss = subjects; TAMG = therapist-administered memory training group; TBI = traumatic brain injury; TLA = temporal lobe abscess; VD = vascular dementia; VE = viral encephalitis; WCST = Wisconsin Card Sort Test; WMS-R = Wechsler Memory Scale—Revised; YCG = younger controls.

APPENDIX 2.2. Intervention

NAMES & DATES	Instructional Approach	Additional Components	Treatment Targets	Tx Dosage	Tx Setting	Tx Providers	Measurement
				ABI			
Glisky et al. (1986a)	MVC vs. EF		I (computer terms & definitions)	8 sessions, 2-3 days apart; additional learning-test session 6 wks later; both learning conditions each session	0	1	# correctly produced (without letter cues) & recognized terms matched to definitions; # of letters required to complete word fragments in presence of definitions
Glisky et al. (1986b)	MVC		I & P (e.g. writing, editing, & executing simple commas)	2x wkly for approx 2 hrs each session; 3 lessons total; long-term retention lessons administered at 1-3 mos	1	1	# of hints & total # of learning trials
Glisky & Schacter (1987)	SIP	Stimuli (varied examples)	P (computer data entry)	Phase 1: 8 sessions; 2x wkly (reached initial mastery in first 6 sessions) Phase 2: 15 sessions, 2-3 day intervals Phase 3: 8 total sessions Phase 4: mostly check-in sessions on the job	1	1	# of hints, error rate & mean time card; task completion time; # of cards entered
Glisky & Schacter (1988)	MVC		I (definitions of computer terms) P (e.g writing simple programs)	2-hr training sessions conducted 2x wkly, until criterion for mastery achieved	1	1	# of trials to criterion; # of hints per trial
Glisky & Schacter (1989)	SIP	Strategy (problem tray for difficult documents) Stimuli (varied examples)	P (complex data entry)	Phase 1: 2x wkly; 18 sessions (5-mos break before final session) Phase 2: 2x wkly transitioning to daily for 3 mos. Phase 3: 9 sessions (used new examples) Phase 4: daily sessions for 5 wks	1	1	# of hints & mean times per trial; total & mean of documents entered; # docs per trial & mean time per doc; # of trials to criterion; # of errors per trial; total # of errors
Leng et al. (1991)	MVC vs. EF		I (computer terms & definitions)	1 hr sessions; alternating between conditions each session. # of total sessions determined by reaching criterion for mastery; 10 sessions total	0	1	# of terms correct
Giang et al. (1992)	SIP	Ss 3 Strategy (self-management) Stimuli (varied examples)	Ss 1 & 2 (math, reading)	2-3x sessions per wk for 6 wks	1	1	% of correct problems; # correct facts per min; % of words correctly repeated/sounds read; % of time on-task following corrective feedback
Glisky (1992)	SIP	Stimuli (varied examples)	I (computer terms & definitions) P (data entry)	Knowledge: 2, 2 hr sessions weekly to criterion Skills: 2, 2 hr sessions weekly	1	1	# trials to criterion; # cues per trial; time to complete each trial; mean time to enter a single record
Butters, Glisky & Schacter (1993)	MVC		I (business terms & definitions)	2-hr, twice weekly sessions until criterion met in each of 3 conditions (under learned 50% correct; learned-100% correct; over-learned-100% correct + 10 trials)	1	1	# of trials to criterion
Baddeley & Wilson (1994)	EL vs. EF		I (words)	1 session	0	0	# of words correct
Van der Linden et al. (1994)	SIP	Stimuli (varied examples)	I (concepts)	Sessions 2-4 times each wk, ranging from 30-60 mins (For Stage 1, training continued until criterion for mastery achieved)	0	0	# of correct concepts identified; # of correctly classified examples of concepts; # correct application of concepts to new examples
Wilson et al. (1994)	EL vs. EF	Strategy (mnemonic)	I (names, objects) P (programming memory aid)	Ss #1-3: 1 session Ss #4: 2x daily sessions over 9 days Ss #5: training sessions over 9 days	0	0	# of names or objects correct; # of steps recalled while programming memory aid; # of time on-task following corrective feedback
Glisky (1995)	MVC		P (word processing)	2x wkly, 2 hr sessions to criterion Exp 1: 2-3 sessions per wk, 1 method per training session; training continued until Ss reached a criterion or a maximum of 20 sessions; 2 additional training sessions, 1 per method 6 wks later Exp 2: 2 sessions per wk; both methods each session; training continued until a criterion or maximum of 12 sessions; 1 additional training session 6 wks later	1	1	# of responses required by patient; # of wks/trials to criterion; # computer/examiner hints per session; amount of time to complete tasks; responses to oral questionnaires
Hunkin & Parkin (1995)	MVC vs. EF		I (computer terms & definitions)	2, 60-min sessions for 8 wks (16 sessions total)	0	0	# of items correctly answered as a proportion of the number of items unknown to the Ss
Schmitter-Edgecombe et al. 1995	SIP	Stimuli (varied examples)	P (external aid)	2, 4-trial sessions per day in each condition, 2x wkly	0	1	Laboratory-based recall (e.g. WMS-R) Laboratory-based everyday memory (e.g., RBMT; EMC)
Thoene & Glisky (1995)	MVC vs. video	Strategy (self-instruction)	I (face-names)	Training continued until criterion achieved or plateaued performance	1	0	# of trials to criterion & # face-names correct
Glisky & Delaney (1996)	EL vs. EF	Stimuli (varied examples)	P (external aid)	Exp 1: 3 sessions with a minimum of 2 hrs between sessions Exp 2: varied # training sessions (range 6-20)	0	0	% words correct
Glisky (1996)	MVC		I (words)	Stage 1: 10 training sessions for 16 days Stage 2: Daily notebook entries prompted by spouse; 8 clinic(?) sessions for 4 wks	0	0	# of paired associates correct using external aid; spouse completed daily checklist of questions
Squires et al. (1996)	SIP	Stimuli (varied examples)	P (external aid)	Exp 1 & 2: 2 sessions, 1 condition per session; 7-day break in between sessions	1	0	# of words correct
Squires et al. (1997)	EL vs. EF		I (words)	Exp 1: 4 sessions; 2 per training condition	0	0	proportion of words correct
Hunkin et al. (1998a)	EL vs. EF		I (words)	Exp 2: 2 sessions; 1 wk apart, 1 session per training condition	0	0	proportion of correct & error responses (i.e., intrusions)
Hunkin et al. (1998b)	SIP		P (word processing tasks)	Total # of sessions = 30, averaging 2 sessions per wk Exp 1: 3 phases baseline=2 sessions; training=6; post-training=4 (6 training sessions were required to reach criterion; 2 wks duration) Exp 2: baseline=4 sessions; training=5; post-training=3 (no criterion set: 5 consecutive training sessions)	0	0	task completion time/timed motor tasks (mouse use/typing tests to factor out motor procedural learning); open-ended questions re: material learned
Parkin et al. (1998)	EL		I (face-names) P (e.g., filing)	pre-work training-1 yr job-site training-25 sessions for 4 mos	0	0	proportion of face-names correct
Andrews & Gielewski (1999)	SIP	Stimuli (varied examples)	I (e.g., face-names)	initial training session via phone:	1	1	# name correct, task completion & level of independence
Ownsworth & McFarld (1999)	SIP	Strategy (self-instruction)	P (external aid)	DO group: 2 wks baseline + 4 wks treatment DSIT group: 6 wks baseline + 4 wks treatment	1	0	mean total # of diary entries, Memory problem score; Ratings of distress, Strategy-use score; Helpfulness & mood ratings
Evans et al. (2000)	EL vs. EF	Study 3 Strategy (imagery)	P (route finding, programming electronic aid)	Exp 1: 4 training sessions per condition: 3 sessions total: 1 wk between sessions Exp 1: 4 training sessions per condition (2x wkly sessions for 2 wks); 1 wk delay between conditions;11 wk duration Exp 2: avg 5-mos break, then 5 additional training sessions over 2* wks	1	0	% or # names or task steps correct
Komatsu et al. (2000)	SIP	Stimuli (initial letter, MVC conditions)	I (face-names)	3 sessions total (1 training condition per session, for the first 2 sessions); 1 wk between sessions	0	1	# of words correctly answered
Riley & Heaton (2000)	SIP		I (facts)		0	0	# of questions correctly answered
Kalla et al. (2001)	EL vs. EF	Stimuli (pre-exposure) Strategy (evaluative questioning)	I (face-names)	All 4 experimental conditions tested during the same session. Sessions lasted approx 1.5 hrs with 10-min breaks between conditions. Each condition was comprised of a "study phase" & a "test phase".	1	0	# of first/last names correct; # of training trials to reach criterion

44

APPENDIX 2.2. (cont.)

NAMES & DATES	Instructional Approach	Additional Components	Treatment Targets	Tx Dosage	Tx Setting	Tx Providers	Measurement
Hillary et al. (2003)	SR/SP		I (words)	1 session	1	0	# of words correct
Talby & Haslam (2003)	EL vs. EF	Strategy (self-generated responses)	I (words)	2 sessions separated by at least 1 wk; 2 conditions presented each session separated by a 20 min break	0	0	# words correct, memory strategies questionnaire
Riley et al. (2004)	MVC vs. EL		I (words)	Study 1: 1 session only / Study 2: 2 sessions separated by 1 wk / Studies 3 & 4: 1 session only	0	0	# of words correct
Ehlhardt et al. (2005)	SIP	Strategy (predict-reflect) Stimuli (varied examples)	P (email)	duration varied; 4-5x wkly; 7-15 sessions required to meet criterion for mastery	1	1	# of email steps correct; # correct responses to goal questions; # of training sessions to mastery; # of training trials to mastery; self-reports of generalization (i.e., goal execution)
Melton & Bourgeois (2005)	SR		I (strategy recall)	Max. 30 mins oer session; daily training until mastery reached on all 3 of their goals, avg of 5.3 sessions per goal.	1	1	% correct responses to goal questions
Stark et al. (2005)	EL vs. EF	Stimuli (varied vs. non-varied examples)	I (sentences)	31 study sessions (control Ss-2 study sessions)	0	1	% sentences correct on visual & auditory recall; participant confidence ratings
Turkstra & Bourgeois (2005)	SR		I (goal questions)	4, 30-min phone sessions a wk until criterion achieved	1	1	# of correct responses to goal questions
Dou et al. (2006)	EL vs. EF	Strategy (mnemonic)	I (memory tasks)	1 mo (20 sessions, 6 days a wk; 45 mins per session) 1 mo f/u assessment	0	1	neuropsych tests
Landis et al.	EL vs. EF		I (facts)	2, 1-hr sessions a wk for 7 wks; 3 of the 7 wks were spent on training declarative knowledge—half of the items were taught with EL & the other half with trial-&-error.; 3 wks of training on unrelated procedural skills.	1	1	# of facts correct
Page et al. (2006)	EL vs. EF		I (words)	Exp #1 &2: 2 sessions separated by 1 wk	0	0	# words correct, recognition test; source memory task
DEMENTIA							
Winter & Hunkin (1999)	EL		I (face-names)	4 training sessions	0	0	# of names correct
Clare et al. (2000)	SIP	Strategy (mnemonic)	I (face-names, facts) P (external memory aid)	Varied across participants	0	0	mean proportion of faces or items correct & frequency of repetitive questioning Neuropsych tests/ratings of behavior mood administered before/after intervention
Clare et al. (2002)	SIP	Strategy (mnemonic)	I (face-names)	6 sessions per name; 1 item trained per session; home practice encouraged during intervention phase & during 1st mo following intervention	0	0	# of names correct
Metzler-Baddeley & Snowden (2005)	EL vs. EF	Strategy (mnemonic)	I (objects; face-names)	8 consec. training sessions for per material set (novel/familiar) for 3 Ss; 4 wks for 1 Ss when learning novel material; Material in both learning conditions repeated 3x daily with 8 days break between learning the familiar & novel material sets	1	0	proportional scoring system based on # of names correct
Ruis & Kessels (2005)	EL vs. EF		I (face-names)	1 session per training condition; 1 wk between sessions	0	0	# of names correct
Haslam et al. (2006)	EL vs. EF		I (high vs. low info; face-names)	2 seasions of 1:1 memory training with 2 wk break between sessions, both learning conditions each session	0	0	# of names correct represented as proportion of "hit rate" vs. "false alarm" rate name familiarity included
Dunn & Clare (2007)	SIP		I (face-names)	6, 1-hr sessions, 2x wkly for 3wks	0	0	# of items correct on each free recall, cued recall, & recognition trials
SCHIZOPHRENIA							
Kern et al. (1996)	EL vs. EF (initial errors)	Stimuli (varied examples)	P (WCST)	training required 1-2 hrs (with breaks); criterion for each phase	1	1	# categories achieved; # perseverative errors; percent conceptual level responses; # card sorting errors; (initial error group: pre/post-treatment administration of WCST)
O'Carroll et al. (1999)	EL vs. EF	Stimuli (varied examples)	I (words)	1 session only	0	1	% word correct
Kern et al. (1999)	EL vs. EF		P (index card filing task, toilet assembly task)	3 learning trials followed by 9 test trials in blocks of 3	1	1	accuracy, speed, overall productivity, on-task performance, & Ss satisfaction with training
Kern et al. (2002)	EL vs. EF	SI group: "calibrated" (i.e. collaborative) strategic instruction DI group: strategic instruction not calibrated	P (index card filing task, toilet assembly task) acquisition	2 training sessions, each lasting 45-60 mins, depending on speed of skill acquisition / 6 sessions on separate days within a 4-wk period (1 pre-test session; 2 Tx sessions; 3rd session-transfer training; 1st post-test)	1	1	neuropsych tests
Young et al. (2002)	SIP	Stimuli (varied examples)	P (WSCT)	2nd post-test session 4 wks later.	1	1	scores on an assessment of personal problem solving
Kern et al. (2005)	EL vs. EF	Stimuli (varied examples)	I (social problem solving skills)	training occurred for a total of 6 hrs across 2 days in groups of 6-8 Ss	1	1	# of words correct; Standardized residualized scores (for experimental group Ss only)
Pope & Kern (2006)	EL vs. EF		I (words)	1 session	1	0	

45

APPENDIX 2.3. Study Design and Outcomes

NAMES & DATES	STUDY DESIGN: Class/ Design	STUDY DESIGN: Statistics	STUDY DESIGN: Reliability/ Validity	STUDY DESIGN: Ecological Validity	OUTCOMES: Immediate Outcomes	OUTCOMES: Generalization	OUTCOMES: Maintenance	OUTCOMES: Author Conclusions
ABI								
Glisky et al. (1986a)	3 within & between-Ss	1	0	0	+	(+) slightly changed definitions; better with MVC	(+) over 6 weeks	Results showed that patients with varying degrees of amnesia were able to learn & retain computer-related vocabulary matched to definitions across both learning conditions but with significantly better performance in the MVC condition, although they depended heavily on first letter cues for successful performance.. They also demonstrated some generalization, matching the computer terms to slightly altered definitions but was significantly less than controls. The control Ss showed no difference between the two learning conditions. The authors suggest that learning was due to priming effects, as Ss reported not remembering the experience of learning.
Glisky et al. (1986b)	4 case comparisons	0	0	0	+	(-) unable to generalize to new examples	(+) at least 1 month	Ss with mild-severe amnesia due to CHI learned & retained complex computer knowledge/procedures commensurate with controls, although their learning was qualitatively different—much less efficient/slower with substantial between-session loss of learning. They required high amounts of repetition before error-free performance was achieved. Also, Ss with amnesia were unable to answer open-ended questions with wording different than that to which they had been exposed during training & could not recall the experience of learning. These results suggest that individuals with amnesia are capable of learning complex skills, although knowledge tends to be "hyper-specific" (i.e., inflexible) & reliant on the specific stimuli to trigger appropriate responses.
Glisky & Schacter (1987)	4 case study	0	0	1	+	(+) workplace	(+) over 5 months	Results show that the MVC was an effective technique for training complex knowledge & skills during the acquisition of phase of learning, while verbal prompts & corrective feedback were effectively applied during later stages in simulated & applied work settings. All skills/procedures were explicitly & directly taught & the participant was provided with high amounts of practice. The authors suggest that the "hyper-specific" nature of MVC & the tasks to which it can be applied are an appropriate fit for individuals with severe amnesia without frontal lobe impairment.
Glisky & Schacter (1988)	4 case comparisons	1	0	0	+		(+) up to 9 mos	Results show that all Ss with memory impairment were capable of learning & long-term retention of domain specific knowledge using MVC; however, their performance differed substantially from controls, requiring many more trials to achieve criterion. The authors suggest that severity of memory impairment may be a better indicator of learning capability than etiology; all patients, regardless of etiology, learned the tasks; however, Ss with more severe impairments required more trials to achieve criterion Also, attentional impairments may also mitigate performance.
Glisky & Schacter (1989)	4 case study	0	0	1	+	(+) novel documents; work setting	(+) maintained full-time employment	Results show that an individual with severe amnesia can learn & perform complex tasks in the work setting & therefore maintain gainful employment. The authors suggest that both impaired & spared memory processes may contribute to performance. They also suggest there are 3 job characteristics critical for success: "1) the job can be broken down into simple components; 2) all relevant knowledge can be trained directly & explicitly; & 3) once learned, the job can be performed repetitively, & does not place on-going demands on memory."
Leng et al. (1991)	4 within-Ss (single case)	1	0	0	+	(+) altered wording & format	(+) 1-month	Results showed that the Ss learned more quickly using the MVC, & some maintenance & generalization were observed across terms trained in both conditions. The authors report that the MVC training program also had a beneficial effect on the Ss's mood due to his success learning a new skill with minimal errors. Using MVC, the Ss later went on to learn a word processing program that enabled him to write articles on preferred topics.
Glang et al. (1992)	3&4 Ss 1: eithin Ss (multiple baseline) Ss 2: case study Ss 3: case study	0	1	1	+	(+) strategy applied to new content	(+) Ss3: 3 mos	Direct instruction techniques were effective in teaching three children with severe TBI selected academic tasks & behavioral (self-management) skills in relatively few (e.g., 12) sessions.
Glisky (1992)	3 within & between Ss	1	0	1	+	(+) minor changes in materials	(+) 4 weeks	Results showed that all patients, regardless of the severity of memory impairment, were able to acquire both factual and procedural knowledge. Declarative knowledge was acquired at a slower rate than procedural knowledge while procedural knowledge was acquired at approximately the same rate across patients and controls. Maintenance and transfer of of performance were also observed across stimulus materials. High amounts of practice were necessary to achieve criterion.
Butters, Glisky & Schacter (1993)	3 within & between Ss	1	0	0	+	(+) alternative version of definitions in passive voice		Patients demonstrated improved transfer of learning with increased learning trials, thus countering previous theory suggesting that extensive repetitions result in inflexible learning. Patients with mild impairments learned more quickly than those with moderate-severe impairments, while the patients as a group required significantly more trials than the controls. These results also suggest that poor generalization in rehabilitation contexts may be attributed to too few learning trials.
Baddeley & Wilson (1994)	3 within & between-Ss	1	0	0	+			This was one of the first studies to evaluate EL compared with EF. EL was superior to EF for word recall, particularly for participants with amnesia. The authors suggest that Ss' impaired explicit memory system forces reliance on implicit memory, which is vulnerable to errors; hence, the need to eliminate errors during the acquisition phase of learning.
Van der Linden et al. (1994)	4 case studies	0	0	0	+	Ss 1: (+) applied novel examples Ss 2: (—) not able to apply to novel examples	(+) Ss 1 & 2: 1 week	Both Ss were capable of some conceptual (i.e., semantic) learning, although performance was significantly impaired compared with non-disabled matched controls and they could not recall the experience of learning. The authors suggest that learning at different stages was sub-served by different memory systems. Specifically, learning via the MVC was likely dependent on the perceptual memory system, whereas the classification tasks were more dependent on semantic memory. Both Sss showed different performance patterns associated with each memory system, suggesting that a common etiology does not imply similar neuropsychological symptoms.
Wilson et al. (1994)	4 case studies	1	0	1	+		(+) Ss #5 1 week	EL was superior to EF across a range of tasks and information (e.g., face-name recall, programming an electronic organizer).
Glisky (1995)	4 case study	0	0	1	+	(+) home use - word processing tasks	(+) at least 10 mos	The MVC was successfully used to train selected word processing skills, though learning rate was slow & error elimination sometimes difficult. The author suggests that an amnesic patient's ability to learn information or procedures may depend to a large extent on the task cues or stimuli that constrain responses. The author also suggests that computer-based training provides a potentially fruitful avenue for skill development leading to vocational opportunities for individuals with severe amnesia.
Hunkin & Parkin (1995)	3 within & between-Ss	1	0	0	/	(—) Exp 1: impaired with wording changes Exp 2: impaired; not influenced by method, modality, wording	(+) Exp 1: after 6-week delay, regardless of method (—) Exp 2: decrease in retention with 6-week delay, more so for the SA method	Learning occurred in both training conditions with no significant advantage of MVC over standard anticipation. In fact, SA showed a significant advantage over MVC in the earlier stages of training in Exp 2, whereas MVC was more facilitative of retention after 6 weeks. Results from a correlational analysis suggest that MVC was perhaps more beneficial for Ss with lower verbal IQ, more severe memory deficits, & compromised frontal lobe functioning, whereas SA was better for less severe Ss. The authors suggest that the lack of significant benefit of MVC over SA likely stems from: (1) the use of explicit recall techniques (i.e., cued recall), where MVC relies more on implicit memory & (2) the task itself—learning novel associations.
Schmitter–Edgecombe et al. (1995)	2 between Ss (randomized control group)	1	1	1	+		(+) 6 months everday memory failures	External memory notebook training in a group setting resulted in significantly lower observed everyday memory problems when compared with supportive group therapy with family & participant observations of memory failures highly correlated. The authors suggest that observational checklists may be more sensitive than laboratory measures in detecting the effects of notebook training.
Thoene & Glisky (1995)	3 within-Ss	1	0	0	/		(+) 3-4 days	The mnemonic condition required significantly fewer trials to reach criterion for mastery and resulted in more names recalled after a long delay compared to the other two training conditions. Furthermore, it was the only condition in which all the participants reached the criterion for mastery. The MVC and video condition did not differ with re: to # of trials to reach criterion. The authors suggest that mnemonic training is an explicit process that promotes meaningful associations facilitative of learning arbitrarily associated information (e.g., name-face pairs). The MVC is less conducive to learning arbitrarily associated information, given that the Ss focus on perceptual-orthographic features.
Glisky & Delaney (1996)	3 &4 Exp 1: within & between-Ss Exp 2: case comparisons	1	0	0	+		Exp 1: NP Exp 2: (+) 5 days; 6-8 weeks	Exp 1: Ss with PTA demonstrated implicit learning/significant priming as evidenced by improved recall for studied words in the implicit stem recall task. Possible reasons for this result include the relatively preserved perceptual (visual) system in pts with CHI. Exp 2: Ss with PTA learned new semantic information, though at a rate slower than normal controls, & partially retained this information after emerging from PTA. Overall, these results suggest that patients with PTA are capable of implicit learning & therefore may benefit from cognitive rehab at an earlier point in recovery than was previously thought.
Squires et al. (1996)	4 Stage 1: within-Ss (single case) Stage 2: case study	1	0	1	+	Stage 1: (—) repetitive questions at home. Stage 2: (+) reduced repetitive questions at home	(+) Stage 1: 7 days (+) Stage 2: timeline not specified	During Stage 1, EL resulted in significantly better paired associate recall using a notebook when compared with EF. Further, these results were applicable to the recall of daily/weekly events in Stage 2, in which the overall amount of questioning was significantly reduced, particularly repetitive questions.
Squires et al. (1997)	3 within-Ss	1	0	0	+			Exp 1: EL was superior to EF in the immediate recall condition. Exp 2: EL was superior to EF in both the immediate & delayed recall conditions. The authors suggest that the superior performance of EL was likely due to the suppression of errors during training, & that the increased effort required to learn novel associations in Exp 2 could explain the significant improvements in favor of EL across both recall conditions. Finally, the authors suggest EL may relay on implicit memory or explicit memory or both.

APPENDIX 2.3. *(cont.)*

NAMES & DATES	STUDY DESIGN				OUTCOMES			
	Class/ Design	Statistics	Reliability/ Validity	Ecological Validity	Immediate Outcomes	Generalization	Maintenance	Author Conclusions
Hunkin et al. (1998a)	3 within-Ss	1	0	0	+		(+) Exp 1: 48 hrs, some decrements in performance	The authors conclude that EL is superior to EF for individuals with moderate-severe memory impairments; however, there is no evidence to suggest that the benefits of EL rely exclusively on implicit memory (as tested through fragment completion in Exp 2) but may instead depend on error prevention associated with residual explicit memory.
Hunkin et al. (1998b)	4 case study	1	0	0	+			EL, spaced repetitions, & high rates of practice were successfully used to teach an individual with severe memory impairment selected word processing tasks. Improved performance could not be explained by parallel improvements in motor function (mouse/typing skills).
Parkin et al. (1998)	4 case study	1	0	1	+	Exp 1: (—) untrained names Exp 2: NP	Exp 1: (+) 5-weeks Exp 2: (+) 2-weeks	EL resulted in significant improvements in face-name recall (politicians, friends) & retention, at 5 & 2 weeks, respectively. A "refresher" test of previously correct names was associated with a high rate of retention throughout training. The authors conclude that EL is a potentially beneficial method of training for individuals with anomia for proper names.
Andrewes & Gielewski (1999)	4 case study	0	0	1	+	(+) work setting	(+) 9 months	The participant successfully learned the targeted work-related tasks using EL techniques. She maintained task independence several months after completing training, resulting in a permanent part-time job. The participant's pre-morbid content (i.e., semantic) knowledge, high IQ, personality, motivation, parental support & pre-vocational training (e.g., diary training) also contributed to success of the program.
Ownsworth & McFarland (1999)	3 between Ss (random assignment, baseline-across-groups)	1	0	1	+	(+)home		Results showed that the DSIT group was more consistent in making diary entries, they reported few memory problems, greater benefit from strategy use & lower ratings of confusion & bewilderment during the treatment phase. All Ss reported improvement in the areas of distress associated with memory problems, degree of strategy-use, depression-defection & fatigue-inertia ratings. The authors suggest these results suggest that self-instructional training has greater ecological validity than task-specific learning.
Evans et al. (2000)	3 within-Ss	1	0	0	/			EL was not consistently superior to trial-&-error learning across experimental conditions/tasks; trial-&-error learning was superior to EL on selected tasks. The tasks & recall conditions that relied on implicit memory seemed to benefit from EL (e.g., name learning with first letter cue), whereas the tasks that relied on explicit recall (e.g., novel associations such as learning a route) did not benefit from EL. Sss with the most severe memory impairments appeared to benefit more from EL & when the interval between learning & recall was relatively short. Finally, the use of an imagery strategy combined with EL facilitated name recall.
Komatsu et al. (2000)	3 within-Ss	1	0	0	+		Exp 2: 2/4 Ss at least a few days	Results showed that the EL conditions, particularly the paired associate in Exp 1, were superior to the errorful conditions. The MVC, anticipated to be an "errorless" but "effortful" condition, did not serve as a completely errorfree task in either experiment. Although Ss in Exp. 2, as a group, did show some improvement in delayed recall with modified MVC. The authors conclude that MVC should be viewed as a "relatively, but not absolutely ELtask." A high number of training trials are also required to facilitate learning. Finally, the authors suggest that there is a trade off between error & effort & that these factors should be distinguished from one another.
Riley & Heaton (2000)	3 within-Ss	1	0	0	/		(+) 1 week depending severity, item difficulty, & condition	Increasing assistance (which promotes effortful recall on training trials) was more effective than decreasing assistance for participants with better memories & for easier questions. Conversely, decreasing assistance (which minimizes training errors) was more effective for participants with more impaired memories & for more difficult questions. The modest increase in errors under increasing assistance was not associated with deterioration in memory performance. The authors suggest teaching strategies should consider the promotion of effortful recall during learning trials as well as the avoidance of errors and that a balance between the two is required so that learning trial recall is effortful but not at the expense of introducing an excess of errors. In practical terms, the level & direction of assistance (increasing or decreasing) will depend on the level of memory severity & task difficulty.
Kalla et al. (2001)	3 within-Ss	1	0	0	+			EL combined with stimulus pre-exposure in the form of elaborative encoding resulted in significantly higher rates of face-name recall than either EL alone or EF. EL alone resulted in significantly better performance than EF, but the magnitude of change wasn't as significant as compared to the pre-exposure conditions. These results suggest that stimulus pre-exposure/evaluative encoding maximizes the benefits derived from EL.
Hillary et al. (2003)	3 within-Ss	1	0	0	+			The spacing effect is a robust finding in the non-disabled population, & in this study resulted in significantly improved word recall & recognition performance by individuals with moderate-severe TBI. These results support use of this technique to improve recall of information in this population.
Tailby & Haslam (2003)	3 within & between-Ss	1	0	0	+			EL utilizing self-generated responses proved superior to EL utilizing examiner-generated responses. EL, regardless of type, was superior to EF across severity groups. Results suggest that implicit memory alone could not account for the benefits derived from using EL—that residual explicit memory may have supported recall performance.
Riley et al. (2004)	3 Studies 1-3: within-Ss Study 4: within & between-Ss	1	0	0	+			Individuals with moderate memory impairments demonstrated superior explicit memory test performance following MVC compared to ELWF. Implicit test recall was best under conditions that were similar to (i.e., "overlapped with") a specific training conditions. These results suggest that MVC may be appropriate when the learner has more preserved explicit memory, the study recall is effortful but still generally successful and the learning task itself is one that can readily be learnt explicitly. ELWF may be preferable to MVC, because of its reduced error rate, when the learner has very impaired explicit memory and/or the task is best learnt implicitly.
Ehlhardt et al. (2005)	3 within Ss (multiple baseline across Ss)	0	1	0	+	(+) non-trained interface	(+) 30 days post	Results showed that 4 individuals with severe cognitive impairment could learn a multi-step procedure using a direct instruction teaching package that included a metacognitive component.
Melton & Bourgeois (2005)	4 case studies	0	1	1	+	(+) reported goal execution in the home & some generalization to non-targeted items	(+) 1 month goal recall & reported goal execution	Spaced retrieval training delivered via phone resulted in high goal attainment & maintenance for verbal recall of compensatory memory strategies & personally relevant facts. In addition, participants reported a high percentage of strategy execution for trained goals. Results suggest that SR delivered via phone (i.e., teletherapy) provides an efficient, cost-effective means of service-delivery & that strategies trained should be specific to an individual's daily need.
Stark et al. (2005)	3 within Ss (Single case) & between-Ss	1	0	0	+	(+) with variance training		The experimental participant demonstrated significantly better visual recognition and recall of probe (i.e, not studied) material as well as overall higher number of items learned following the EL with variance training condition; however, overall learning was slow and impaired compared to normal controls. The authors suggest that variance reduces hyper-specificity of learning and supports generalization. Interestingly, confidence ratings were not commensurate with performance (i.e., trend toward higher confidence ratings given for items that were incorrect) and reactions were times equivalent across correct/incorrect responses. In addition, the participant had no recollection of previous exposure to the material, suggesting he was not using residual medial temporal lobe (MTL). Rather, EL served as an external proxy for what the MTL normally does to help integrate information into the neocortex.
Turkstra & Bourgeois (2005)	4 case study	0	0	0	+	(—) No behavior changes		SRT via phone resulted in improved verbal recall of personally relevant goals statements; however, behavior change (i.e., following through on these goals) did not occur. (Anecdotally, post-study implementation of SRT targeting action-based responses to therapist questions did result in behavioral change.) The authors suggest that implicit learning, which underlies SRT, is hyper-specific and therefore generalization to stimuli beyond the features associated with the learned behavior is limited. Frontal lobe impairments & inconsistent staff follow through with goal-related behaviors contribute to lack of generalization.
Akhtar et al. 2006	3 within & between-Ss	1	0	0	+			The results showed that EL was significantly better than EF across both groups & replicates findings from previous EL research with a new population: individuals with mild cognitive impairment (MCI). The MCI group made significantly lower JOL overall, suggesting that they were aware of their memory difficulties. JOL across groups were higher in the EL condition. Finally, inter-list recall analysis suggested EL facilititates both acquisition & consolidation of new information.
Dou et al. (2006)	3 between-Ss (Randomized)	1	0	0	+			Results from this pilot study showed the potential benefits of using CAMG: an enriched computer program using EL principles; however, in general, no significant differences between CAMG & TAMG were found. The authors acknowledge weaknesses in the study including lack of a comparison to other treatment approaches. They also discuss some of the challenges in implementing computer-based technology in China, including therapists' preferences for face-to-face clinical contact.
Landis et al. (2006)	3 within-Ss (retrospective)	1	0	0	-		(+) varied according to age, severity, & condition	Results do not support EL as a generalized intervention for youth with memory impairments due to TBI. No clear patterns were identified indicating specific age or severity groups that might benefit from this technique. For example, younger children with moderate impairments performed significantly better with trial & error at the 7-day interval, whereas younger children with mild & severe impairments showed an advantage with EL. The authors hypothesize that differences in the neural mechanisms mediating initial learning & delayed retention may explain the dissociation in treatment effects. Study limitations include the use of examiners not blinded to condition evaluating retention of material & the small number of participants.
Page et al (2006)	3 within-Ss	1	0	0	+			Results from both experiments support the EL advantage across severity levels & demonstrate that the use of implicit memory across groups is sufficient for EL advantage to occur. These findings were supported by testing which revealed minimal to no source memory across severity groups.

APPENDIX 2.3. *(cont.)*

NAMES & DATES	STUDY DESIGN							OUTCOMES
	Class/ Design	Statistics	Reliability/ Validity	Ecological Validity	Immediate Outcomes	Generalization	Maintenance	Author Conclusions

DEMENTIA

NAMES & DATES	Class/Design	Statistics	Reliability/Validity	Ecological Validity	Immediate Outcomes	Generalization	Maintenance	Author Conclusions
Winter & Hunkin (1999)	4 case study	0	0	0	+			The authors suggest that EL has potential for patients with AD.
Clare et al. (2000)	3&4 within Ss (multiple baseline & single case)	1	0	1	+	(+) face-name recall to real-life setting (2 Ss); memory strategies in new situations reported by 1Ss	(+) 6 mos.	Individually tailored instructional packages based on EL resulted in significantly improved and maintained face-name/information recall and external aid and memory use for 5 of 6 participants with DAT. Generalization was observed in at least 2 participants.
Clare et al. (2002)	3 within-Ss	1	0	0	/		(+) 6 & 12 mos	Results showed significant improvements in face-name recall with training; however, not all participants benefited equally. The authors suggest that this was likely due to individual variability in neuropsychological profiles/processes underlying performance. Participants with greater awareness of deficits and less severe AD performed better and variations in medication protocols did not affect outcomes. Finally, the treatment protocol showed no negative impact on well-being (e.g., anxiety & depression).
Metzler-Baddeley & Snowden (2005)	3 within-Ss	1	0	0	/			Aggregate results supported EL over EF in learning familiar and novel information; however, significance was not reached on the individual level and participants also learned in the EF condition. The authors suggest that the small sample size may have contributed to these results in addition to their particular approach to EF learning in which participants were not set up to make an error on each trial as is the case in previous studies comparing EL with EF. Training effects were also mitigated by use of mnemonic strategies across conditions for selected participants, suggesting that EL might be more beneficial when mnemonics are less useful as an approach to treatment combining EL with mnemonics and/or expanded rehearsal.
Ruis & Kessels (2005)	3 within-Ss	1	0	0	/			EL resulted in better face-name recall immediately following repeated learning trials, but there was a decline in performance after 10-minutes. The authors suggest that EL is of limited benefit to individuals with moderate-severe dementia and that it is likely other cognitive processes besides implicit memory explain the effects of EL shown in less impaired populations (e.g., early dementia).
Haslam et al. (2006)	3 Study 1: within & betweens Ss; Studies 2 & 3: within-Ss	1	0	0	/			Results from Studies 1 & 3 show a significant advantage for EL over EF when learning specific (i.e., 'low' level information); however, individual variability among participants across all 3 studies was evident, including instances of equal, if not better performance in the EF condition. The authors speculate that lack of consistent benefit of EL over EF across all participants may be related to several factors, including the presence of floor & ceiling performance effects, individual differences in cognitive profiles, specifically, differences in attention-concentration, with impairments in this domain potentially diminishing benefits from EL. These results suggest that EL is not equally beneficial for all patients with memory impairment.
Dunn & Clare (2007)	3 within-Ss	1	0	0	-			Results showed that participants learned both novel and familiar face-name pairs across all conditions (errorless/errorful & effortless/effortful) with no significant differences between conditions, excepting the slightly higher mean scores in errorful conditions. The authors qualify that non-significant group differences may have masked individual differences suggesting benefit from different methods.

SCHIZOPHRENIA

NAMES & DATES	Class/Design	Statistics	Reliability/Validity	Ecological Validity	Immediate Outcomes	Generalization	Maintenance	Author Conclusions
Kern et al. (1996)	2 between Ss (randomized)	1	0	0	+		(+) Both groups maintained at 1, 2, & 4 weeks	Results showed that EL was associated with significantly improved performance pre- vs. post-treatment for the Initial Error group, and there were no significant differences between the Initial Error and No Error groups related to error history. Both groups maintained performance levels post-training.
O'Carroll et al. (1999)	2 between Ss (non-randomized control group)	1	0	0	+			EL was superior to EF for individuals with schizophrenia and impaired memory. Results could not be explained by differences in age, gender, IQ, education, etc. The authors suggest these results may be due to the relatively preserved implicit memory system. An alternative explanation could be that individuals with schizophrenia have difficulty source monitoring in EF conditions (i.e. difficulty determining self-generated vs. externally generated stimuli).
Kern et al. (2002)	2 between Ss (randomized control group)	1	1	0	/		(--) decline in performance for both groups at 3 mos	Significant group differences were found in favor of EL on measures of accuracy and productivity but not speed or on-task behavior with declines in performance noted after 3 months. The effectiveness of EL in this population may be attributed to the neurocognitive impairments associated with schizophrenia in which explicit memory is generally more impaired than implicit memory.
Young et al. (2002)	2 within & between-Ss (randomized control group)	1	1	0	+	(+) SI group; selected measures (object sorting task)	(+) 1 mos	Scaffolded instruction resulted in significant improvements across several of the dependent variables. The authors suggest that the collaborative focus/calibrated input associated with this technique contributed to its success. There were no significant differences between the SI and control groups on the # of WCST categories achieved (considered the 'essence' of the task), and the DI group may have engaged in a form of 'discovery learning' not available to the SI group. The authors suggest that, similar to the SI group, the control group may have been overtaxed.
Kern et al. (2005)	2 between Ss (randomized control group)	1	1	1	+	(+) different problem solving scenarios	(+) 3 mos	The participants in the EL condition performed significantly better than their matched controls on a measure of social problem solving ability, immediately post-treatment and at 3 months. A social validity measure (10-point Likert scale) showed no significant differences in participants' ratings of instructors across conditions. These results show that EL can be applied to complex skills as well as simple, discrete tasks.
Pope & Kern (2006)	2 within & between-Ss (non-randomized group)	1	0	0	+			Participants with schizophrenia/schizoaffective disorder performed significantly worse than healthy controls in the errorful condition and approached significance in the errorless conditions. These results suggest that individuals with schizophrenia benefit from eliminating or reducing errors when learning new skills, although errorless learning does not completely eliminate the learning deficit experienced by this population. Specifically, problems with 'signal to noise' (i.e., distinguishing correct vs. incorrect input) discrimination in part account for differences in performance.

CHAPTER 3

The Learning Context

Beyond Practice
(What They Didn't Teach You in Graduate School)

with RIK LEMONCELLO and EVA VAN LEER

Rehabilitation does not occur in a vacuum. Contextual variables such as personal, environmental, and therapy program characteristics affect the learning process and determine learning outcomes. Examples abound. For the student who has failed math, future learning may be compromised by reduced self-efficacy or expectations. Improvement after taking tennis lessons on a grass court may not transfer to a clay tennis court. Daily dance lessons will produce different outcomes than lessons held once per week. How can we leverage positive contextual factors and mitigate barriers in order to improve our rehabilitation outcomes? In this chapter, we address this question by reviewing concepts important to consider when designing an optimal behavioral intervention.

WHAT HAVE WE LEARNED
FROM THE MOTOR-LEARNING LITERATURE?

The motor-learning literature provides a number of theoretical and clinical principles that are relevant to designing behavioral intervention. Although this literature was

Rik Lemoncello, PhD, CCC-SLP, is an Assistant Professor in the Department of Speech and Hearing Sciences at Portland State University. His research focuses on the use of assistive technologies to support community participation for individuals with acquired brain injury.

Eva van Leer, PhD, CCC-SLP, is an Assistant Professor in the Department of Otolaryngology at the University of Cincinnati Hospital. Her clinical and research interests focus on voice disorder, with a specific focus on treatment adherence.

intended for application to physical exercises (e.g., for leg and arm movements, speech, or swallowing), many of the principles extend to cognition and behavior. We do not know whether impaired systems are sensitive to the same principles of learning as intact systems; nevertheless, the principles of learning in healthy motor systems provide a useful framework for our treatment efforts (Maas et al., 2008). We draw upon this literature in our discussion of contextual factors that need to be considered when planning optimal instruction.

Perhaps the most important element of a successful treatment program is whether the client follows through with treatment recommendations. The term *compliance* is often used to describe a person's fulfillment of a prescribed treatment or exercise regimen (Dishman, 1994a). This term implies that a clinician sets therapy goals and judges whether the client meets them. A more collaborative therapeutic relationship might be achieved by using terms such as therapy *participation, adherence, cooperation,* or *completion* (Chen, Neufeld, Feely, & Skinner, 1999; Dishman, 1994a; Friedrich, Gittler, Halberstadt, Cermak, & Heiller, 1998). In the remainder of this chapter we use the term *participation* and review factors that can improve this aspect of therapy.

There is a large body of literature on factors that influence participation in exercise programs. Researchers have attempted to predict or explain exercise program participation in healthy adults (e.g., Dzewaltowski, 1994; King, 1994; Robison & Rogers, 1994), elderly adults (e.g., Dishman, 1994b; Henry, Rosemond, & Eckert, 1998), and patient populations receiving physical therapy (e.g., Campbell et al., 2001; Friedrich et al., 1998), occupational therapy (e.g., Chen et al., 1999), or speech therapy (e.g., Easterling, Grande, Kern, Sears, & Shaker, 2005). Across studies, over 200 variables contributing to exercise adherence have been identified (Meichenbaum & Turk, 1987). It is clear that a variety of interacting factors contribute to short- and long-term adherence to exercise programs, and no single factor consistently predicts adherence. A review of the literature, however, suggests that influences on program participation can be categorized into three factors: personal characteristics, environmental factors, and program characteristics.

Most of the research on participation comes from studies of motor learning. The results, however, are also relevant to behavioral programs that do not contain a substantial motor-learning or exercise component, such as medication adherence, diet, psychotherapy, and smoking cessation (Alexander, Sleath, Golin, & Kalinowski, 2006; Bastian, Molner, Fish, & McBride, 2006; Dominick & Morey, 2006; Haynes, Ackloo, Sahota, McDonald, & Yao, 2008; Horvath & Luborsky, 1993; Yancy & Boan, 2006). The overlap likely occurs because any type of behavioral intervention requires purposeful, volitional, active participation and self-regulation by the patient, both within and between treatment sessions, as opposed to treatments in which the patient plays a largely passive role (e.g., surgery, massage, hemodialysis, or electroconvulsive therapy). Variables that support success in behavioral interventions typically do so for three reasons: (1) They either support independent self-regulation of behavior or reduce the demand for self-regulation; (2) they support motivation to stick with the program; and (3) they enhance the therapeutic relationship between the client and clinician. In the next sections, we describe personal, environmental, and program features that support these three aspects of a successful rehabilitation program.

PERSONAL CHARACTERISTICS THAT INFLUENCE LEARNING

The first group of factors influencing participation in a therapy program consists of characteristics of the individual client. The six personal characteristics below have been shown to predict participation in behavior-change programs.

Self-Efficacy

Self-efficacy is the most widely accepted and discussed personal characteristic that influences participation in behavior change programs. The term *self-efficacy* refers to the belief that one can perform a particular task; it is related to self-confidence (Chen et al., 1999; Driver, 2006; Dzewaltowski, 1994; Robison & Rogers, 1994) and based on the assumption that individuals can determine and control their own behavior (Dzewaltowski, 1994). A related concept proposed by Driver (2006) is *self-regulatory efficacy*, the belief that one can perform a particular task despite the presence of barriers. Self-efficacy can be influenced by previous experiences with performing a task, observation of others performing a task, social context, and physiological reactions to exercise, such as pain (Driver, 2006). Some studies have shown positive correlations between self-efficacy, affect, and participation in exercise programs (e.g., Chen et al., 1999; Driver, 2006). Others have suggested that high self-efficacy may be more important to beginning an exercise program than to sustaining it (e.g., Jette et al., 1998). Research in the area of TBI suggests that both previous success with related tasks and also collaboration in goal setting and the therapy process can enhance self-efficacy among individuals with cognitive impairments (Ylvisaker & Feeney, 1998).

Locus of Control

Research has shown that an internal versus external locus of control, particularly in relation to health responsibility and control over change, predicts completion of exercise programs (Dzewaltowski, 1994; Jette et al., 1998; Robison & Rogers, 1994). With an internal locus of control, individuals believe that they have control over change and take responsibility for making active behavioral changes. An internal locus of control predicts greater short-term completion of exercise routines (Campbell et al., 2001; Friedrich et al., 1998). In general, older persons perceive less control over their activity levels than do younger counterparts (Dishman, 1994b). Holmes, Fletcher, Blaschak, and Schenk (1997) suggested that reducing the frequency of therapy visits could encourage self-monitoring and internalize the locus of control for adults receiving occupational therapy outpatient services. Encouraging client collaboration in the therapy process also may encourage an internal locus of control.

Beliefs and Expectations about the Therapy Program

An individual's beliefs and expectations about the benefits of exercising or participating in a therapy program also influence participation (Berg, Dischler, Wagner, Raia, & Palmer-Shevlin, 1993; Dzewaltowski, 1994; Robison & Rogers, 1994). For example, positive attitudes toward exercise predict greater willingness to accommodate exercise into daily routines (Campbell et al., 2001). The role of expectations may vary depending on the disease course. A large study of patients receiving physical therapy, for example, showed that expected recovery influenced participation more for individuals with acute onset of symptoms than for those with chronic impairments (Sluijs, Kok, & van der Zee, 1993). This finding is understandable, as motivation can be difficult to sustain when immediate benefits are unlikely (Friedrich et al., 1998). In any case, the perceived benefits need to outweigh the perceived barriers of following a therapy plan (Kosma, Cardinal, & McCubbin, 2005).

There is a two-way relationship between beliefs and exercise, evidenced by the finding that persons with better participation in exercise programs were more likely to believe that exercises were effective (Campbell et al., 2001). Evidence-based practice reminds us to consider the client's values, preferences, and beliefs when deciding on any therapeutic recommendations (Sackett, Straus, Richardson, Rosenberg, & Haynes, 2001), and also when monitoring participation over time.

Disease Characteristics

Disease characteristics may also help predict participation. For example, individuals with physical problems who are symptomatic, experience pain, or present with greater functional limitations may be more likely to participate in physical therapy exercise programs (Campbell et al., 2001; Jette et al., 1998). This may be true based only on perception of symptoms rather than objective criteria for disease severity (Berg et al., 1993; Sluijs, 1991; Warren, Fey, & Yoder, 2007). The influence of disease characteristics clearly overlaps with other motivation-related factors previously discussed, such as self-efficacy and individual expectations (e.g., if a disease carries a positive prognosis, the patient may feel more or less in control of recovery).

Cognitive Status

The individual must possess knowledge of how to complete a therapy regimen properly if there is an expectation for independent execution (Logemann, 2005; Morris, Taub, & Mark, 2006; Robison & Rogers, 1994). For example, Jette and colleagues (1998) found that elderly participants with confusion demonstrated lower participation, "likely because they were not certain what was expected of them" (p. 419). In addition, prospective memory failures may cause individuals to fail to complete exercises daily, even when patients recall exercise techniques (Sohlberg & Mateer, 2001b). Individuals with severe cognitive impairment may also become internally distracted, agitated, or lack sufficient vigilance to actively participate in some rehabilitation tasks (Sohlberg & Mateer, 2001b). Chapter 2 discussed specific factors related to the etiology of cognitive impairments and candidacy for treatment. In successive chapters, we make specific instructional recommendations to enhance program completion for individuals with a variety of cognitive impairments.

Psychosocial Status

It is well known that psychosocial and emotional factors can influence the ability to process, encode, store, and retrieve new information (Gazzaniga, Ivry, & Mangun, 2002).

Factors that enhance learning include motivation, support, and engagement. Factors that inhibit learning include disinterest, depression, grief, and stress or anxiety. The animal research discussed in Chapter 1 clearly shows that learning is better when tasks are meaningful and relevant to the organism, supporting the importance of engagement in the task.

Recommendations to Enhance Learning: Personal Variables

There are a number of strategies clinicians can employ to optimize client engagement. Many of these are outlined in Audrey Holland's 2007 text *Counseling in Communication Disorders: A Wellness Perspective*, which provides techniques for enhancing client participation while working on rehabilitation goals. On the basis of that publication and the current literature, the following eight strategies can be used to promote participation in behavioral programs:

1. Encourage high self-efficacy and an internal locus of control by supporting clients to participate in and ultimately manage their own program; make decisions to fit recommendations into their belief system and facilitate early success during therapy (Berg et al., 1993; Driver, 2006; Morris & Schulz, 1992).
2. Provide clients with tools that will allow them to evaluate their potential ability relative to their current status (with disability), rather than to their before-injury status, to reduce chances of negative affect and decreased self-efficacy (Driver, 2006).
3. Encourage motivation by exposing clients to successful examples, such as individuals who are similar in terms of age, gender, and ability (Driver, 2006).
4. Use behavioral incentives, rewards, and reinforcements (verbal or tangible) to encourage motivation, as necessary (Robison & Rogers, 1994).
5. Remind clients *early and often* of the benefits and goals of the therapy program (Chen et al., 1999; Dishman, 1994b; Robison & Rogers, 1994; Sluijs, 1991).
6. Prepare clients to cope with temporary lapses by making alternative plans in case challenges arise (Chen et al., 1999; Dishman, 1994b; Dzewaltowski, 1994).
7. Reduce potential anxiety by instructing clients about upcoming therapy activities and possible physiological or psychological responses (e.g., frustration, pain, or fatigue) (Driver, 2006).
8. Conduct a thorough cognitive assessment to ensure that clients possess the requisite abilities to actively participate, such as basic vigilance and awareness of the environment (Sohlberg & Mateer, 2001b).
9. Insert variety during learning regimen to increase client engagement (Dishman, 1994b).

ENVIRONMENTAL CHARACTERISTICS THAT INFLUENCE LEARNING

The second category of factors that influence participation in behavioral therapy programs includes three environmental characteristics: the facilities, the social or cultural context, and the extent to which treatment is developed collaboratively with the client and other stakeholders.

Facilities

Characteristics of the therapy facility, such as proximity, convenience, appearance, and comfort, can influence participation (Kirwan, Tooth, & Harkin, 2002; Robison & Rogers, 1994; Sluijs et al., 1993). In fact, Dishman (1994b) reported that access to exercise facilities was an important influence on participation for older adults. The number of people present and wait times can also influence participation (Kirwan et al., 2002). We also know that the environment can serve as a facilitator or a distracter to individuals. The same cue may work both ways. For example, a beeping alarm might be an effective cue to check a daily planner when the client is taking a break, but may be a significant distractor when the client is engaged in a complex task.

Social and Cultural Influences

Positive persuasion from immediate family members or close significant others has been linked to increased participation (Robison & Rogers, 1994). This may be particularly true when the persuader is perceived to be an expert (Driver, 2006). The influence of social context is one reason why group exercise classes can augment adherence to a fitness regimen (Olney et al., 2006). Communities that endorse and support participation may also be a positive influence (King, 1994), as do external reminders of the benefits of continued participation, such as advertisements or brochures (Berg et al., 1993).

Support does not necessarily have to be provided face-to-face. One example of successful telephone-based support for behavior change is the quit line for smoking cessation ("A Clinical Practice," 2008). Social supports also can be provided via the Internet (Gustafson et al., 2002); this delivery route is particularly useful for patients who have logistical barriers to attending face-to-face sessions, or for whom therapy is not reimbursed.

Collaboration

Collaboration refers to a process in which family/significant other expertise is acknowledged and used explicitly to direct the selection, implementation, and evaluation of treatment plans. Expertise is shared across disciplines, and the patient and important others in his or her life are active and equal participants in intervention planning. To achieve this collaboration, however, the professionals on the team must have strong interpersonal communication skills and be willing to "release" their role as the only experts on the team (Sohlberg & Mateer, 2001b).

This approach may seem difficult to achieve in the current health care climate, where there is little time or infrastructure for interactions with others in the client's life. Collaboration is of increasing importance, however, as lengths of stay become shorter and resources scarcer, and important people in an individual's life assume more of the burden of long-term care and sustained support. The work of Mark Ylvisaker has provided the field of brain injury rehabilitation with evidence of the power of collaborating with community sources of support in order to enhance rehabilitation outcomes (e.g., Feeney & Ylvisaker, 1997) and shown that this model can lower care costs (Ylvisaker, Feeney, & Capo, 2007). Although collaboration is often given lip service and held as an ideal in rehabilitation, most therapists tend to work from an individual perspective that emphasizes client education, client compliance, and the professional's responsibility in fostering client progress, rather than an equal, collaborative role. An effective collaborative intervention model incorporates the clients' and families' perspective to determine rehabilitation priorities, and teaches families to systematically observe events related to issues of concern, provide feedback on noted trends, and offer suggestions for management strategies (Sohlberg & Mateer, 2001b). Sohlberg and Mateer (2001b) developed a model for collaborating with families that includes the following components:

- Interviewing to learn the family's background, needs, and concerns
- Helping families determine their priorities
- Teaching families to systematically observe events in their environment relevant to the issues of concern
- Providing feedback on trends noted in family observations
- Offering suggestions for strategies and helping families generate methods to monitor strategy success
- Revising goals and monitoring issues of concern on an ongoing basis.

Collaborative rehabilitation requires that the clinician determine what works for the client and associated support people. For example, if the clinician has assigned homework to track "forgetting experiences," but the homework is frequently not completed, perhaps the clinician needs to work with the family to identify a different tracking method. Alternatively, the clinician could gather the information via structured interview and facilitate client/family insight using an interview process rather than a written log. The idea is to work in partnership and not fall into a clinician-directed mode of therapy. Ultimately, collaboration will yield the most meaningful and lasting therapeutic outcomes.

Recommendations to Enhance Learning: Environmental Variables

As is the case with all clinical recommendations, the needs and circumstances of each client must be considered individually. For example, some people do not work well in groups, whereas others benefit greatly from peer input and support. Below we list seven considerations regarding environmental factors that may enhance the learning milieu for individual clients.

1. Be cognizant of how the therapy setting can facilitate or even enhance learning. Consider alterations to the environment, schedule, or transportation to maximize program participation and allow patients to have easy access to services (Dishman, 1994b; Robison & Rogers, 1994).
2. Where appropriate, use environmental cues such as stickers, reminder notes, and calendars to prompt target behavior (Morris & Schulz, 1992; Sluijs & Knibbe, 1991).
3. Consider the client's ability to focus on the learning task. Are environmental distractors influencing performance? Be sure the client is able to focus on the

learning task without internal or external distraction if this is an issue for the client (Sohlberg & Mateer, 2001b).

4. Collaborate with families and other stakeholders as rehabilitation partners. When appropriate, ask them to assist with observations, generation of management strategies, and provision of feedback. Train support people in systematic observation techniques (Sohlberg & Mateer, 2001b).

5. Consider the role of the patient's family or other stakeholders, and how they might provide meaningful feedback to the patient. For example, it might be helpful for some individuals to establish a relaxed but positive environment (Driver, 2006, p. 158).

6. When possible, important people in that person's life should offer positive praise and support for participating in therapy programs (Driver, 2006).

7. Include social supports and encourage the patient to complete therapy activities with others (Chen et al., 1999; Dishman, 1994b; Robison & Rogers, 1994).

PROGRAM CHARACTERISTICS THAT INFLUENCE LEARNING

Characteristics of the therapy program itself may be the greatest determiner of rehabilitation outcomes, especially related to practice conditions. Many of these factors are under direct control of the clinician. The literature describes nine critical program characteristics that influence therapy participation and enhance learning outcomes.

Program Intensity

The intensity of the exercise or therapy program influences participation. In Chapter 1, we discussed the importance of intensity and repetition in the context of neural plasticity and the strong evidence that supports the benefits of intensive therapy programs across rehabilitation domains. For example, systematic research recommends intensive treatment programs for impairments in attention (e.g., Sohlberg et al., 2003), language (e.g., Cherney, Patterson, Raymer, Frymark, & Schooling, 2008; Robey, 1998), and physical functioning (e.g., Sirtori, Corbetta, Moja, & Gatti, 2009; Smidt, de Vet, Bouter, & Dekker, 2005) following ABI. Therapies addressing motor impairments, such as limb muscle weakness, voice disorders, and swallowing disorders, rely heavily on frequent drills and exercise. Less is written about the schedules of treatment that support improvements in cognition and language, although as seen in Chapter 2, increased practice generally is associated with better learning outcomes. The number of repetitions, duration of an attention training exercise, amount of time between sets, and number of days per week or total duration of exercises are all examples of variables that can be manipulated to increase the amount of practice (Burkhead, Sapienza, & Rosenbek, 2007; Clark, 2003). However, it is important to consider that the recommended level of intensity and duration of the program may deter some individuals from completing behavioral programs (Jan et al., 2004; Morris & Schulz, 1992; Robison & Rogers, 1994). Clinicians may also be challenged to keep an intensive intervention "fresh, interesting, and fun" (Jette et al., 1998, p. 75) to maintain the client's motivation and interest. Clinicians should be creative about possible ways to augment limited therapy visits to maximize program intensity, perhaps implementing strategies such as intensive home practice programs and making use of natural supports in the client's everyday life.

Timing of Intervention

Another key principle of neural plasticity relates to the timing of rehabilitation. Kleim and Jones (2008) suggested that intervention in the early stage postinjury may contribute to neuroprotection (i.e., preventing neural loss) and prevent formation of maladaptive neural connections. They added the important caveat, however, that in animal studies, very early, intensive therapy exacerbated brain damage via excitotoxicity, leading to increased lesion size and poorer outcomes. Human studies have been somewhat contradictory on this issue. In their review of multidisciplinary strength training interventions poststroke, Ada, Dorsch, and Canning (2006) reported similar effect sizes posttraining for stroke survivors in acute and chronic periods of recovery. Bonaiuti, Rebasti, and Sioli (2007) reviewed the evidence supporting a specific physical therapy exercise program (constraint-induced movement therapy [CIMT]) and concluded that CIMT resulted in positive outcomes across studies that evaluated patients in acute (<1 month), subacute (1–6 months), and chronic (>1 year) periods of poststroke recovery. A recently published single-blind randomized clinical trial of occupational therapy after stroke, however, had different results (Dromerick et al., 2009). In this study, patients with unilateral stroke and persistent hemiparesis were randomized at 9 days poststroke to one of three treatment conditions: standard occupational therapy, low-intensity CIMT (2 hours of therapy per day + mittening, or hand movement constrained by a mitten, for 6 hours per day), or high-intensity CIMT (3 hours of therapy + 90% mittening per day). There was no difference in outcome at 90 days for the low-intensity versus standard therapy groups, and the high-intensity group had worse outcome than either of the other two groups. In evidence reviews of the cognitive rehabilitation literature conducted by the Academy of Neurogenic Communication Disorders and Sciences (see *www.ancds.org*), including the study described in Chapter 2, few controlled studies of acute therapies were identified. Among these, however, there was no evidence that acute therapy—at least, drill-type therapy—provided benefits beyond what would be associated with spontaneous recovery. This was in contrast to the strong evidence in support of intervention in the chronic stage. There also are compelling psychosocial reasons for limiting the requirement for intensive practice while the individual recovers medically and begins to adjust to new cognitive impairments (Holland & Fridriksson, 2001). As noted above, engagement is an important element of treatment adherence, and many people are not ready to participate fully in rehabilitation until they have had the opportunity to experience the real-life consequences of their injuries. Thus, the timing of intervention must be carefully considered, particularly intervention that aims to change discrete behaviors through high-frequency practice.

Task Complexity

The complexity of therapeutic activities also influences completion (Berg et al., 1993; Sluijs et al., 1993). For example, patients who find exercises too difficult may stop doing them (Campbell et al., 2001), and providing clear instructions may augment participation (Berg et al., 1993; Sluijs, 1991; Sluijs et al., 1993). Henry and colleagues (1998) showed that older adults were better able to perform exercises when assigned two at a time, versus eight at a time, suggesting that dosage recommendations should consider the individual's ability to manage complex tasks. Related research from special education recommends teaching prerequisite skills prior to engaging learners in complex tasks, as well as breaking down complex or multistep behaviors into smaller chunks that the clinician chains together in order to facilitate learning (Engelman & Carnine, 1982). This has the added benefit of building what Feeney and Ylvisaker (1997) referred to as "positive behavioral momentum," a version of "success breeds success," as learners are likely to feel more motivated, engaged, and confident approaching a complex task if they have mastered components of that task. Whether teaching motor skills or cognitive processes, the decision of whether to aim for simple or more complex skills and the method used to teach them will be related to the type of skill being taught and the learner's cognitive strengths and limitations.

Practice Regimen

A critical review of the motor-learning and speech rehabilitation literature provides a framework for understanding the conditions of practice that need to be considered when developing a therapy program to teach or reteach skills (Maas et al., 2008). The following three practice conditions have relevance across rehabilitation domains (Lemoncello, 2008; Maas et al., 2008).

Errors

As reviewed in Chapter 2, individuals with moderate-to-severe declarative memory impairments show enhanced learning when errors are minimized during the initial acquisition of a target fact, skill, or strategy. By contrast, individuals with good declarative memory may have greater long-term retention of new information if they learned it via *trial-and-error*, which may enhance effortful processing (Lesgold, 2001). The critical distinction is that individuals with declarative memory impairments may not be able to effectively learn from mistakes; that is, they may learn primarily via classical conditioning so that mistakes made during target acquisition become entrenched. *Error-minimization techniques* (the focus of this manual) are preferred when teaching new information, skills, or strategies to individuals with declarative memory impairments.

Practice Distribution

The phrase *distribution of practice* refers to the spacing of practice over a set period of time, as discussed in Chapter 2. *Massed* practice occurs when an exercise or skill is practiced for a given number of trials or session in a relatively small time period (e.g., 10 repetitions in a row). *Distributed* practice occurs when the spacing of practice trials or exercises occurs over a longer period of time, with varying intervals of unrelated events between practices (e.g., 10 repetitions with a 2-minute interval between each, in which the client practices a different task). The literature pertaining to motor learning (Maas et al., 2008) and specifically to neurogenic rehabilitation (Ehlhardt et al., 2008) suggests that distributed practice enhances long-term learning. However, the nature of the task may influence the selection of practice regimen. For cognitively complex tasks, massed practice may be more effective in the initial phases of learning (Donovan & Radosevich, 1999).

Stimulus Variability

The specificity of practice is another important therapy condition. *Constant* practice occurs when the same, specific stimulus is used to elicit the target (e.g., entering the same doctor's appointment into a PDA multiple times). By contrast, *variable* practice provides a wider range of context in which to practice the target skill (e.g., entering a variety of medical, social, and vocational appointments into the PDA). The literature suggests that it may be beneficial to initially provide very specific, constant practice to establish a target behavior, but then provide more variability as skills are mastered in order to enhance generalization (Ehlhardt et al., 2008; Maas et al., 2008).

Cueing and Feedback

Two additional factors that clinicians can directly manipulate to enhance learning are cueing and feedback. *Cueing*, or prompting, refers to the information that a clinician gives *before* the client responds, in order to enhance the likelihood of a correct response. Cues may vary in terms of the level of support they provide, their timing, their schedule, and their modality, each of which can be systematically manipulated.

Level of Support

Cues are often delivered along a hierarchy of support. When using an error-control approach, the clinician begins by providing full support, then gradually fading support through guided practice to eventually enable the client to produce the target independently. Levels of support include the following:

- Physical assistance, in which the clinician manipulates the client's muscles to complete a task (e.g., hand-over-hand manipulation to write a letter).
- Modeling, in which the clinician demonstrates how to complete the target task (e.g., demonstrates steps to check e-mail on computer).
- Specific cues, in which the clinician provides detailed information to allow the client to complete a task (e.g., "Next, click on the word *send*").
- General cues, in which the clinician prompts the client to perform a behavior, but without giving specific information, such as telling a client to "begin now" or prompting him or her to use a metacognitive strategy (e.g., "What will you do next?"). These may also be referred to as "content-free cues" (e.g., an occasional alarm noise at unpredictable times to prompt a person to pay attention; Selznick & Savage, 2000).
- Opportunity cues or implicit cues, in which the clinician provides a subtle prompt, such as a pause or expectant gaze, to encourage clients to generate a response.

Timing

The clinician may elect to provide immediate or delayed cues when asking a client to respond. Cues should become progressively more delayed as clients become more independent.

- *Immediate cues* occur just prior to the client's response. (For example, "I want to practice your routine for standing from the wheelchair. Remember that the first step is to lock your brakes.")
- *Delayed cues* are separated from the client's response. (For example, "Your occupational therapist's name is Zander. He works with you on arm exercises and bathing. Who is your occupational therapist?").

Schedule

The frequency of cueing can also influence clients' performance. Constant cues might be needed in the initial learning phase, but to encourage more independent use of target skills or information, the clinician must fade cues over time (i.e., give them less frequently and with less information), thereby reducing the level of support. Types of cueing include:

- *Constant cueing*, which occurs before every response.
- *Scheduled cueing*, which occurs before a preestablished interval (e.g., every third trial).
- *Random cueing*, which occurs intermittently before a response.

Modality

Cues can occur via any sensory modality, but most commonly are physical, verbal, or visual.

- Physical cues require contact with the learner (e.g., the physical therapist helps the client move his or her leg when taking a step).
- Verbal cues are spoken by the clinician (e.g., "Think about what you need to do when you get to the next intersection"). As discussed in Chapter 8, clinicians can also teach clients to self-cue by verbalizing the steps of a task as a metacognitive strategy (e.g., "Check my work"; Whitman, Spence, & Maxwell, 1987).
- Visual cues can be hand gestures (e.g., a gesture to slow speech rate) or environmental signals (e.g., Post-it notes).
- Information in other modalities can also serve as useful triggers to begin a task, such as the vibration of a pager, the feeling of hunger, or the smell of smoke. We refer to these environmental triggers as *associative cues*.

When first mastering a rehabilitation target, the learner may require physical prompts, but again these should be gradually faded. For clients with impairments in prospective memory or initiation, naturalistic associative cues will be particularly important.

Feedback refers to the information that a clinician gives after a client's response and, like cueing, can shape a client's learning. The most critical feedback variables are content and timing.

Content

There are two main types of content feedback:

- *Knowledge of performance* refers specifically to descriptions of how the target response was produced (e.g., when practicing home safety precautions, telling the client that his or her oxygen cord was tangled around his walker). Feedback about performance is most critical during initial acquisition, when the learner has not yet internalized a reliable representation of the target, to ensure that the learner encodes the target correctly (Maas et al., 2008).

- *Knowledge of results* refers to the overall accuracy of a target response (e.g., correct or incorrect, complete or missing steps). Feedback about results may best be implemented after the learner has established a clear understanding of the intended target concept or skill.

Timing

Feedback can also vary in terms of the timing of delivery.

- *Immediate feedback* is provided directly after the learner produces a response. Although immediate feedback may be important during initial target acquisition, it may be not only impractical but also detrimental to maintenance and generalization during later stages of learning by discouraging self-evaluation (Maas et al., 2008).
- *Delayed feedback* is provided after a latent period in which the learner is expected to reflect on and evaluate his or her own performance. When a learner has the requisite ability to do this, delayed feedback that encourages self-reflection can enhance durability of learning (Maas et al., 2008).

Maintenance and Generalization

The ultimate goal of rehabilitation is to improve the learner's everyday function and quality of life outside of the therapy room, and maintain these improvements after therapy has ended. Clinicians are often focused on facilitating learning during initial target acquisition, but may not be in the habit of systematically programming the process to foster retention of the learning or generalization to everyday settings. There is an important distinction between performance during the initial acquisition, or early practice period, and maintenance and transfer of the newly acquired skill to other contexts and conditions. Performance during practice often is not a good predictor of maintenance and generalization (Maas et al., 2008). It is important to plan for retention and transfer when planning practice conditions. As a skill is learned, the clinician can enhance maintenance effects by systematically manipulating factors such as program intensity, practice regimen, cumulative review and booster sessions, and use of cueing and feedback. Generalization can be enhanced by systematic manipulations of task complexity, practice tasks, and faded cueing and feedback. The greatest gains for a particular activity are seen when the training goal most closely resembles the end goal (Burkhead et al., 2007).

Therapeutic Relationships

The development and fostering of interpersonal relationships between the therapist and client greatly influence program participation (Berg et al., 1993; Sluijs, 1991). This includes client–clinician agreement about the goals and tasks of therapy (Horvath & Luborsky, 1993; Horvath & Symonds, 1991). Therapeutic relationships are enhanced when the clinician understands the client's individual needs, enables open communication to allow for mutual goal setting and problem solving, and provides feedback and encouragement (Kirwan et al., 2002).

One approach to attaining goal agreement and supporting patient motivation is motivational interviewing (Miller & Rollnick, 2002).[1] This client-centered therapeutic intervention has been effective in increasing patient adherence to a variety of behavioral programs, even when it is conducted only briefly, preceding a traditional treatment program (Hettema, Steele, & Miller, 2005). The motivational interviewing approach contrasts with a more traditional medical approach of "prescribe and persuade," in which the clinician recommends a goal or plan of action and subsequently attempts to persuade the client to comply. In contrast, motivational interviewing uses reflective listening and open-ended questions to elicit the client's goals and self-supportive pro-change statements.

Whereas reflective listening and open-ended questions are familiar to many clinicians, the elicitation of pro-change statements may not be. The process can be guided by a "readiness ruler," a simple visual analogue graphic on which clients rate (0–10) the importance of homework tasks and their confidence in completing them (Rollnick, Mason, & Butler, 1999). Discussion of ratings can elicit pro-change statements. By asking why an importance rating for a task is high, the clinician can elicit statements in favor of change, such as, "Well, I've done something like this before, it's really important to me, and I think my friend might be able to help me with this." By asking why confidence ratings are low and discussing what could be done to make the rating higher, barriers and goal statements are likely to be elicited (e.g., "I'd have to reschedule some of my day or ask my friend to remind me") and a reasonable plan of action can then be devised.

Supervision/Accountability

The level of supervision provided in a therapy program can also influence program participation (Robison & Rogers, 1994; Sluijs & Knibbe, 1991; Sluijs et al., 1993). Supervised programs that provide sufficient monitoring and feedback by professionals are associated with higher participation rates (Olney et al., 2006; Sluijs et al., 1993). Adherence to prescribed therapy activities decreases when supervision stops, presumably because of lack of feedback or motivation (Friedrich et al., 1998; Sluijs & Knibbe, 1991). Infrequent maintenance programs—or booster sessions—may help promote long-term adherence (Fatouros et al., 2005; Trappe, Williamson, & Godard, 2002).

Use of Technology

With the advent of increasingly affordable, accessible, and often mobile technology, some of the elements that support treatment can be provided via information and communication technology. By providing the client with supports for practice between sessions, such technologies can help us move from an episodic to a continuous model of care. Web-based and text-message interventions (Norman et al., 2007) and programs using PDAs (e.g., Burke et al., 2009) are two possible options. For a more complete review of available assistive technologies for cognition, see Scherer, Hart, Kirsch, and Schulthesis (2005).

Technologies to enhance program participation may focus group or individualized support. Group peer support can be provided through client and disorder-specific social

---

[1]The term *interviewing* is used to denote the task of the clinician in the field of counseling; this approach could also be thought of as *motivation counseling*.

networking websites, which can be password protected to ensure privacy. Individual support can be provided via mobile technologies (e.g., cell phones, smart phones, and portable media players), which can be used to store cues, reminders, clinician examples, and video self-models to enhance motivation and program participation. Video self-monitoring, in particular, has growing potential for improving patient participation, given advances in inexpensive video technology. There is evidence to suggest that observing a video recording of one's own mastery of a skill can enhance motivation, treatment adherence, and task performance across a variety of tasks (Bellini & Akullian, 2007; Dowrick, 1999; Hitchcock, Dowrick, & Prater, 2003; Law & Ste-Marie, 2005; McGraw-Hunter, Faw, & Davis, 2006; Ram & McCullagh, 2003; Rickards-Schlichting, Kehle, & Bray, 2004), and it can be used in either face-to-face therapy or remotely. As a concrete example, in speech therapy for stuttering, clients' twice daily observation of their own fluent speech production reversed relapses of dysfluency in those who had previously completed therapy successfully, and use of self-modeling videos was more effective than a standard-of-care maintenance program in relapse prevention (Cream, O'Brian, Onslow, Packman, & Menzies, 2009). Perhaps observing oneself master a skill provides the ultimate "mastery experience" to support self-efficacy.

It should be emphasized that use of technology requires systematic instruction in device use, as lack of training is a major contributor to failure to use technology in everyday life. This includes not only instruction in technical aspects of the device, but also systematic instruction in *when* to use it. Instructional strategies for device use are discussed in Chapter 7.

Recommendations to Enhance Learning: Program Variables

Program participation will likely be enhanced by the use of multiple strategies. For example, the medication adherence literature suggests that the combined use of counseling, reminders, brochures, and peer support is more effective in increasing participation than the use of any single strategy (Haynes et al., 2008; McDonald, Garg, & Haynes, 2002). Individuals have different preferences, and these preferences may change over time; hence, it is important to evaluate the most effective combination of strategies for a particular client at a given point in time (Burbank, Padula, & Nigg, 2000; Elley, Dean, & Kerse, 2007; Resnicow et al., 2008; Sohl & Moyer, 2007; Velicer, Prochaska, & Redding, 2006). Specific options for maximizing program success are as follows:

1. Individualize therapy programs and try multiple strategies.
2. To increase motivation and participation and reduce boredom, collaborate with the client to create programs that accommodate to that client's lifestyle (Jette et al., 1998; Logemann, 2005). Consider using motivational interviewing strategies to facilitate this discussion (Hettema et al., 2005). If available, consider using the client's existing technology to support practice via use of logs, timers, self-reminder messages, or sample videos.
3. Ensure that activities and materials are age-appropriate (Dishman, 1994b).
4. Help the client establish a therapy routine that fits into his or her schedule (Chen et al., 1999; Robison & Rogers, 1994; Sluijs, 1991).
5. Provide clear, ongoing instructions and feedback about therapy performance and progress (Chen et al., 1999; Dzewaltowski, 1994; Lysack, Dama, Neufeld, & Andreassi, 2005; Weeks et al., 2002).

6. Ensure that activities are not too difficult or tiring for the client to complete independently, if independent practice is a goal (Easterling et al., 2005). Consider error-control techniques (Chapter 2) and teaching prerequisite knowledge or skills and breaking down multistep tasks into component steps using task analysis (see examples in Chapter 6) (Ehlhardt et al., 2008). Examples for home practice can be digitally recorded and provided to the patient on mobile technology borrowed from the clinic, sent via e-mail,[2] or recorded on a CD or DVD.

7. Use written goal logs and provide regular feedback on completion of goals to increase accountability (Robison & Rogers, 1994; Sluijs, 1991).

8. Monitor participation regularly and attempt to resolve challenges to program participation (Dishman, 1994b; Sluijs, 1991).

9. Provide personalized attention, education, and support as needed (Dzewaltowski, 1994; Robison & Rogers, 1994).

10. Record and review examples of successful in-session mastery of tasks with the client as a "self-as-model" intervention. Consider providing a copy of this video for home review and self-encouragement (Cream et al., 2010).

SUMMARY

In this chapter we presented a review of personal, environmental, and program factors that can influence learning outcomes and increase program participation. No factor alone can predict therapy task completion or guarantee learning outcomes, and the evidence to date suggests that targeting a *combination* of factors is more effective than focusing on only one.

Although the bulk of the research evidence is from studies of individuals without cognitive impairments, it is based on psychosocial principles that are relevant to individuals with cognitive disorders, such as the need for volitional, active participation and self-regulation. Thus, we have attempted to relate the information to recommendations for intervention with individuals who have cognitive impairments. This research also focuses on physical rehabilitation, but again the general principles are relevant to cognitive intervention, particularly for clients with declarative memory impairments whose cognitive gains will rely primarily on procedural learning.

Factors that influence purposeful behavior and self-regulation have a significant impact on participation in treatment programs and therefore on treatment outcomes. The clinician should remain cognizant of these factors when working in a rehabilitation setting and teaching clients new facts, concepts, skills, behaviors, and strategies.

---

[2] If e-mail or web-based communication is used, verify that the privacy and security settings of the site and server meet standards set by your institution. All sites should be able to provide this information for review by your institution's Internet technology (IT) experts or human subjects institutional review committee. For example, Internet-based programs such as Gmail have chosen to voluntarily comply with the Department of Commerce "Safe Harbor" guidelines (*www.export.gov/safeharbor*), which restrict sharing of personal information but do not meet privacy standards of the Health Information Portability and Accountability Act (HIPAA). You must also ensure that the client has signed a release to use e-mail for health-care-related communication.

CHAPTER 4

The Training Framework
Plan, Implement, and Evaluate (PIE)

Previous chapters provided the theoretical and conceptual foundations supporting training practices in neurorehabilitation. Chapter 2 described research evidence for different instructional techniques, and Chapter 3 reviewed patient, environment, and therapy program characteristics that have been shown to influence rehabilitation outcomes. The next task is to incorporate these foundations into a systematic, efficient rehabilitation process. This chapter describes a general therapy practice framework, PIE, with which to Plan, Implement and Evaluate therapy. The PIE framework serves as the basis for designing and implementing the different types of therapies outlined in the remaining chapters of this manual.

OVERVIEW OF PIE

The three phases of the PIE framework are shown in Figure 4.1. *Planning* the therapy process has an enormous bearing on its success. Many critical clinical decisions are made *outside of the therapy session*. Initial planning decisions must consider the learner, the environment, and the treatment program itself. A careful needs assessment facilitates the selection of appropriate functional therapy targets that the client can and will use in everyday life. *Implementation* refers to methods that maximize the efficiency and durability of learning. Important clinical considerations *during the session* include characteristics of stimulus presentation, the practice regimen, and the client's level of engagement and strategy use, all of which have profound effects on therapy outcomes. Finally, *Evaluation* of client performance within and outside of the session is critical for both measuring outcome and making decisions about future therapy. These clinical data are essential to evidence-based decision making. Data gathered on the learning process *during therapy* and on the impact of the training *outside of therapy* will drive clinical decisions. The three PIE phases—Plan, Implement and Evaluate—provide the scaffolding for effective instruction.

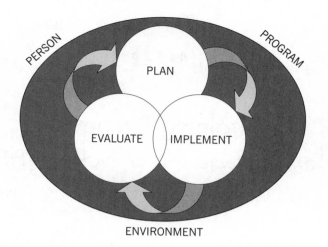

FIGURE 4.1. The three phrases of the PIE framework in relation to person, environment, and program factors.

PIE: PLANNING EFFECTIVE INSTRUCTION

We begin with a discussion of the planning phase. Effective instruction requires careful advanced planning. Table 4.1 shows the four steps that are critical to planning effective training. Each step is linked to one of the key questions that must be answered in treatment planning: *who, what, where, when, why,* and *how.*

Rehabilitation professionals are familiar with a variety of assessment methods, including standardized, norm-referenced, or criterion-referenced tests; interview scripts; systematic observation methods; and dynamic assessment methods. Depending upon the type of therapy target, the clinician may also engage in a formal needs assessment (see Chapter 7 for examples). In this chapter, we provide the general planning framework that can be refined for specific needs assessments relevant to a range of rehabilitation targets.

TABLE 4.1. Basic Steps in Planning Treatment and Key Questions to Ask at Each Step

Step	Key questions
1. Identify key learner characteristics.	*WHO* is the learner?
2. Define treatment target.	*WHAT* am I teaching that will support life participation for this learner?
	WHERE is the target environment?
	WHEN will the learner implement it?
3. Specify desired outcome.	*WHY* am I training this target?
4. Design individualized training plan.	*HOW* will I teach the target?

Planning Step 1: Identifying Key Learner Characteristics

The first critical question is WHO *is the learner*? Based on the results of the initial rehabilitation assessment, the clinician will have a sense of a learner's strengths and weaknesses. Consideration of learner characteristics is critical to candidacy, selection of appropriate targets, and design of the instructional plan. Listed below are the five learner domains that need to be considered for each client.

1. *Cognitive–linguistic functions*: The cognitive processes of attention, memory, executive functions, and self-awareness; the communication functions of speech and language comprehension and expression (including reading and writing); and the related ability to interact socially will all affect the design of therapy.
2. *Physical functions*: Mobility, endurance, and fine and gross motor skills need to be assessed, including not only limb functions but also physical functions related to speech and swallowing.
3. *Sensory abilities*: Vision, hearing, balance, somatosensory function, and sense of smell are important learner characteristics. Intake screening assessments routinely underestimate the prevalence and influence of impairments in hearing and visuomotor functions. These must be evaluated carefully.
4. *Psychological status*: A client's interests, motivation, awareness of deficits, and perceived locus of control and self-efficacy; his or her beliefs and expectations about treatment; and factors that increase or decrease his or her motivation for therapy all play a role in the design and implementation of therapy. The client's emotional state, including feelings of anger, grief, or depression and the presence of emotional lability, will also be important to consider.
5. *Social connection*: It is important to identify family, friends, and community sources of support who might play a role in treatment, along with the client's level of connectedness to these individuals.

Each of these five learner domains can influence candidacy for treatment. For example, clients with severe cognitive impairments (i.e., at Rancho los Amigos Levels of Cognitive Function I–V) may not be good candidates for systematic instruction. Reduced self-awareness, another cognitive consideration, may limit the client's engagement in therapy and the carryover of instruction to everyday life, and require an increase in external sources of supports (Scherer, Jutai, Fuhrer, Demers, & DeRuyter, 2007). Clients with language impairments (e.g., aphasia) may require adapted inputs to ensure comprehension of instructions. Physical and sensory abilities will especially influence the prescription of external aids (Sohlberg, 2006). Clients who are still adjusting to postinjury challenges may require counseling before beginning intensive rehabilitation (Holland & Fridriksson, 2001). Finally, the clinician must also consider social connections, which are critical to planning for ongoing supports and are a predictor of long-term outcomes for both the person with the brain injury and for his or her careers (Douglas & Spellacy, 2000; Wood & Rutterford, 2006). Table 4.2 provides a case example of how these five domains can affect planning for instructing an individual in the use of a memory system.

In some cases, learners may be people who support that client rather than the client him- or herself. A common example is the training of conversational partners for people with aphasia, in which significant others or volunteers are trained in techniques to

TABLE 4.2. Case Example: Possible Effects of Learner Characteristics on Planning Training in the Use of a Memory Aid

Sample learner characteristic	Possible effect on target selection	Possible effect on design of training plan
Cognitive–linguistic functions: *Female learner has impaired declarative learning but relatively intact procedural memory and recall of previous declarative knowledge*	System should be simple to use with easily set alarm/alert features. Consider use of calendar application on her cell phone, which she already carries and is familiar with the basic device.	Acquisition phase will require systematic instruction with EL (errorless learning) that chains together steps for entering reminders and alarms; distributed practice and cumulative review will be important for maintenance and generalization.
Physical functions: *Learner has left upper-extremity hemiparesis*	Need to evaluate ability to easily press buttons with dominant hand while holding phone with weaker hand.	In task analysis, need to include step indicating in which hand to hold device.
Sensory abilities: *Learner has binaural high-frequency hearing loss*	Need to evaluate whether alarm tone is in hearing range.	In tasks analysis, need to include step evaluating ability to hear alarm in quiet versus noisy environments.
Psychological status: *Learner not interested in improving independence in home management; time with grandchildren is very reinforcing*	Show learner how memory tools can facilitate grandchild-related activities. Demonstrate grandchildren calling on phone to arrange a visit and entering visit date on the cell phone calendar.	Collect examples of activities/interactions typical with grandchildren and use these as the primary training stimuli. Insert other target household routines after initial device use established.
Social connection: *Local adult daughter involved in care; friends have fallen away*	Interview daughter about learner's current cell-phone use and priorities for scheduling.	Provide daughter with task analysis and collaborate on a practice routine. Ask daughter to help reinforce use during acquisition and maintenance phases by having grandchildren supply scheduling targets.

increase engagement and participation of affected individuals (Kagan, Black, Duchan, Mackie, & Square, 2001; McVicker, Parr, Pound, & Duchan, 2009). In the case in Table 4.2 the client's language skills are not the target; rather the people in the environment are taught methods to accommodate her impairments. Partner-focused instruction is a growing part of intervention for many neurological disorders, including dementia (Robison et al., 2007) and TBI (Togher, McDonald, Code, & Grant, 2004). Although support people typically do not have cognitive impairments affecting their learning, their training can benefit from many of the same systematic instructional procedures described in this manual for clients. Clinicians must recognize, however, that training the caregiver to use strategies and supports may come at a cost of increased burden for that caregiver (Hoepner & Turkstra, 2010).

Planning Step 2: Defining the Training Target

Having defined the key learner characteristics, the next step is to define the instructional target(s) and learning context. To do this, we use a modified version of the framework

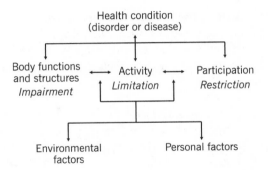

FIGURE 4.2. Defining the instructional target(s) and learning context using the International Classification of Functioning, Disability, and Health (CF; 2001).

for classifying health outcomes proposed by the World Health Organization (2001): the International Classification of Functioning, Disability, and Health (ICF), shown in Figure 4.2. According to this framework, a health condition (e.g., stroke, hemiparesis, aphasia) may result in impairments in body structures and functions, limitations in performance of activities (e.g., using the telephone), and restrictions in the ability to participate fully in social or occupational roles (e.g., unemployment). A key feature of this framework is that the link between an impairment and participation-level outcome is not linear, but rather is influenced by a variety of personal and environmental factors. These latter factors include those discussed in Chapter 3, such as motivation, mood, and access or barriers to services. The ICF framework represents a shift in the philosophy of rehabilitation from a *medical model* to a model of *social disability*, in which the clinician shares responsibility for improving life participation beyond the clinic. This shift has led to the creation of new tools to measure life participation and perceived quality of life, including measures such as the Community Integration Questionnaire (Willer, Rosenthal, Kreutzer, & Gordon, 1993), the Quality of Communication Life Scale (Paul et al., 2005), and the Impact on Participation and Autonomy scale (Cardol et al., 2002).

To illustrate the use of the ICF framework in planning, consider two males age 70 years, both with hypoxic brain damage after a heart attack and moderate anterograde amnesia. Bob is retired, educated, generally healthy, has a supportive family living nearby, and has hobbies that require mostly procedural memory. Doug lives alone, has medication-dependent diabetes, is estranged from his children, is employed as a chief financial officer of a company, and depends on his work income for his living expenses. These are two men with the same degree of cognitive impairment, but the effects on their life participation are likely to be strikingly different.

It is important to recognize that most patients' goals—even goals at the level of impairment—ultimately are about life participation ("I want to get back to being myself") rather than fixing that specific impairment for its own sake. Thus, our treatment planning is "outcome-driven" rather than "impairment driven," and our first step is a thorough evaluation of, and collaboration with, the client[1] to identify treatment targets that will be relevant to his or her everyday life. This evaluation may include stan-

---

[1]The term *client* is used here to refer to the client and to other stakeholders—that is, individuals in that person's life who will be part of the rehabilitation process.

dardized questionnaires (such as those noted above) and interviews with the client, his or her care providers, and other rehabilitation staff. To maximize generalization, from the very beginning planning must consider not only the target but also the context in which it will be used. Three specific questions related to defining the training target are discussed below.

- *WHAT are you teaching that will improve life participation?* This is an important question because it sets the stage for the entire treatment plan. The goal must be meaningful not only to the client, but also to third-party payers, who require clear, concise goal statements that will lead to meaningful changes in the individual's ability to function in everyday life. Frequently the answer to this question is obvious and straightforward (e.g., choosing the goal of remembering names of important customers because it's a condition of employment in a specific workplace). Some therapy objectives, however, require more specification and detail (e.g., use a planner notebook to organize a daily agenda for meetings). Each client may have several treatment targets. The decision of which target to address first depends on the client's preferences, the potential impact of a particular target on activities and participation, and the time required to train that target.

In this manual we present training guidelines for five types of targets that are common in rehabilitation:

1. *Facts and concepts* (Chapter 5), which include information such as face–name associations and autobiographical information.
2. *Multistep procedures* (Chapter 6), which are complex actions such as the routines involved in activities of daily living, functional sequences such as operating an appliance, work skills, or exercise programs.
3. *External aids* (Chapter 7), which include a wide range of low- to high-tech devices and cognitive prostheses (e.g., a planner, notebook, calendar, watch, or cell phone) to assist clients with completing desired tasks.
4. *Cognitive strategies* (Chapter 8), which include self-instructional routines or procedures to help individuals monitor and adjust performance, general strategies to facilitate goal completion, as well as domain-specific strategies such as academic strategies to improve study skills.
5. *Social skills* (Chapter 9), which include both skills for positive interactions in social settings and also strategies for managing behavior problems.

Although there are overlapping characteristics among these different categories, and they share training principles, each has unique features that merit discussion. Thus, each chapter begins with a brief review of constructs that are particular to that category of instructional target.

After working with a client to identify the specific therapy target(s), the clinician needs to define two additional components. The first is whether there are *prerequisite* behaviors or information that need to be trained prior to addressing the target. For example, when training a person to follow a phone procedure to call for emergency help, it may first be necessary to teach him or her what constitutes an emergency. In addition to ascertaining any prerequisite knowledge, the clinician must also work with the client to *identify all of the components or steps* necessary for successful use of that target. In our example, the clinician and client need to generate a task analysis for the emergency phone procedure before beginning the actual training. The specific sequence of steps relevant to that person's unique call procedure is then identified so that each step can be trained.

- *WHERE is the target environment?* Having defined the treatment target(s), prerequisites, and necessary components, the clinician and client next must identify the target environment. Analyzing the environment where the treatment target will be used allows for the identification of training examples that apply to the desired environments. The plan should specify the environment(s) where the targeted skill will occur, including (1) natural contexts in which to conduct sessions, to program for generalization beyond the therapy room; and (2) environmental facilitators or barriers that need to be considered when designing the training.

Defining the ultimate target environment(s) at the beginning of intervention allows the clinician to identify the different training examples and contextual variability that need to be programmed into therapy to ensure generalization. For example, consider a student with a memory impairment who needs to write down school assignments in a homework planner. The clinician could create training stimuli by recording the school bell and using it as a cue for the student to practice writing in her homework planner. In terms of stimulus variability, treatment may begin with one type of assignment, such as a math assignment modeled after the format implemented in the student's math class. As the client is successful, other types of homework assignments (e.g., from the student's language arts class) may be added to the instructional plan. The field of direct instruction (Engelmann & Carnine, 1991) refers to this as *general case programming*. Treatment begins with the most general case example and then extends it in order to capture a sufficient number of scenarios that will allow the client to generalize.

It is also important to identify environmental facilitators or barriers, including people who interact with the client in the environment, competing demands on the client's time and attention, and facilitators or triggers of the desired client behavior. For example, there may be a natural prompt in the environment for a person whose goal is to initiate using a specific memory aid, such as the school bell in the previous example (an environmental facilitator). An example of a barrier might be the limited time between class, which does not allow sufficient time to write down assignments, necessitating the development of a template or checklist to decrease writing time.

There may be more than one target environment. Some rehabilitation goals have *sequential* target environments. For example, the initial target environment may be the hospital or therapy room, whereas home is the ultimate target environment. Similarly, there may be *simultaneous* target environments. For example, the goal for training a memory prosthesis may be to use it at home and in the community. An effective treatment plan considers each of these environmental factors from the outset.

- *WHEN will the learner implement the training target?* The third question relevant to defining the treatment target involves describing the timing context during which it needs to occur—that is, determining the context or event that will trigger the use of that target. This trigger may be another action (e.g., start cooking dinner after turning off local news), a condition (e.g., use escape routine when angry), or a specific time (e.g., prepare dinner at 6:00 P.M.). Evaluation of natural environmental supports can assist in this decision making.

In summary, defining the treatment target requires that the clinician and client collaborate to identify the type of target, operationally define the targeted behavior, and specify both environmental and timing contexts for the treatment plan. Chapters 5–9 contain a wide range of targets, treatments, and contexts as examples.

Planning Step 3: Specifying the Desired Outcome

At this point in designing an instruction plan, the clinician has identified key learner characteristics, defined the treatment target, and specified contextual factors. The next planning question to consider is *WHY instruct or train this target?* As noted, when defining the specific intervention target, the clinician must ensure that targets are functional. To ensure the ecological validity of the training and the incorporation of the client's needs and values, it is also important to determine the desired impact of a training program at the outset of the intervention. Determining impact also helps the clinician to plan effective therapy. Clinicians can contribute significantly to the accumulating evidence base by tracking and reporting on clinical data, a process that is referred to as *practice-based evidence* (Wambaugh, 2007).

Before beginning the actual training or instruction, the clinician and client collaborate in defining the ultimate goal of therapy and in identifying the steps that will lead to this goal. With the client, the clinician plans how to evaluate the effects of the therapy throughout the learning process, including measuring both the learning of the target and the implementation of that target in natural contexts. A framework for evaluating the effectiveness of such instruction is provided in the evaluation section below.

Collaborating with the patient and his or her family may be especially difficult in an acute rehabilitation setting, as they are coping with a potentially life-threatening event with which they likely have no previous experience (Holland, 2007) and have not yet experienced the impact of their impairments in everyday contexts (Baughman & Thomas, 2008). Clinicians in acute settings should consider choosing learning targets that (1) are critical for independent functioning in the structured hospital setting; (2) are important for transfer to postdischarge settings; and (3) help educate the patient and family about the patient's strengths, limitations, and gains made during this early stage of recovery (Holland & Fridriksson, 2001).

Planning Step 4: Designing an Individualized Training Plan

The development of the training plan, or determining *HOW the rehabilitation target will be trained*, relies heavily on information gathered in response to the previous three questions. The clinician has identified the learner's characteristics and has worked with him or her to define the rehabilitation target and context and specify the desired outcome. Treatment planning is based on these factors in conjunction with environmental factors such as the availability of services. The training plan integrates the information gathered and specifies the following:

- Who is the learner? Specify whether this is the client or another support person. The clinician has now considered the key learner characteristics.
- What am I teaching? Specify the treatment target, defined operationally with a "do" statement, and include a "what for" statement—that is, how it will improve daily functioning.

- Where is the target environment? Specify the desired context(s) in which the learner will complete the targeted behavior.
- When will the learner implement the target? Specify any associative or contextual prompts that will trigger the target behavior.
- Why am I training this target? Specify how you will measure the outcome and the criterion for meeting the desired outcome.
- How will I teach the target? Specify the training approach. The approach discussed in this manual is *systematic instruction*.

Form 4.1 in the Appendix (an enlarged version is on the book's page on The Guilford Press website) provides a generic worksheet designed to facilitate the construction of a training plan. The worksheet provides questions to ensure that the clinician has considered the relevant factors related to the learner, training target, learning context, and outcome measurement. The next critical factor to consider is how to implement effective systematic instruction in order to move the learner through the learning stages of initial acquisition, mastery, and maintenance.

PIE: IMPLEMENTATION OF INSTRUCTION

This section describes the variables important to consider during the actual instructional process, across three phases: acquisition, mastery, and maintenance. In all training sessions, the clinician should be thoughtful about matching the training stimuli, practice regimen, level of cognitive engagement, and outcome measurement to the client's specific needs and the learning phase.

Three Phases of Training

Implementation Phase 1: Initial Acquisition

The term *acquisition phase* refers to the initial learning (or relearning) of the rehabilitation target. As discussed in Chapter 3, when first teaching a target concept, skill, or behavior, it is important to consider the training stimuli, practice regimen, and client's level of cognitive engagement.

TRAINING STIMULI

At this stage, the clinician has identified the target, training materials, cues and prompts, and context in which training will occur, and is ready to begin training. The first step is to make sure that the learner has the prerequisite knowledge and skills, and to determine whether the training target is new to the learner or if he or she has premorbid knowledge of it. Clients who have preinjury experience or knowledge of the training target may require less initial acquisition training and more practice for mastery or generalization. On the other hand, previously learned procedures may be difficult to change: A client who used a complex electronic planner to organize meetings and travel might have to unlearn some procedures in order to use a simple digital aid for tracking medications. Unlearning, or *extinguishing*, previous behaviors may be as important in treatment as learning and must be addressed systematically.

The second step when teaching a concept (e.g., safety awareness) is to provide a range of both positive examples (e.g., lock brakes on wheelchair before standing) and negative examples (e.g., do not walk in slippery socks) to establish the concept.

The third step is to select a range of training stimuli that will elicit the training target. Ensuring this "stimulus variability" helps ensure that the skill will generalize to the variety of task requirements in the client's daily life. For example, when training a client to use an external aid to record appointments, the clinician would have the client practice with a variety of functional appointments (i.e., different types of appointments, different times, different information).

PRACTICE REGIMEN

When a person with declarative memory impairments is first acquiring a target concept, skill, or behavior, three training conditions will maximize learning potential:

Error-Control Methods. The clinician is attempting to *establish* the target. While it may not be possible to prevent all errors from occurring, errors are minimized during acquisition by the use of errorless instruction techniques. These techniques include ensuring an appropriate level of task difficulty; clinician modeling with gradually fading prompts or cues; and use of immediate corrective feedback with knowledge of performance when an error is made.

Massed Practice. When first establishing the target, the clinician engages the learner in massed practice trials. The goal of these trials is to ensure that the learner is able to successfully produce the target in response to the cue, without assistance from the clinician—which might take several repetitions of the target in a row. This intensive schedule has been shown to enhance initial target learning (Huckans et al., 2010). If the target has multiple steps or components, the clinician chains them together, but may need to isolate difficult steps or concepts and provide specific intensive practice on them. This acquisition training is systematic and relatively fast-paced in order to provide sufficient learning opportunities and keep the client engaged.

Intensive Practice. In addition to massed practice, it is also critical to provide sufficient repetition of practice when first establishing the target. For some clients and instructional targets, the acquisition phase may be very short—a portion of one session. Other training scenarios may take considerable time. For example, teaching a person with a severe memory impairment a behavioral sequence (e.g., doing laundry) may require several weeks of acquisition training. Home programs can play a crucial role in providing ample practice opportunities; however, it is important to keep in mind that errors in the home environment will have to be controlled, and the support person in the learner's home environment should receive training to do this. The importance of error control outside of the therapy session cannot be overestimated: Many training programs fail because learning conditions at home "undo" what has been trained in therapy. Although there currently are no evidence-based guidelines for caregiver training in cognitive rehabilitation (Boschen, Gargaro, Gan, Gerber, & Brandys, 2007), there is growing evidence that caregivers can learn to manage cognitive impairments in children and adults (Judge, Menne, & Whitlatch, 2009; Sander, Clark, Atchison, &

Rueda, 2009; Wade, Carey, & Wolfe, 2006), and that this can significantly decrease stress and burden at home (Sander et al., 2009; Wade et al., 2006). It is noteworthy that successful caregiver training programs offer *ongoing* support by health care professionals. Without this support, caregivers may experience increased burden, because they feel that they are "on their own" managing both maintenance of treatment gains and also new problem behaviors (Hoepner & Turkstra, 2010).

LEVEL OF COGNITIVE ENGAGEMENT

The third consideration during initial target acquisition is the level of learner engagement. This engagement (or lack thereof) has been considered in the selection of the target and training stimuli and, in some cases, might require the use of external reinforcers. Effortful processing techniques (e.g., semantic elaboration, visualization, self-generation of responses) as well as metacognitive strategies (e.g., prediction/reflection) have been shown to enhance engagement and therefore learning. There is a necessary tension between minimizing errors and encouraging effortful processing; ultimately, it is necessary to use clinical judgment to strike a balance for an individual learner. Most importantly, clinicians should avoid passive learning. For example, if training a patient in a cooking routine, a clinician might have the client periodically taste the recipe and evaluate whether it needs more flavor rather than only reviewing and practicing the recipe steps.

Implementation Phase 2: Mastery ("Fluency") and Generalization

The goal of the mastery and generalization phases is to consolidate new learning so that the client can use it reliably. For example, a person may be able to use a strategy in a quiet room but not when distracted or tired, or may still need cues at times. The clinician should probe the client's performance at the start of each session. When the client demonstrates the ability to complete the target behavior during a session, but does not necessarily recall the complete target later in that session or in the next session, or does not implement the target consistently in the desired contexts, it is time to move into the mastery phase of training. It should be noted that failure to establish mastery of new skills is a common occurrence in rehabilitation, where lengths of stay are becoming progressively shorter and opportunities for practice in everyday contexts are limited. This phase, however, is critical for generalization and maintenance and requires careful attention in rehabilitation. Establishing target mastery and generalization requires manipulation of the same three factors discussed in Phase 1, as described next.

TRAINING STIMULI

Incorporating stimulus and contextual variability is critical at this point. During the planning process, the clinician and client identify the environments and contexts in which the target will be implemented, which in turn allows for the identification of antecedents in each context that can trigger the desired skill or concept. During the acquisition phase, a general response has been established. During the mastery phase, target responses for all of the conditions are practiced, requiring the clinician to provide more varied training stimuli and move out of the clinic into the client's natural environments.

While this may seem impractical, the characteristics of procedural learning require that the learning context be similar to the context in which the skills will be used. Therapy that does not consider this basic learning rule is unlikely to generalize and thus is not a cost-effective use of rehabilitation.

PRACTICE REGIMEN

The clinician makes active modifications to these three elements:

Errorless Methods. The clinician continues to use errorless instruction methods. Given that the learner has already acquired the target, modeling is limited to instances in which the client makes errors, to prevent *drift*—the tendency to move away from the target response over time. The clinician should continue to provide guided practice through occasional prompting with general or opportunity cues, while gradually fading cues based on learner performance. Feedback also can be adjusted to move from immediate corrective feedback to delayed general feedback, using knowledge of results (e.g., "Did you complete all the steps?").

Distributed Practice. Fundamental to the mastery phase is the introduction and gradual lengthening of distributed practice trials so that the learner is able to implement the target independently over increasingly longer periods of time. It may be that as training conditions are altered (e.g., by changes in the prompt or environment), it will be necessary to drop back to acquisition training and provide some massed practice. Keeping careful session data will reveal this need. As described in Chapter 2, spaced retrieval (SR) training is a specific treatment procedure that provides structure to distributed practice trials; it is discussed further in Chapter 5.

Intensive Practice. The clinician maintains high levels of practice during the mastery phase to establish fluency with the instructional target. The goal is for the target to become automatic and natural in a variety of contexts. Continued practice is essential. The clinician should continue to monitor and document home practice, to ensure that correct practice is completed with sufficient intensity.

LEVEL OF COGNITIVE ENGAGEMENT

During the mastery phase, the clinician incorporates additional metacognitive components to facilitate active engagement during practice sessions. Examples of metacognitive techniques include having the learner predict and then reflect on accuracy of performance by taking session data, and comparing his or her own performance across trials and sessions. The client also may predict which aspects will be easy or challenging, then reflect on how those factors operated during performance. The clinician and client may choose to modify the target or the environment based on this assessment. It should be noted that there is a necessary tension between enhancing learner involvement and limiting errors. As the learner gains more control in the process, there will be more opportunities for error; hence, the clinician must gauge whether error responses will be intrusive or instructive as the client is learning the therapy targets. Errorless responses are most critical during initial acquisition. It is also important to keep in mind that previous declarative knowledge and reasoning skills may be preserved in individuals with profound anterograde memory impairments. That is, the person's ability to tell you what he or she *would* do in a given situation often is not correlated with actual performance. Thus, for this population we recommend minimizing discussion of target behavior and instead focusing on rehearsal of correct responses.

Implementation Phase 3: Maintenance

The maintenance phase occurs once the learner has demonstrated the ability to complete the training target reliably and fluently in his or her desired contexts. Distributed practice trials and probe data during the mastery phase will have revealed this ability. However, recidivism and abandonment of targeted strategies or behaviors is a common rehabilitation problem that clinicians must mitigate. In the maintenance phase, the clinician utilizes methods that increase the likelihood that a rehabilitation target will be retained beyond the cessation of therapy. In most cases, this phase of therapy is not conducted by the clinician in a therapy setting. Below we list factors that the clinician should build into the training process to promote durability of learning. This can take considerable planning, as often the clinician enters the maintenance phase for one target while beginning the acquisition phase for another.

TRAINING STIMULI

Once the learner has mastered the target and consistently demonstrates it in the desired contexts, the clinician and client are ready to move to the maintenance phase. During this phase, the clinician may train natural supports, which are the people and contexts that promote ongoing use of the instructional target. These supports may have been previously identified and trained during therapy; for example, an educational assistant may be trained to encourage ongoing use of an assignment completion strategy, or a colleague may be trained to support the use of a memory system in a supported work environment. There may also be factors that are part of the learner's natural environment that have been exploited to provide ongoing facilitation, such as the school bell noted earlier as a signal to use a memory aid. Careful investigation of opportunities and people in a person's natural environment can be the key to his or her long-term use of a target skill.

PRACTICE REGIMEN

The need for cumulative review of instructional targets is often overlooked. Even without a cognitive impairment, people do not behave as robots and automatically continue implementing all intended behaviors. The implementation of diets, exercise programs, and mental health strategies all have peaks and valleys, and most people need ongoing support and adjustments to maintain desired habits. People with cognitive impairments need periodic review and support. "Booster sessions" have been shown to facilitate maintenance of gains after therapies such as SR for memory impairments in adults with dementia (Cherry et al., 2009), and often are cited as a necessary ingredient in effective clinical treatment trials (e.g., Bourgeois et al., 2007; van Hout, Wekking, Berg, & Deelman, 2008). People and their contexts and goals will change, and adjustments in a schedule, routine, or behavior are likely to be necessary. Clinicians must consider how follow-up and adjustments might take place and who will be involved in this process. Planning for cumulative review should be part of the therapy process and built into the training of natural supports.

LEVEL OF COGNITIVE ENGAGEMENT

During the mastery phase, the clinician introduced metacognitive strategies to enhance engagement. The ongoing use of metacognitive strategies can reinforce the learner's ownership of target skills or behaviors, ability to reflect on his or her own performance, and ability to monitor the need for adjusted levels of support. For clients with reduced self-awareness, the clinician should identify natural support persons to monitor the need for target adjustments or booster sessions.

THERAPY SESSION: HAVING AN AGENDA

Clinicians need efficiency and systems that can be replicated across clients in order to realistically implement effective instruction. Having a session plan or agenda can help streamline decisions and information. The typical instructional session consists of three parts:

1. *Probe.* Most sessions begin with a probe to determine durability of previously taught concepts, skills, or behaviors and to pinpoint where to begin in the training sequence in that session.
2. *Practice.* Based on performance during the initial probe, the clinician engages the learner in practicing therapy targets, which comprises the bulk of the therapy session. As outlined above, the amount and type of practice vary with the learning phase.
3. *Review.* Sessions typically end with a review and perhaps homework or planning.

   In the chapters that follow, sample session agendas specific to different types of instructional targets are provided. Having a protocol for implementing effective instructional methods during therapy sessions increases the ease with which a clinician can implement therapy and may thereby improve effectiveness and productivity.

PIE: EVALUATION OF OUTCOME

The clinician considers evaluation during initial planning by working with the client to identify the desired outcome and criterion for target performance. This planning then results in specific training objectives. In collaboration with the client, the clinician conducts ongoing evaluation of learning throughout the implementation phase.

   As shown in the ICF model in Figure 4.2, the client's outcome may be measured at the level of body structure and function, activity, or participation. Most rehabilitation programs are focused at the level of impairment, and, if there are sufficient resources and time, activity-based outcomes also are included. Instructional targets are selected because they serve a functional purpose for the client (although often the client is not included in the planning process), and outcome is measured by a metric indicating whether the client has learned the target skill or knowledge with a specified degree of support. Typically, clinicians, third-party payers, and institutions define and determine this level of outcome. There is growing evidence, however, that participation-level factors are critical to rehabilitation outcomes, including factors such as the impact of the intervention on that person's ability to be independent (Olswang & Bain, 1994), return to school (Kennedy et al., 2008) or work (Corrigan & Bogner, 2004), or maintain friendships (Engberg, 2004). Thus, participation-level outcomes are included as "impact" data below.

In this section, we provide a five-tiered model for evaluating clinical outcomes relevant to instruction. Because each type of data contributes to ongoing clinical decision making and the direction of therapy sessions, clinicians should consider collecting data across the five dimensions outlined below.

Session Data

The bulk of time during training sessions is spent providing practice opportunities for the learner. The clinician should keep data on the number of correct practice trials and the associated level of support provided. Analysis of these data can provide insights into adherence to the recommended practice regimen. For example, data may reveal that prompts were faded too quickly to allow for errorless instruction or that there were not enough practice opportunities to allow for target acquisition. These session data are most critical during the massed practice trials of the initial acquisition phase.

Generalization Probes

The clinician should also determine whether the skill or information taught is used in the identified naturalistic environments. This can be accomplished through periodic use of naturalistic *probes*, which are samples of the target behavior in the relevant context (e.g., testing a face–name association in that person's workplace). Probe data do not have to be taken during every session, but they should be collected systematically to avoid error bias (e.g., only probing on "good" days or in certain contexts). These data are important for testing generalization and can both reveal the need for additional training in a specific context and also influence selection of treatment stimuli.

Maintenance Probes

It is also important to collect probe data to determine if the learning is durable over time. As mentioned in the session agenda section above, each session generally begins with the administration of a learning probe. These accumulated data points are critical for making clinical decisions about moving from the acquisition to mastery or maintenance phases of training.

Impact Data

A critical clinical question is, if the skill or information is learned and implemented in natural settings, how will it improve the client's daily functioning? Improvement in daily functioning is the ultimate goal of learning and motivates the initial choice of training targets. Recall that this focus contrasts with the medical model, in which impact is considered post hoc, also referred to as "train and hope" (Kennedy & Turkstra, 2006), rather than planned for in advance. Impact data are generally collected at two points in time: pretreatment (baseline) and at the conclusion of treatment. For example, if the goal of training swallowing strategies is to permit a mechanical soft diet without increasing the risk of aspiration, what is the person's diet and pneumonia history now compared to pretraining? There is little point to independent use of swallowing exercises if there is no functional impact on swallowing. Further, third-party payers routinely deny coverage for impairment-level cognitive goals (e.g., "Improve short-term recall to 90% accuracy"), and instead expect goals that are directly linked to improvements in everyday outcomes, such as independence and employment (e.g., "Use a memory aid to complete work tasks with 90% accuracy," providing that meets the minimum standard for the workplace).

Efficacy Data

In the era of evidence-based practice, it is important for clinicians to document that time spent in skilled treatment sessions contributes to positive targeted outcomes. In the medical rehabilitation profession, this is often confounded by spontaneous recovery. The key efficacy question is, how do we know that the intervention, and not some other factor, is responsible for the observed gains? In order to document evidence of efficacy, clinicians should consider collecting pre–posttreatment *control* data (Olswang & Bain, 1994). Control data are measures of performance on targets that were not treated directly and are unrelated to the intervention, and thus should *not* change during the treatment period (Beeson & Robey, 2006). If the clinician observed improvement on control data, he or she could not necessarily conclude that gains in session, generalization, maintenance, or impact data were due directly to the clinician's instruction. In our experience, control data are the most difficult for students and clinicians to grasp; we have generally not been trained to collect these data. However, they can contribute significantly to the strength of one's own clinical data as a source of practice-based evidence.

Consider a case example to illustrate the potential use of control data for decision making. A clinician teaches a client with TBI the names of therapy staff. The goal of the intervention is not to improve underlying declarative memory processes, but rather to help the client locate his scheduled therapist independently. In this case, session data show that the client is able to verbalize staff names when shown pictures without prompts. Generalization probes show that the client is able to name staff when encountered during therapy sessions or in the hallway. Maintenance data reveal that the learner continues to correctly name staff during visits after discharge from therapy. Impact data reveal that the client demonstrates improved self-efficacy due to resultant positive social interactions. How might we document that these observed effects were due to our intervention and not to some other factor, such as spontaneous recovery? We can take control data. The clinician takes a pre–posttherapy measure of declarative memory (e.g., scores on a word-learning test). If this measure shows no change, or changes significantly less than performance on face–name associations, then the clinician would have strong evidence that the treatment was responsible for the client's ability to remember staff names. However, if the declarative memory assessment revealed significant improvement at posttest, the clinician could attribute observed gains to spontaneous recovery. The clinician could also measure recall on names that were not trained as part of therapy. If learning occurs for trained names only, it is likely the result of therapy.

Uses of Clinical Data

Table 4.3 provides specific clinical examples illustrating the different domains of outcome measurement and their use in clinical decision making across four types of instructional targets. First, consider training the rehabilitation target "using a PDA to record appointments" for a client with moderate–severe cognitive impairment following an anoxic event. Session data reveal the client's ability to use the PDA as taught during therapy, measured by either number of PDA entries or by steps in the PDA procedure completed independently when observed. Another level of measurement is whether the skills to use the PDA are implemented outside of therapy in real-world contexts (i.e., generalization probes). This could be assessed by client or care provider report of real-world use. The clinician also uses probe data at the beginning of sessions during the mastery phase to demonstrate maintenance following distributed practice training. Ultimately, assuming PDA use is mastered and implemented in daily life, the clinician measures the functional impact of the training to determine whether there is an increase in the frequency of getting to appointments. Collecting pre- and postimpact data through logging appointment successes and failures demonstrates potential impact. Finally, clinical case evidence is strengthened by control data demonstrating that the client is unable to successfully use an untrained PDA for appointment management. Collection and analysis of data at these different levels during the therapy process allow the clinician to adjust intervention and targets accordingly.

SUMMARY

This chapter has reviewed the PIE framework that can be used to create a customized therapy plan for teaching a wide variety of targets to a wide variety of clients. The framework incorporates methods of instruction that have been empirically shown to result in learning in children and adults with cognitive impairments. Figure 4.3 provides a graphic summary of the PIE components. In the chapters that follow, the PIE framework is applied to specific intervention targets, and materials are provided for clinical use when instructing on each type of target.

TABLE 4.3. Sample Evaluation of Outcome before, during, and following Intervention for Different Instructional Target Categories

Sample targets	Sample session data	Sample generalization probe data	Sample maintenance probe data	Sample pre- and postimpact data	Sample pre- and posteffcacy data
Facts and concepts: *Orientation to circumstance*	Longest time interval learner can correctly answer the question "What happened to you?" (SR training)	Number of times client provides correct orientation information during a conversation about his injury with mother and father	Correctly answers the question "What happened to you?" on three occasions 2 weeks after stopping direct training, with no review	Mother reports decreased caregiver burden due to cessation of questions about "What happened to me?"	Retrieval of autobiographical information not targeted in therapy does not improve at the same rate or to same extent as the trained orientation information
Multistep procedures: *Bill paying*	Number of steps in task analysis completed with full cues	Independently and correctly completes bill-paying sequence when at home if spouse organizes materials and gives prompt to initiate task	Continues to complete bill-paying sequence 2 months following withdrawal of direct training	Client reports improved sense of independence on rating scale	Observation of client completing an untrained cooking routine does not show change
External aids: *Voice organizer for logging daily diary*	Number of practice trials in which learner independently listens to prior recordings and makes a new recording	Number of new entries made at home between therapy sessions	Number of new recordings each day for 2-week period following treatment withdrawal	Client reports improved memory for daily events on a memory rating scale	Recall when voice organizer not utilized is less than when device is implemented
Strategies: *Goal completion strategy*	Number of steps in strategy learner can demonstrate during therapy with opportunity cues	Number of times learner uses strategy at home, as recorded on strategy log	Number of times learner uses strategy at home, as recorded on strategy log 2 weeks after treatment completed	Care provider reports improvements on burden questionnaire	Executive function battery shows selective improvement only on a subtest involving goal completion

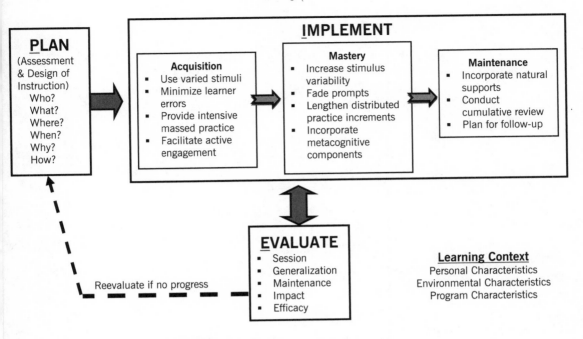

FIGURE 4.3. Summary of the PIE framework.

PART II

THE TRAINING PROCEDURES

CHAPTER 5

Training Facts and Concepts

Occasional memory lapses happen to most of us: It's not uncommon to forget the name of a new acquaintance, or a phone number or password. In fact, it's so common that there are legions of books and tricks available to help remember important bits of information. These memory lapses may be merely inconvenient for most of us, but for those with acquired memory disorders, they are a source of major frustration and have significant effects on independence, employment, and education.

In this chapter, we discuss an approach to training facts and concepts when clients have impairments in the acquisition of information. A *fact* can be defined as something that has objective reality, that is done and can be proven; a *concept* is an idea or notion that exists in the mind, a unit of knowledge linked to a symbol that can be shared, such as a word.[1] As is discussed below, training facts and concepts typically is part of a larger intervention plan that also includes methods such as strategy instruction or training multistep procedures, depending on the client's goals. The overall aim is to minimize demands on impaired memory processes, mostly declarative learning and retrieval from long-term memory, so that the client may participate more fully in his or her desired activities; that is, we are working to make access to information and routines more automatic and thereby increase the probability that the client will be successful.

The chapter begins with a brief overview of the characteristics of facts and concepts that should be considered when choosing therapy targets. We then use the PIE (Planning, Implementation, Evaluation) framework to explain and organize the key instructional components important for learning and retrieving facts and concepts.

THE NATURE OF FACTS AND CONCEPTS

How Are Facts and Concepts Learned?

There is ongoing debate about how facts and concepts are learned, particularly the extent to which different types of memory are involved (see Martins, Guillery-Girard,

---

[1] We recognize that these definitions, from *Merriam-Webster* (1986), are hotly debated among philosophers, but we accept them for the purposes of this discussion.

Jambaque, Dulac, & Eustache, 2006). Based on the discussion in Chapter 1, you might imagine that the learning of facts and concepts relies heavily on declarative (explicit) memory processes—that is, conscious attention to the information as it is learned. This learning involves both episodic and semantic memory, as information that begins as an episodic memory (e.g., remembering that you heard about HIPAA laws in staff orientation) may become a semantic memory (e.g., knowledge of HIPAA laws) over repeated exposure and time. The extent to which declarative memory is required, however, depends on *how* the information is learned and remembered. Declarative memory is necessary when using strategies that focus on conscious learning, such as elaboration, mnemonics, and visual imagery. By contrast, implicit memory underlies learning through repetition of correct responses and associations, such as in spaced retrieval training (SRT). These are not all-or-none processes: A person will use some combination of implicit and declarative memory on any given task, depending on the nature of his or her memory impairment.

The type of memory involved also depends on what is meant by *remembered*. Declarative memory appears to be necessary for the *recollection* of facts and concepts; that is, the ability to recall information in response to a question that triggers a conscious memory search, such as "What is the name of your speech therapist?" Implicit learning leads to a sense of *familiarity*, which is tested by prompts, such as "Guess the name of your speech therapist," or by providing a cue that triggers an automatic response—for example, "Your speech therapist's name is ... " if the patient was trained to say "Susan" when he or she heard that sentence stem (Anderson & Craik, 2006).

In everyday learning situations, declarative and implicit memory interact with other cognitive processes, and this interaction can be a challenge to disentangle when setting treatment goals. As an example, consider the staff meeting mentioned previously. The day after the meeting, you recall some details of the event (e.g., how one team member monopolized the HIPAA discussion), which is episodic memory. You also learned facts about how HIPAA applied to a particular patient, which is a combination of episodic and semantic memory, depending on the type of information you remember. Both of these pieces of information contribute to your general impressions of that team member and patient (e.g., the team member is obnoxious, the patient values privacy), so regardless of how you learned them, they might both become semantic memories. To complicate matters, at the same time as these declarative memory processes are engaged, you might be unconsciously influenced by previous negative feelings about the team member (implicit memory for emotional associations). The meeting also provided the opportunity to rehearse interpersonal negotiation skills (implicit memory for procedures). At the end of the day, your future behavior is shaped by all of these processes together, integrated by your skills in executive function and attention. A large part of the process of memory training is deconstructing tasks just this way: figuring out which type of cognitive functions are used and when, so that we can capitalize on preserved skills to make learning more efficient and effective for each person.

Because new learning can be implicit, patients with memory disorders can learn facts and concepts without ever remembering the learning event itself; that is, *semantic* memory (memory for facts and concepts) can be dissociated from *episodic* memory (memory for events linked to a time and place). This disconnection has been shown in many studies of individuals with episodic memory impairments (see review by Dewar, Patterson, Wilson, & Graham, 2009). For example, Vargha-Khadem and colleagues

(1997) found that children with severe memory impairments from a young age had nevertheless learned new concepts over several years of schooling, although they had no conscious memory of the learning events per se. This dissociation between semantic and episodic memory has been hypothesized to reflect the different roles of hippocampal structures versus nearby brain regions in these two types of learning (Tulving & Markowitsch, 1998; Vargha-Khadem et al., 1997), and has led to several studies showing good semantic learning in patients with little memory for events. In practical terms, this finding might lead us to change our assessment questions, so that we do not rely on clients' recall of the learning events (e.g., asking "What did you learn from the nutritionist today?") but instead look for evidence that the person can use the new information (e.g., by changing his or her food choices).

Approaches to Training Facts and Concepts

When we examine different memory training methods, we see that the key feature distinguishing them from each other is the extent to which they rely on intact declarative memory. Training techniques also vary in the extent to which they require executive function. At the most conscious, controlled end of the spectrum (i.e., high declarative memory and executive function demands) are strategies such as elaboration, visualization (or visual imagery), and mnemonics, whereby a patient learns to consciously use a strategy during the initial learning stage to make the information more memorable. As mentioned previously, internal strategies that the client uses independently to control or monitor his or her own thinking and behavior are referred to as *metacognitive strategies*. Methods for training clients to use metacognitive strategies are discussed in detail in Chapter 8. In this chapter we focus on strategies the *clinician* can use to help structure information so that clients with memory problems can learn and remember facts and concepts. For these targets, elaboration can be done in a variety of ways, but the most common is to link the target to other semantically, acoustically, or visually related information. For example, if the client works at a grocery store and needs to remember that peanut butter is shelved next to jelly and bread in the store, he or she might be trained to think of peanut butter and jelly sandwiches. A mnemonic strategy for this information might be to learn the acronym "PB&J," and a visualization strategy might be to imagine him- or herself taking items from those shelves to make a sandwich. The notion of visualization can be made concrete by inviting the client to "make a picture or video in your mind of what you want to remember" (O'Neil-Pirozzi et al., 2010). If the items don't go together easily, the client might make up a very short story to help remember them (O'Neil-Pirozzi et al., 2010), such as thinking about whether Lincoln liked cheesecake as a way to remember to look up the Lincoln Memorial and find a cheesecake recipe when he or she gets home.

At the other end of the spectrum are techniques that rely primarily on implicit or procedural memory and do not require conscious effort by the patient (i.e., low declarative memory and executive function demands). These include the method of vanishing cues (MVC) and SRT, introduced in Chapter 2. MVC is a method for facilitating the initial acquisition of a target, and SR is a method for both learning and retaining memory of a target. To illustrate the use of each of these methods, consider the example of a man with severe declarative learning impairments who wants to learn the name (Tina) of a caregiver who works in his group home. On the first trial, the clinician presents the client with a photograph of Tina and a card on which her name is written.[2] The client names the person in the photograph by reading the card aloud. On Trial 2, the clinician presents the photograph with the card again, but this time the card has one less letter (Tin_). If the client answers correctly (*Tina*), the clinician removes one letter (Ti_ _) and asks again, ultimately presenting the photograph with no card. If the client gives an incorrect response on any trial, the clinician returns to the previous successful stimulus length and begins again. Typically, the learning proceeds until there are no visible cues, then distracters are introduced systematically until the name can be recalled in contexts similar to the client's daily life.

The same target could be taught using SR alone. In this case, the clinician would point to the photo and say "Tina" (or "Her name is Tina"), then ask the client to repeat the name immediately. If the client answers correctly, the clinician distracts him or her for 30 seconds and then shows the photo again. If the client correctly says "Tina," the clinician doubles the time interval to 1 minute, with a distracter activity in the interim, and then shows the photograph again. Time intervals are doubled until either some practical upper limit is reached (e.g., the end of a 30-minute therapy session) or the client makes an error. If the latter occurs, the clinician immediately models the correct stimulus–response pairing, asks the client to repeat it, then returns to the last delay interval at which the client was successful. The response is considered learned when some criterion time has passed and the client can produce the correct response to the stimulus. In traditional SR training (Brush & Camp, 1998), the training is considered successful when the client can produce the response accurately the following day.

The critical element of these two approaches is error minimization: The client is actively discouraged from using strategies or searching explicitly for the answer. If the correct response is not produced immediately after the stimulus, the clinician interrupts the procedure, models the correct response and asks the client to repeat it, then returns to the last delay at which the person was successful. If the client cannot produce a correct response after the shortest delay (30 seconds), then MVC can be used for initial acquisition of the stimulus–response pairing, again with the goal of minimizing errors. At the end of the session, the client must have produced more correct responses than errors. The process requires some skill in identifying stimulus–response pairs that are important in the client's everyday life, are natural for the client to produce, and occur in natural settings with enough frequency and consistency that there is sufficient opportunity for practice.

Forms 5.1 and 5.2 in the Appendix (enlarged versions are on the book's page on The Guilford Press website) are two worksheets for tracking client data, reproduced from the SR training manual (Brush & Camp, 1998; the manual can be ordered online at *store.myersresearch.org*) with permission of the authors. The SR manual is highly recommended for helping screen candidates, plan therapy, and track progress over time.

In summary, facts and concepts can be taught using any of these methods, depending on the stage of intervention (e.g., identifying a target, initial learning, retention over time, or generalization), the target itself, and the patient's memory strengths and weaknesses. If the facts or concepts are likely to change over time, the best approach might be not to teach the fact or concept at all, but instead to teach the person to access an external memory aid such as a planner, where facts or concepts are written down (see

---

[2] Methods were adapted from Haslam et al. (2010).

Chapter 7). The process for choosing the best approach is discussed below in Consideration 2: Selecting a Target and Training Method.

PIE: PLANNING FOR TRAINING FACTS AND CONCEPTS

By now you will be familiar with the four considerations critical to the therapy planning process. In this section, we review the key planning considerations specific to the training of facts and concepts.

Consideration 1: Who Is the Learner?

The clinician first considers the neuropsychological profile of the learner, as well as personal factors, such as motivation and premorbid knowledge base, and environmental factors, such as available supports. Assessment of learner characteristics should include formal memory testing, given the importance of this information to treatment planning. Observation in everyday performance also is critical: Standardized tests often reveal optimal performance, which may differ substantially from performance after a half day of mental effort in a busy office. Interviews with the learner and important others in that person's life will direct the selection of goals and also provide insight into that person's awareness of, and motivation for, therapy.

Because memory-training methods such as visualization and elaboration require conscious effort, they are better suited for individuals with some insight into their limitations. These techniques are initiated by the learner and thus require an understanding of when to implement a particular technique and a sense of how it will be helpful (Sohlberg & Mateer, 2001b). Systematic instruction methods such as SR require limited insight, although the person must be sufficiently motivated to participate in treatment. A highly motivated individual with relatively good awareness, who has a job that demands independent recall of facts, may be a better candidate for an explicit strategy such as visualization. By contrast, a person with the same employment demands but limited awareness might be a better candidate for an implicit learning strategy such as SR, with the goal of training him or her to use external aids (Chapter 9) or highly structured procedural routines (Chapter 6), both of which can be trained as automatic behavioral sequences without relying on significant client insight.

Consideration 2: Selecting the Target and Training Method (What? Where? When? How?)

The main considerations in selecting a learning target and training approach are summarized in Figure 5.1. The questions to be answered are as follows:

What Is the Specific Need?

There is no point in teaching information for its own sake. Because all learning must be in the service of achieving a life participation goal, the clinician should begin by identifying the client's overall goal and then analyzing activities related to that goal to identify places where learning facts and concepts would be helpful. For example, if the

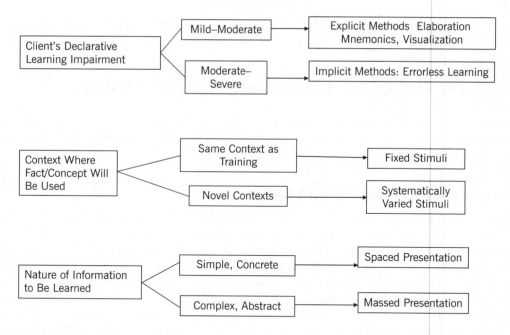

FIGURE 5.1. Considerations when choosing a method for initial acquisition of facts and concepts.

goal is for the client to have a social conversation, the client might wish to recall autobiographical information to share with others, or he or she might like to tell a joke or talk about world events. If the goal is independence, the client might need to know his or her address and phone number and the name of an emergency contact person. If the goal is related to work, face–name associations or job titles might be relevant information. For school, it may be academic knowledge or vocabulary. As noted above, training of facts and concepts likely will be part of plan that includes other training methods and targets as well. A social conversation might require turn-taking strategies as well as acquisition of facts to share, and independence in activities of daily living likely will require not only facts and concepts but also multistep procedures and strategies. Thus, identifying the specific need means determining which facts and concepts should be taught as well as identifying other training methods that will be needed.

Where Is the Information Going to Be Used?

As is discussed below in the section on training procedures, the context is going to serve as an important cue to the retrieval of the newly learned facts and concepts. Therefore, it is important to identify the situation in which targets will need to be recalled. The "situation" includes the *physical* context, such as a classroom or office; the *person* context, such as with a family member or stranger; and the *activity* context, such as at mealtime or in response to a question from another person. The importance of context cues increases in proportion to the severity of the client's declarative memory impairment: Individuals with more severe declarative memory impairments are going to rely more on procedural learning, which is highly context-specific. In this case, generalization to novel contexts is going to occur only to the extent that the novel context resembles the context in which the fact or concept was taught. For example, a person with profound anterograde amnesia might learn to give a brief description of his or her injury in response to the question "What happened to you?" If the question changes, however, to "Tell me about your injury," the new phrasing might not serve as a cue to the trained response. Likewise, a student learning a new vocabulary word in school might not automatically use that word in a variety of different ways (see Case 1, below, for an example). Later in this section we discuss how to plan for generalization in therapy, because generalization *is* possible even with individuals who have profound memory impairments, but it is important to know in advance how flexibly the client will have to use the fact or concept to be trained.

When Is the Information Going to Be Used?

The most important question in training is whether the target fact or concept is going to change in the future. Facts and concepts, once learned, may be very difficult to extinguish, particularly for individuals with severe anterograde memory impairments. For example, in a previous study (Bourgeois et al., 2007), we were asked by care staff to teach a group home resident that bowling was scheduled for Wednesdays. The aim was to reduce the resident's repetitive questions about the date for bowling, which had been on Tuesdays the previous year. This resident had dense anterograde amnesia, so she learned primarily by implicit methods. We used SR training to teach the new bowling day, but after three or four sessions it was proving difficult to extinguish the previous Tuesday response, and the resident was learning a response of "Tuesday … No … Wednesday"—which was confusing to everyone. The care staff then told us that bowling would be changing to Thursdays the next month! Clearly, the best approach in this case was to teach the strategy of checking a planner for the bowling date. That way, the routine would stay the same despite changes in the facts. One general rule of thumb is that if the facts or concepts are likely to change in the future, train a strategy or procedure to *access* the information, rather than training the information itself.

How Will the Fact or Concept Be Trained?

There are competing views in the literature about the best method for training facts and concepts, but two general themes are worth noting:

- *For patients with severe episodic and semantic memory impairments, error-control methods with SR may be the most effective approach.* There is strong support for this practice from the literature in dementia (Hopper et al., 2005) and TBI (Ehlhardt et al., 2008), and growing evidence from other clinical populations (e.g., alcoholics with impaired declarative learning; Pitel et al., 2010). Trial-and-error techniques might be as effective as error-control techniques for those with less severe memory impairments; for example, there was no EL advantage in a study of concept learning in children with memory impairments ranging from mild to severe (Landis et al., 2006), although benefits have been demonstrated in adults with milder impairments (Bourgeois et al., 2007).

- *Internal memory strategies may be effective for patients with mild-to-moderate memory impairments.* In general, although there is evidence to support the use of such strategies for memory rehabilitation (see review in O'Neil-Pirozzi et al., 2010), to date this literature has had many methodological limitations, including the combining of internal strategies with the use of external aids, so it's not possible to tell which is benefiting the learner. Internal strategies are discussed in detail in Chapter 8.

When choosing treatment targets, it might be helpful to consider a few key principles (see summary in Table 5.1). If the clinician chooses to use a strategy that relies on *declarative* memory, particularly semantic memory, the following principles apply:

• *Information that is more meaningful to the learner is learned and retained better.* This includes information that the person believes is important and also information that can be connected to the learner's previous knowledge. For example, a tennis player would be expected to learn new tennis terms more easily than geology terms, because he or she has an existing knowledge context for the new information. This is particularly true for declarative training strategies, because the person's previous knowledge about that target will provide meaningful links for new information (Dewar et al., 2009).

• *Abstract concepts are more difficult to learn than concrete concepts.* For example, the concept of *executive dysfunction* is more difficult to learn than the concept of *failing school if you don't get your work done*, because the notion of executive function is abstract, whereas failing in school has concrete repercussions. Even abstract concepts can be made concrete, however, as in the use of metaphors described by Ylvisaker and Feeney (2000). These authors collaborated with adults with TBI to develop personally relevant metaphors, often in the form of people they admired, that captured complex behavior and personality profiles desired by each client. For example, one client, Jason, had severe behavior problems, which he learned to control by internalizing a self-image of "Jason the Marine" and "Jason as Clint Eastwood." This was a way to make very abstract concepts, such as control, independence, and competence, concrete and accessible to the learner.

TABLE 5.1. Tips for Choosing Learning Targets

When training with declarative learning techniques (e.g., elaboration, visualization, association), keep in mind the following points:

• Facts and concepts that are more meaningful to the learner are learned and retained better.
• Abstract concepts are more difficult to learn than concrete concepts.
• Concepts that the learner can visualize are learned and remembered better than concepts that are more difficult to visualize.
• Facts and concepts from highly populated categories are more difficult to recall than those from less-populated categories.
• Face–name associations are particularly difficult to learn.

When training with implicit learning techniques (e.g., SR, MVC), keep in mind the following points:

• Simpler is better.
• Because learning is specific to the stimulus and context, generalization is limited unless stimulus variability is built into the training program.

For both declarative and implicit learning techniques, if facts or concepts are likely to change in the future, train a strategy or procedure to access the information, rather than training the information itself.

• *Concepts that the learner can visualize are learned and remembered better* than ideas that are more difficult to visualize (e.g., *traffic accident* is an easier concept to learn than *defensive driving*). This point is related to the previous principle: Concepts that are easier to visualize are generally more concrete, although not always (e.g., the client might have a memory of a person performing a brave act, which can help him or her visualize courage).

• *Facts and concepts that come from highly populated categories are more difficult to recall than those from less-populated categories.* The number of closely related items in a given category is referred to as *neighborhood density*: The more highly similar items there are within that category, the more difficult it may be for a person with a memory problem to retrieve the specific item he or she needs. For example, *small dogs* is a highly populated category—157 dog breeds were officially recognized by the American Kennel Club in 2009 (*www.akc.org*), and about half of these are small dogs. By contrast, *famous Scottish philosophers* is a relatively small category: There are about 20 who are internationally recognized, but most people have heard of only two, David Hume and Adam Smith. If a person who is not an expert is trying to recall the name of a single category member, the name of a small dog breed will be harder to remember than the name of a Scottish philosopher because there are more potential competitors from among small dog names than among Scottish philosopher names.

In addition to semantic "neighbors," other types of neighbors influence the probability of correct recall of a given fact or concept. These include sound-alike (i.e., phonologically similar) neighbors (e.g., *dog*, *clog*, *cog*), look-alike neighbors (e.g., similar-appearing dogs), and written words with similar forms (e.g., *harrier* vs. *terrier*). Neighborhood density effects are probably why *unicorn* is easier to learn and recall as a distinct concept than *Romano* cheese, although they are similar in frequency of occurrence in written English. There is only one type of unicorn, but Romano is one of many similar-looking types of cheese that are used with the same foods. Romano also has competition from a commonly used phonologically and graphemically similar neighbor: *parmesano* cheese. Thus, a person trying to learn Romano cheese might recall parmesano cheese in error.

Most of us have experienced neighborhood density effects with numbers and passwords, which are proliferating in our everyday lives and becoming more and more difficult to sort out from each other. Neighborhood density effects should be kept in mind when choosing targets for training: Targets from high-density neighborhoods might be more difficult to learn and recall accurately, depending on the individual patient's knowledge and expertise and the type of training approach to be used.

• *Face–name associations are particularly difficult to learn.* As noted in Chapter 2, face–name associations are completely arbitrary and require the person to learn not only the association between a name and a face but also the association between a first and last name (Thoene & Glisky, 1995). Face–name learning methods that work for individuals without memory problems, such as connecting the name to a characteristic of that person (e.g., Bob bobs his head when he says "yes"), are generally not practical for people with memory disorders, mostly because they forget to use them. Also, although there is evidence that mnemonic techniques can work if the clinician provides the image and the link (Manasse, Hux, & Snell, 2005; Thoene & Glisky, 1995), this not the same as generating a mnemonic independently. The requirement to first generate an image, then link it with a name, then retrieve both when needed is taxing for an already impaired cognitive system and is unlikely to be used in everyday life. The literature on treatment of adults with dementia suggests that the most effective approach for training face–name associations is SR training (Hawley et al., 2008; Hopper, Drefs, Bayles, Tomoeda, & Dinu, 2010). There is some evidence that this is true for individuals with TBI as well (Bourgeois et al., 2007).

For training methods that rely more on *implicit* memory processes, the following principles have emerged from the literature:

• *Simpler is better.* SR and other error-minimization methods are based on classical conditioning, wherein the clinician and client identify a stimulus that will trigger a specific response, and the response must be produced correctly each time. Based on our own experience (Bourgeois et al., 2007), we recommend that the stimulus and response be kept as simple as possible. The probability of producing a long, complex piece of information correctly is lower than if the information is short and simple, and the likelihood of learning is lower as well. Recall that implicit learning methods require that the correct response be produced more often than errors, so it is critical to identify a response that the patient can produce successfully and consistently. If the information to be learned is complex, it might be more efficient and effective to train a procedure that the client can use to access that information (e.g., putting an autobiographical statement in a notebook, and training the client to access the notebook when asked about his or her personal history). Complex facts and concepts can be broken down into pieces and trained via chaining (discussed in Chapter 6), but the client must be able to produce each piece successfully.

• *Generalization of implicit learning is limited.* The results of many studies of implicit learning in people with amnesia have shown that this type of learning is *hyperspecific*: That is, it is specific not only to the information learned but also to surface features such as the materials used and the physical context. The following, paraphrased from an example provided by Stark and colleagues (2005), shows how declarative learning might operate:

> It is relatively easy to learn the fact that *the New Orleans Saints beat the Indianapolis Colts in the U.S. 2010 Superbowl.* Having learned this piece of information, you immediately understand that it is also true that "the Colts lost to the Saints" and "the Saints won." This knowledge is available to your conscious recollection, and, if your declarative memory is intact, will automatically be linked to related facts such as knowledge about Hurricane Katrina and how important a Saints win was to the people of New Orleans, and perhaps memories of previous Superbowl games that were less exciting.

The processes engaged in declarative learning such as this are automatic and underlie the flexible use of new semantic information in a variety of contexts. By contrast, a person who learns only via implicit mechanisms will learn, literally, the statement *"The New Orleans Saints beat the Indianapolis Colts in the U.S. 2010 Superbowl."* This response will be triggered only by the cue with which it was trained, and the information will not automatically be linked to previous knowledge. For this reason, when training persons with declarative memory impairments, each link to previous knowledge must be taught directly, and the clinician can make no assumptions about generalization to other contexts (e.g., other persons asking the prompt question or other, even similar, prompt questions). From a rehabilitation perspective, this hyperspecificity is perhaps the most critical feature of implicit learning, because it has serious implications not only for where training is conducted, but also for counseling stakeholders about the limits of new learning. Most patients have some residual declarative learning, as true anterograde amnesia is relatively rare. Even for individuals with milder declarative memory impairments, however, generalization must be planned early in the training process, and the clinician should consider conducting training in the context where the learning ultimately will be used, and with the materials and people that will be involved in its everyday use.

Consideration 3: Specifying the Desired Outcomes (Why?)

Setting Goals

Facts and concepts are among the easiest treatment targets in terms of outcome measurement: The goal is for the person to recollect the information independently, use the information in a given context, or produce an answer when cued. Goal-writing components include statements about the treatment approach, treatment target, objective performance measurement, criterion for success, level of independence, and conditions/context.

Multilevel Evaluation

The clinician must measure the client's understanding of, and ability to use, the fact or concept both in the clinic and in the target context. As described in Chapter 4, five types of clinical data should be collected: (1) session data, such as the percent of targets accurately recalled; (2) generalization probes, typically percent accuracy on related facts and concepts; (3) maintenance probes; (4) impact data that reflect the effect on the learner's life-participation goal; and (5) efficacy data, which show that changes in the target are not due to untreated factors such as spontaneous recovery. These data sources are necessary for the clinician to monitor learning during the treatment process, evaluate how facts and concepts are used in the desired context, and assess the effects of target use on the participation goals of the learner. Table 4.3 provides examples of these different types of data for facts and concepts.

Consideration 4: Designing the Individualized Plan

By now the clinician, having gathered all the information necessary to design an individualized training plan, integrates the information collected during the client evaluation with the needs assessment, in order to outline an instructional plan. Form 5.3 in the Appendix (an enlarged version is on the book's page on The Guilford Press website) is a sample planning sheet; Figure 5.2 shows a completed planning sheet for a client's goal of learning a joke to tell at parties.

WHAT will I teach the client?

Long-Term Goal: | Learn joke to tell at parties

Initial Acquisition
Objectives: | Tell joke in therapy session with "Anyone know a joke?" cue

(Specify target, approach, objective performance, independence, criterion, and context/conditions.)

HOW will I train the fact/concept?

(Specify method; e.g., MVC, SR, elaboration, visualization, mnemonics, strategy training.)

SR with MVC

☑ It is a functional target
☑ It is customized to client
☑ The context is specified
☑ Progress measurement specified in long-term goal and/or short-term acquisition objectives

Plan to enhance client motivation/engagement: | Client chose goal and joke

WHEN will I teach the target?

Therapy Frequency: _____ 6X _____ / week
Session Duration: _____ 30 _____ min
Therapy Duration: _____ 2 _____ Sessions, (Weeks,) Months

☑ There is opportunity for sufficient practice within sessions
☑ There is opportunity for sufficient practice across sessions

To be used in same context or novel context?
Same context: Fixed stimuli = _____
Novel contexts: Varied stimuli = Will vary cues and pratice with novel partners

Nature of information to be learned
Simple: Plan for spaced presentation is _____
Complex: Plan for massed presentation is _____

WHO will implement training outside of session?
☑ Support person identified to provide additional practice between sessions   aide
☑ Sufficient variety of people identified to provide stimuli to allow generalization

Describe plan to *train* support person/people: Aide will attend three Rx sessions

FIGURE 5.2. Sample completed instructional planning worksheet for facts and concepts.

PIE: IMPLEMENTING SYSTEMATIC INSTRUCTION FOR FACTS AND CONCEPTS

The planning process reviewed in the above section lays the groundwork for effective and efficient training carried out in the implementation phase. The planning process generates the target fact or concept and the context in which it will be used, as well as measurable goals and objectives with which to monitor performance. The next phase is to *implement* the training. This section details the different training phases. The therapy dose (frequency and duration) needed to train facts and concepts varies greatly, depending on factors such as the complexity of the information to be trained, severity of the patient's memory impairment, type of training approached used, and concomitant cognitive impairments (e.g., in language, attention, or executive function). The studies reviewed in Chapter 2 contain a wide range of treatment doses, from three or four 30-minute sessions to more than 3 months of weekly group meetings; this range will depend on each individual client.

Initial Acquisition Phase of Training

Methods used in the initial acquisition phase of training are dictated by answers to the considerations noted above. The decision chart in Figure 5.1 can be helpful in choosing the approach that best fits the client's memory profile and the goal and context.

Mastery and Generalization Phase of Training

The mastery phase occurs when the fact or concept has been demonstrated fluently and automatically in optimal conditions (e.g., in the therapy room), but use has not generalized to the natural environment or is not yet used consistently and automatically in that environment. When the factor or concept is used consistently in everyday conditions, generalization has occurred. Again, for clients who have executive function impairments but relatively intact memory, moving to the generalization phase may occur after one session or demonstration. Ironically, this also might be true for clients with profound declarative learning impairments who learn by implicit mechanisms only: These individuals have no "interference" from declarative learning and may master some facts and concepts in a single session using errorless learning methods (Bourgeois et al., 2007). For these individuals, however, generalization will be completely dependent on the similarity of the target context to the one in which they were trained. If they are expected to use their new learning in an even slightly different context, it will be critical to follow the procedures outlined below for systematically varying stimuli.

In general, mastery and generalization of the target strategy are accomplished by attending to three variables:

1. *Fading learning supports.* Depending on which learning supports were introduced and the severity of the client's memory and executive function impairments, the mastery phase will involve fading the supports and helping the client gain automatic recall of the target information. Using the example in Figure 5.2, the clinician's cue of "Anyone know a joke?" may be faded to just the word *joke*, then to an expectant look, then to no cue.

2. *Incorporating or increasing stimulus variability.* If the target needs to be used in a variety of contexts, this is addressed during the generalization phase. The important context variables to manipulate will depend on the target. For the example in Figure 5.2, the "context" might be different people, so the client might practice with different people at the rehabilitation facility, then different people in everyday life. The more severe the impairment in declarative learning, the more that patient will rely on environmental cues to trigger recall.

3. *Maximizing engagement.* Individuals with limited awareness of their deficits can still learn new information, particularly with errorless techniques such as SR training, but the therapy process is likely to be more successful if the client is actively engaged in the selection of goals and can see evidence that the therapy is working. We have found it helpful to create a visual goal breakdown to show clients where the specific learning target fits into their long-term goals. A sample is presented in Figure 5.3; it was developed for one of the two adolescents described in the case at the end of this chapter.

Maintenance Phase

The maintenance phase begins after target information has been consolidated in long-term memory. Patients with memory problems need practice to remember new learning over time, and the clinician must actively plan how to help the patient retain new facts and concepts once therapy is no longer available. Practicing does not mean testing, but rather presenting opportunities for the information to be recalled. The clinician should look at the patient's environment and everyday routines for opportunities to practice recall. For example, if a diabetic patient with brain injury learned names of low-carbohydrate foods, could the patient do his or her own grocery shopping or meal

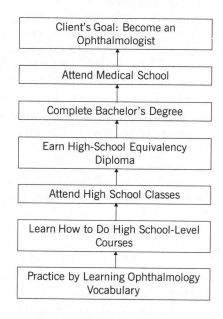

FIGURE 5.3. Sample visual goal hierarchy.

selection so that he or she has the opportunity to label items? If not, can the opportunity to make food choices be added to his or her everyday routine? It is much more effective to use natural cues to trigger recall of the information in context than to ask a hypothetical question in a drill format. Very few people enjoy being tested! The use of diaries, logs, and "check-ins" can be helpful for tracking maintenance of learning, provided support people in everyday life are trained in how to use them: It is unrealistic to expect a person with a memory impairment to remember to note when he or she forgets!

In terms of long-term retention of facts and concepts, it is important to acknowledge that contexts and information change; mechanisms need to be in place for reevaluating learning targets and adding new targets as the need arises. The optimal model for long-term service delivery may be a "train the trainer" approach, in which the caregiver learns how to train new facts and concepts, with guidance from a clinician. In this way, new information can be added as the need arises, with the added benefit that the caregiver is in the target context so that generalization is efficient.

PIE: EVALUATING THE LEARNING OF FACTS AND CONCEPTS

As shown in Form 5.3, the planning process results in a long-term outcome goal and also short-term acquisition objectives. Success in achieving the goal and objectives should be evaluated at multiple levels. Examples of different types of data needed to evaluate outcomes are shown in Table 4.3 and provided in the case example at the end of this chapter.

The first step is to record progress in the most structured and supportive context. For some patients, this is the therapy session, where there are no distractions and the clinician is providing cues. For others, particularly patients with severe declarative memory impairments, training must take place in the context in which the fact or concept will be used—in which case the "context" is where, when, and with whom the patient will be using the target information. For example, if the patient is learning a face–name association for a caregiver, the session might be in a therapy room using a photograph of that person. If the patient is learning to put his or her car keys in a regular spot in the kitchen, however, the session may be in his or her home. The most common measures of progress are percent accuracy of recall, type and amount of cueing needed, and response latency (i.e., how long it takes the patient to produce a response after a cue is given). These are the *session data*. If the training takes place somewhere other than the target context, or there are multiple contexts in which the information will be used, then the clinician needs to collect *generalization data*, which are measures of how the information is used in progressively less structured and supported contexts (e.g., with no cues, different partners, or the real person vs. a photograph). If the training took place in the context where the facts and concepts are to be used, then generalization is automatic.

Facts and concepts are only useful if they are remembered over time. Thus, the third type of data to be collected is *maintenance data*. Often, patients are discharged from therapy soon after they master a goal, and the clinician never knows if the information is used over time. Long-term retention cannot be assumed, however, so it is important to find some mechanism for checking that the patient can still remember the target information when he or she needs it. This information not only helps that individual patient, but also informs the therapist's future clinical practice.

Perhaps the most important outcome measure is whether the training had a positive impact on the patient's everyday functioning. If the patient learned the bus route to the hospital, could he or she find her way back for outpatient visits? If the patient learned to describe his or her own memory impairments, could he or she use this information effectively to self-advocate for accommodations at work? These *impact data* can be obtained via interviews with stakeholders or from memory logs or other types of journals recorded by the patient, with data compared to baseline evaluation before training began.

The collection of *efficacy data* is also an important evaluation component. Although patients with mild memory impairments may show improvements on novel targets if they begin to use learning strategies independently (see examples in O'Neil-Pirozzi et al., 2010), training of facts and concepts is not expected to result in higher memory scores on standardized tests. Thus, treatment efficacy might be measured by comparing recall for trained versus untrained items, or trained items versus scores on a standardized memory test, or trained items versus measures of other cognitive functions (e.g., language or attention). For example, if the client is trained to recall his or her address and phone number, the clinician can compare this to pre- versus posttreatment recall of an unrelated address and phone number. Because changes in mood and motivation also might contribute to treatment benefits, it is important to measure these factors as well if there is any suspicion that they have influenced treatment outcome. If mood and motivation can improve recall, it may be more efficient to treat these first.

PUTTING IT ALL TOGETHER: CASE APPLICATIONS

The following section provides two client examples that show the use of the PIE model in training facts and concepts. The first example is from the research literature (Oberg & Turkstra, 1998) and uses elaborative encoding for two adolescents with TBI. We chose this study because it reveals the strengths and limitations of semantic learning in individuals with declarative memory problems and also illustrates the process of choosing functional goals. The second example is a recent client seen in a university outpatient clinic.

An Example from the Literature

Description of Clients

BW and SN were two adolescents with severe TBI who participated in a study of elaborative encoding for learning new vocabulary. BW was a male, age 18 years old, who was injured at age 5 years. A recent computer tomography (CT) scan showed evidence of bilateral necrosis of the prefrontal cortex, left more than right. He had below-average scores on all tests of cognitive function, including memory and language, particularly abstract language comprehension and use. SN, also an 18-year-old male, had been injured 12 months prior to his enrollment in the study. He had a right frontal hematoma and required a left temporal lobectomy at the time of the accident; a follow-up CT scan showed encephalomalacia (softening of the brain) in the left temporal region.

Like those of BW, SN's scores on tests of language and memory were below average. He also showed perseveration in words, gestures, and ideas. For example, his definitions for *brave*, *precise*, and *strenuous*—when he was asked to define one after the other—were "honest and power inside," "happenings within," and "strength used within." Perseveration would prove to be a challenge when choosing and training vocabulary items (recall the discussion of *neighborhood density*, above). Important for the purposes of this chapter, both of these adolescents were outgoing, sociable individuals who were interested in learning new words that would help them in school. Also relevant, in retrospect both had excellent procedural learning and memory, which turned out to be a significant factor in the study results.

Choosing Treatment Targets

For each adolescent, the authors chose 100 hundred words that were needed at work or in school. For BW, these were newspaper and school-text words that were relevant to his curriculum; for SN they were words related to his goal of working in the field of ophthalmology. Each participant was asked to generate definitions for the 100 words, and of those defined incorrectly, 40 target words were chosen. These were divided into 20 treatment words and 20 control words that would be used to test efficacy.

Implementation Phase

In the acquisition phase, treatment included the following elaborative encoding strategies:

- Reviewing words and definitions
- Matching words to synonyms
- Matching words to definitions
- Filling in the blanks in sentences with target words
- Generating definitions with help from the dictionary
- Generating synonyms with help from the dictionary
- Using each word in a self-generated sentence
- Giving self-generated definitions to a classmate for feedback

Based on previous studies of elaborative encoding in TBI, stimuli were spaced rather than massed (e.g., each word was reviewed once, then the list was repeated, rather than repeating the same word several times before moving on to the next). To maximize generalization, the investigators emphasized multiple word meanings and using the words in a variety of sentences. BW completed ten 30-minute sessions over a 5-week period, and SN completed eighteen 30-minute sessions over 6 weeks.

Evaluation

Both participants learned 11 of the trained items versus one to two of the control items, and both maintained these gains after 1 month without treatment. Even after 1 year, SN was able to produce the exact definitions he had learned in treatment. In addition, both acquired partial knowledge about additional words on the training list. Most often, this partial knowledge was the ability to use the word in a syntactically correct sentence but with the wrong meaning. For example, SN was taught the word *formation* in the context of geology. Over the course of therapy, he produced these definitions:

- "In Utah there are a lot of Jurassic formations."
- "Triceratops is found in Jurassic, that's a good formation."
- "Triceratops are found a bunch in the Jurassic formation."
- "The formation of the Santa Rita Mountains has some matrix upon it."
- "The formation in those one mountains are really prolific."
- "Iron is the most important formation in my vehicle."

Matrix and *prolific* were other items on the training list and appeared above as perseverations. When asked to use the word *assume* in different sentences, SN provided these definitions:

- "I assume too much."
- "Out of life I assume way too much."
- "You assume too much is going to happen when in reality it won't."
- "I assume too much out of life."
- "Some vehicle places assume too much with engine products."
- "She assumed a lot of money from her job."

These examples show that SN extracted syntactic information about the items—appropriately, as this is the implicit aspect of language—and learned some associations with the items (e.g., one meaning of *assume* is to take on, and being paid for a job might be linked to taking on money). BW showed the same pattern. This was perhaps the most important message of the study: Correct production of the trained concept did not equal full understanding of, and ability to use, that concept in all contexts. For patients with declarative memory impairments this severe, "what you see" might be "what you get."

Case Application: Dave

Consideration 1: Who Is the Learner?

Dave was a college student, 22 years old, who sustained a severe TBI in a motorcycle accident after his freshman year. A CT scan showed bilateral frontal lobe lesions. Previously a gifted student, postinjury Dave had a moderate declarative memory impairment and severe executive dysfunction, including impairments in focusing attention, resisting distraction, identifying the most important information to be learned, organizing information for learning, and inhibiting irrelevant thoughts and words. Like many individuals with ABI (Kennedy, Linhart, & Brady, 2006), Dave had poor awareness of his cognitive and behavior problems at the time they were occurring; he had very good general awareness of his strengths and limitations, however, and recognized the need to do things differently than he had preinjury. He also was highly motivated to succeed in school and had supportive parents who lived close by.

Consideration 2: Selecting the Target and Training Method (What? Where? When? How?)

WHAT IS THE SPECIFIC NEED?

After several months of in- and outpatient rehabilitation, Dave stated at 1 year postinjury that he was ready to go back to school. He had been a history major, but his injury inspired him to switch to psychology so that he could learn more about the brain. In collaboration with his speech–language pathologist, he chose an introductory psychology course, which would give him an overview of the areas included in psychology and help him decide if he was interested in pursuing this as a career. Dave was strongly interested in this area and perceived the course to be advancing his personal goals; therefore he was highly engaged in the therapy process. The importance of personal choice and relevance was particularly salient with Dave, as, consistent with his executive function impairments, he had almost no ability to delay gratification. If therapy goals and strategies did not have face validity, he would not attempt them. Two further considerations in choosing this course were that the classes were short (50 minutes each), and the instructor was highly organized and provided lecture handouts and study guides to the students (i.e., the instructor could provide executive function supports). Dave chose to begin by attending class without accommodations, but after a few weeks he was significantly behind and sought help learning the basic constructs in the course.

WHERE IS THE INFORMATION GOING TO BE USED?

In the short term, the information would need to be recalled (in short-answer questions) or recollected (in multiple-choice questions) on a written midterm examination. Facts and concepts from this course also would serve as the foundation for learning in subsequent courses.

WHEN IS THE INFORMATION GOING TO BE USED?

Facts and concepts for this course were well suited for training because they would not change in the near future. Thus, targets to be trained could be used both in the near term, for the current course, and also in future courses.

To meet Dave's needs as a student, in addition to training facts and concepts he received strategy instruction training and support for time management, using procedures such as those described in Chapters 6 and 8. The following sections focus on facts and concepts, but these other intervention techniques were included in each session as well.

Consideration 3: Specifying the Desired Outcomes (Why?)

MULTILEVEL EVALUATION

Evaluation of treatment outcomes included several types of measures. As Dave had good insight into his learning after the fact, the *session outcome* measures were recall and recollection of facts taught in each session and his confidence in mastery of the concepts in therapy sessions. Confidence estimates involved a metacognitive strategy (see Chapter 8) that was intended to help Dave learn to calibrate his perception of learning to actual learning data, so that he could independently choose study targets. The *generalization* measure was his grade on the midterm examination. The *maintenance* measure was his grade on the cumulative final examination. The *impact* data were his overall course grade and his beliefs about success in the course, and *efficacy* data were his grades from a previous semester in which he had not received therapy.

Consideration 4: Designing the Individualized Plan

Dave attended therapy twice weekly, with both sessions scheduled in the morning before his class. The first obstacle was therapy attendance: Because of his impairments in executive function, Dave often got distracted doing other tasks and forgot to come to therapy. This distraction was addressed by sending him a text message 30 minutes prior to therapy, which was his choice of prompt. With this cue, Dave arrived within 10 minutes of the designated start time for 90% of therapy sessions. By contrast, without a prompt he missed more than 80% of his scheduled meetings with others, including his academic advisor. Use of the texting prompt provided Dave with an opportunity for errorless learning of session times and days of the week, so that eventually he would not need a prompt. Note that sessions had to occur at the same time and location each week, so the pairing of time and attendance was consistent.

In the acquisition phase of training, concepts were taught using two main strategies. First, the therapist used the course handouts provided in advance of each lecture to develop graphic organizers for the content in that lecture. Graphic organizers are visual depictions of content, showing links among related concepts and facts; they also are referred to as *mind maps*, *concept maps*, *storyboards*, and *flowcharts*. An example from one lecture is shown in Figure 5.4. Second, Dave and the therapist reviewed the

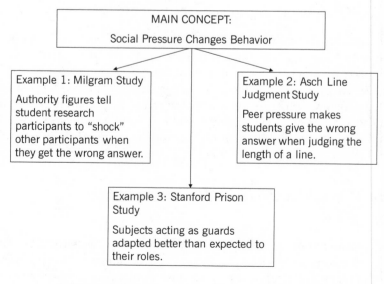

FIGURE 5.4. Example of a graphic organizer.

course handouts to identify essential content that Dave did not understand. This collaborative approach maximized Dave's engagement in training sessions, which was a significant concern given his distractibility. Concept definitions then were trained using the SR techniques described earlier in this chapter. Therapy sessions were on Mondays, Wednesdays, and Fridays, and session outcomes were determined by recall at the beginning of the following session. Along with new facts, elaboration and association were used to help Dave learn explicit links among newly learned concepts and also to connect new information to his previous knowledge and interests. In the generalization phase, newly learned targets were connected explicitly to other concepts in the course, again using graphic organizers and SR training, along with other association and elaboration strategies. In the maintenance phase, concepts from previous weeks were reviewed briefly as a check on learning.

Dave took his first midterm exam after 3 weeks of therapy. He earned a grade of 60%. The professor offered to test Dave's knowledge via an oral examination, and in that format he earned a grade of 72%. This finding was relevant to treatment planning, as SR training session outcomes had been measured by oral testing, which would not be expected to generalize to written tests. These midterm results suggested that intervention should be modified to include written exam-like question formats. Dave continued treatment until the end of the semester and earned a grade of B in the course, with no exam modifications other than testing in a quiet room. This accomplishment allowed Dave to continue on to the next course in his study plan and was a significant boost to his confidence.

Treatment efficacy was revealed in an unfortunate way: After two semesters of supports and passing grades, Dave chose to take two courses without assistance. This choice was understandable given that his goal was to be an independent learner, and it was hoped that he had established sufficient study skills to succeed. After the first month of the semester, however, he was sufficiently behind that the workload appeared unmanageable, and he dropped both courses. He transferred to a community college where classes were taught at a slower pace, and he achieved success in that setting.

SUMMARY

This chapter applied the PIE framework training components to teaching new knowledge and skills to individuals with significant cognitive impairments. Treatment techniques discussed in this chapter vary from those that are highly metacognitive, such as internal memory strategies, to those that require little or no awareness on the part of the patient, such as SRT. To select the technique that will best serve an individual patient, the clinician must have a thorough understanding of that patient's cognitive profile, particularly in the domains of executive functions and memory. As shown in Figure 5.2, the best technique for a given patient also depends on factors such as the contexts in which target knowledge and skills will be used and the complexity of the treatment target. We presented several considerations that are unique to learning facts, such as the benefit of choosing personally meaningful targets, the difficulty of learning abstract information compared to concrete information that can be visualized, the effects of interference when targets are similar to each other in meaning, and the difficulty of learning face–name associations. Throughout this chapter, the importance of planned generalization was emphasized, rather than a "train-and-hope" approach, particularly for patients with moderate-to-severe declarative memory impairments. By starting with the target context, we can maximize the potential for treatment to result in meaningful improvements in the patient's everyday life.

APPLICATION EXERCISES

1. Consider a work task you must complete each week. Identify facts and concepts a new staff member would be required to learn to successfully complete this task. The goal of this exercise is to recognize the importance of facts and concepts in everyday life and also to practice deconstructing tasks into treatment targets.

2. Identify a fact or concept you would like to learn. With a partner, create a training stimulus and response for that treatment target and have your partner train you to recall it using MVS and SR methods. Use a blank SR worksheet to track progress and make sure you measure maintenance at some future time, such as the same time the following day. The goal of this exercise is to practice framing appropriate treatment targets for MVC and SR techniques, which is one of the most challenging aspects of using these techniques. This exercise also provides practice with timing repetitions and recording session data. A countdown timer is helpful, so that the trainer can focus fully on nontarget distracters in the intertrial intervals, rather than looking at a watch or clock.

CHAPTER 6

Training Functional Multistep Routines

This chapter applies the PIE framework to the instruction of multistep procedures for people with cognitive impairments. As reviewed in Chapter 4, effective training or instruction depends on thorough *planning*, *implementation* of systematic training, and conducting multilevel *evaluation*. In this chapter, we consider each of these PIE components as they relate to the training of multistep routines, behaviors, or actions.

Many rehabilitation goals can be parsed into a sequence of steps. These include training in the use of strategies (Chapter 8) and of external aids or devices (Chapter 7). We do not consider these two specific training targets here, because they are discussed in detail in their respective chapters, but the same general principles will apply. Table 6.1 provides examples of multistep routines in different functional domains that could serve as rehabilitation targets.

PIE: PLANNING FOR TRAINING MULTISTEP ROUTINES

Consideration 1: Who Is the Learner?

When planning for effective instruction, the clinician must first consider the learner. Assessment of the client across a range of cognitive–linguistic, physical, and sensory abilities provides critical information about the client's individual strengths and weaknesses. Understanding the profile of learner characteristics often occurs simultaneously with planning consideration 2 (below), as the learner profile will necessarily dictate the instructional steps and level of detail needed when designing the routine. Assessment also reveals potential emotional or social barriers to learning, as discussed in Chapter 3. Assessment may include standardized testing (e.g., testing cognitive abilities, such as executive functions, that play a role in complex behavioral routines), observation of behaviors in the target environment, and interviews with the client and relevant support people. Most learners or clients who require training of multistep routines have moderate–severe memory or learning challenges that necessitate a structured, systematic intervention approach with cognitive supports (e.g., explicit prompts and cues).

In terms of candidacy, clients must have sufficient procedural memory skills to learn routines. However, clients do not necessarily need to have awareness of, or explicit memory for, the routines being learned and may be able to learn them as automatic sequences in conjunction with a cue or prompt to initiate the action (Glisky, 1992; Glisky & Schacter, 1987, 1988; Sohlberg, Mateer, Penkman, Glang, & Todis, 1998).

TABLE 6.1. Sample Multistep Routines

Functional domain	Sample routines ("therapy targets")	Related research
Activities of daily living	• Bathing and grooming • Dressing • Cooking • Laundry • Bill paying • House cleaning • Medication management • Gardening	Mastos, Miller, Eliasson, & Imms (2007); Giles, Ridley, Dill, & Frye (1997); McGraw-Hunter, Faw, & Davis (2006)
Exercise/motoric sequences	• Swallowing exercises • Physical therapy exercises • Fitness routine • Speech exercises • Visual tracking exercises • Inhaler use routine	Mastos, Miller, Eliasson, & Imms (2007); Logsdon, McCurry, Pike, & Teri (2009)
Community activities	• Bus-riding routine (known route) • Pedestrian navigation route (known route) • Using library • Banking • Grocery shopping	Newbigging & Laskey (1995); Gumpel & Nativ-Ari-Am (2001)
Vocational tasks	• Bookkeeping task • Phone routine • Filing routine • Janitorial routine	Manley, Collins, Stenhoff, & Kleinert (2008); Kern, Green, Mintz, & Liberman (2003)
School activities	• Accessing locker • Bringing class materials • Assignment completion • Schedule management • Recess routine	
Recreational activities	• Computer game sequence • Knitting routine • Drawing routine • Softball procedures	
Social communication/ behavior	• Use of social network site (e.g., Facebook) • Social greeting routine • Lunchroom routine • Telephone scripts • Conversational scripts	Taber, Alberto, Seltzer, & Hughes (2003); Lekeu, Wojtasik, Van Der Linden, & Salmon (2002)

Consideration 2: Generating the Task Analysis (What? Where? When?)

Designing the multistep routine requires the clinician to define the series of steps that constitute the routine for the individual client—in other words, the clinician must perform a task analysis that is both *individualized* and *comprehensive*. This analysis should answer four interrelated questions:

1. Who am I teaching?
2. What am I teaching?
3. Where is the target environment?
4. When will the client implement the routine?

To answer these planning questions, the clinician conducts a *needs assessment*. Depending on the client, the needs assessment may consist of an interview with the client or a relevant support person. As was the case for assessment of the client's strengths and limitations, task analysis also may involve a home or community visit to evaluate the target environment; in fact, a site visit is highly recommended, given the context-specificity of procedural learning. The clinician's task is to determine what information is needed for the design of an appropriate multistep routine, and how this information can be obtained. Options for collecting the necessary information are outlined in Table 6.2.

Delineating the correct steps *before* teaching a multistep routine is vital to the success of therapy. This planning process does not need to take a large amount of therapy time. The time needed will depend, in large part, on how reliable and knowledgeable the client and significant others are in relation to the clinical goal, and how well the clinician knows the client's profile. After answering the four planning questions above, the clinician will be ready to "list" the steps in an individualized task analysis, making sure that it is sufficiently detailed and tailored to the individual client and circumstances.

Although there is significant overlap between training procedures reviewed in this chapter and those in related chapters, there are two unique considerations to training functional multistep routines. The task analysis must contain *sufficient detail* and be *customized*.

Sufficient Detail

The clinician must ensure that the to-be-learned sequence is broken down into defined, discrete steps that are sufficiently detailed to teach the routine but not onerous for the client. The specifics of the sequence will be determined by the client's learning profile. By considering this profile in the planning process, the clinician forms an idea of the amount of detail required. At this phase, the clinician must also consider the need to teach any prerequisite concepts (Chapter 5) or subskills (Chapters 7–9). When identifying the specific steps to be taught, the clinician should also consider selecting specific keywords that can reduce memory load and facilitate learning. Consider the example of teaching a three-step routine for a client to "go to a new public place": (1) "Enter building and note a landmark near the front door to remind you of the exit; (2) locate the restroom; and (3) locate a bench or open seating for when you need to rest." When

TABLE 6.2. Options for Collecting Information to Develop Task Analysis for Routines

Planning question	Related interview topics	Other assessment options
Who is the client? • Cognitive–linguistic abilities? • Physical abilities? • Sensory abilities? • Affective issues? • Social connection issues?	• When client attempts this routine or related routines, are there any (cognitive, physical, psychoemotional, social, or other) barriers to successful performance? • Have you tried anything that lessens the impact of these barriers? • Is the client motivated or interested in performing this routine? • Are there any preferences for style, steps, or methods for carrying out the routine?	• Cognitive testing • Physical testing • Sensory testing • Psychological evaluation
What am I teaching the client?	• What is the desired goal or outcome? • Is it functional for the client's everyday life? • What was the client's prior experience (if any) with this routine?	
Where is the routine to be performed?	• Will the routine take place in one or multiple environments? • What else is going on in this environment in terms of activity, noise, or competing demands? • How is the space organized? • Who else would be involved or present when this routine is performed?	• Site visit
When will the client implement the routine?	• Can the routine happen at set times or in association with another activity? • What will the client likely be doing prior to the routine? • What could trigger or facilitate initiation of the activity?	• Site visit

training, the clinician might say or write the keywords *landmark, restroom, bench* to facilitate learning (the *PIE* acronym is another example of using keywords).

Customization

Customization is the tailoring of the steps to the individual client profile and circumstances and is also critical for success. Every client has different strengths, limitations, and needs, and as a result, there are very few generic routines that can be used across clients. Certain exercises or motor sequences might be standard, but even these will need to be modified to incorporate individual client characteristics, such as decreased motivation, impulsivity, or decreased initiation. An important aspect of customization is to specify what will *trigger*—or be the antecedent to initiating—the routine. Perhaps there will be no prompt other than a specific time, place, or person. In many instances, however, there may be environmental conditions that trigger the behavior (e.g., an alarm, a prompt by a caregiver), or the new routine may be linked to an existing one (e.g., learning to take pills after brushing one's teeth or during a morning coffee routine). These antecedents are key components of training and need to be identified in the task analysis.

Table 6.3 provides an illustration of the importance of specificity and customization, based on answers to the *What, When,* and *Where* questions used to create the task analysis. Sample routines are shown for two different client profiles. Client 1 presented with severe cognitive impairments, including a severe impairment in declarative learning and reduced awareness of her strengths and limitations. Client 2 had moderate cognitive impairments, including dysexecutive syndrome and a mild impairment in declarative learning. Both clients had normal procedural learning and memory, and Client 2 also had previous declarative knowledge about the target task. The task analysis for the *washing dishes routine* is more specific and contains additional steps for Client 1. This person not only had a significant memory impairment but also no previous knowledge, and therefore needed a more fine-grained task analysis. Client 2 had retained the basic construct for washing dishes and could follow procedures with multiple components, but needed a checklist posted on a white board to facilitate sequencing and to curb impulsivity. Different environmental factors also necessitated different routines: Client 1 would be washing dishes in the sink, whereas Client 2 was using an automatic dishwasher.

Similar considerations led to the generation of different task analyses for the *bus-riding routines,* also included in Table 6.3. Because of her severe cognitive impairments, Client 1 needed external prompts to initiate her routine; thus, her task analysis needed to incorporate attending to these initial prompts. The task analysis also had to integrate support people available in the natural environment, as it was not realistic that the client would become independent in the entire routine. In contrast, the planning interview for Client 2 revealed that behavioral control issues were a major barrier to using the bus, because the client was inappropriate in conversing with passengers and had been asked to disembark on several occasions due to complaints. His assessment process required in-depth interviewing to identify a preferred activity that could replace social interaction. The client shared that he loved pop culture and looking at magazines with pictures and stories on current pop stars. Hence, his bus-riding routine included taking and reading his magazine as a replacement for talking to (i.e., disrupting) other passengers.

A comparison of routines generated for the same functional skill set for two different clients illustrates the importance of careful planning and consideration of the *Who, What, When,* and *Where* planning questions. Having defined the overall treatment target and specified the relevant client and environmental characteristics, the clinician is ready to generate the detailed, customized task analysis. The task analysis can be outlined on the instructional planning worksheet, as illustrated in Figure 6.1. The "check boxes" identify therapy planning elements that should be addressed when designing the intervention. Of note is the importance of collaborating with the client and his or her care providers in establishing the overall treatment goals, the steps of the routines, and the prompts that will be utilized.

In addition to creating the specific, customized task analysis, planning for instruction of multistep routines also requires the clinician to prepare a range of teaching stimuli to promote generalization. For example, when training Client 2 in the bus-riding routine noted in Table 6.3, the clinician generated a range of scripts derived from actual reports of the client getting into trouble when he bothered other riders on the bus. The clinician used those scripts in the clinic to train the client to focus on reading his magazines and practice ignoring other passengers. The clinician had strangers (colleagues) come in periodically and simulate passengers (using the scripts), to make sure that the client understood the routine and could execute it in a controlled environment before practicing on the actual bus.

TABLE 6.3. Illustration of Need to Modify Routines based on Environmental and Learner Characteristics

Sample routines	Task analysis for Client 1	Task analysis for Client 2
	Client profile: Severe cognitive impairments, including impaired declarative learning and reduced self-awareness of deficits	*Client profile*: Moderate cognitive impairments, including mild declarative learning impairment and dysexecutive syndrome (problems with organization, sequencing, and impulse control)

Washing dishes routine	*Context*: Has no dishwasher
	1. Fill half of sink with warm, soapy water.
	2. Place dirty dishes in soapy water.
	3. Select a dish and scrub with brush.
	4. Rinse dish on other side of sink.
	5. Place dish on drying rack.
	6. Select a new dish to scrub.
	7. Scrub.
	8. Rinse.
	9. Place in drying rack.
	10. Repeat until all dishes are done.
	11. Let out water.
	12. Wipe off counters.
		Context: Has automatic dishwasher and intact previous declarative and procedural knowledge about dishwasher use.
		1. Stack dirty dishes on left side of sink.
		  1a. Check off step.
		2. Put silverware in largest pan with water to soak.
		  2a. Check off step.
		3. Begin with the glasses and rinse each glass one at a time.
		4. Place glasses in top rack of dishwasher.
		  4a. Check off step when all glasses are done.
		5. Move to plates and rinse each plate one at a time.
		6. Place plates in bottom rack.
		  6a. Check off step when all plates are done.
		7. Rinse and place silverware in holder.
		  7a. Check off step.
		8. Wash any large pans with soap and scrubber; set in rack to dry.
		  8a. Check off step.

Bus-riding routine	*Context*: Uses cane for mobility assistance. 1. Acknowledge morning cell phone alarm. 2. Grab daypack that was packed by your aide and is hung on your cane. 3. Press side button on cell phone when you have put on daypack and have cane. 4. Walk to bus stop outside apartment when cell phone beeps. 5. Show driver bus pass with destination indicator. 6. Sit in disabled seating behind bus driver. 7. Get off when bus driver indicates you have arrived at stop for your work station.	*Context*: Initiates inappropriate conversations with strangers. 1. Check "key items list" by door at 7:10 A.M. 2. Make sure all items are in bag (keys, planner, lunch, bus pass, wallet, magazine). 3. Leave house at 7:20 A.M. and walk to bus stop. 4. If people at stop say, "Good morning," respond to their greeting; do not ask questions. 5. Board Bus #5. 6. Sit at first available seat as you get on. 7. If seat next to you is occupied, may greet with "Good morning" or "How's it going?" Do not ask questions. 8. Look at magazine in pack during ride. 9. Get off at Harris stop.

Long-Term Goal:	JR will independently dress himself with the clothes laid out by morning aide for three out of four consecutive mornings within 15 minutes of aide's verbal prompt to get started dressing.
Initial Acquisition Objectives:	Following systematic instruction, JR will independently complete a six-step dressing routine at bedside with OT present and written checklist posted on bedside table for three consecutive days.

(Specify target, approach, objective performance, independence, criterion, and context/conditions.)

Prerequisite Skills:	

WHAT will I teach the client to do?

Task Analysis (List Steps)

1. Acknowledge prompt "time to get dressed" with verbal response or nod
2. Press "play" on CD player for morning motivational music
3. Remove pajama shirt and replace with daytime shirt
4. Remove pajama pants and replace with boxers
5. Put on pants
6. Put on sandals
7. Note whether morning song completed or ongoing on checklist

☑ It is a functional target
☑ It is customized to client
☑ Context/antecedent specified
☑ Progress measurement specified in long-term goal and/or acquisition objectives

Plan to enhance client motivation/engagement:

Use self-selected morning motivational song, with goal to complete dressing prior to CD completion.

WHEN and HOW will I teach the instructional target?

Therapy Frequency:	5	/ week
Session Duration:	1	min
Therapy Duration:	4	Sessions, Weeks, (Months)

☑ There is opportunity for sufficient practice within sessions
☑ There is opportunity for sufficient practice across sessions

(cont.)

FIGURE 6.1. Sample completed instructional planning worksheet for a dressing routine. OT = occupational therapist.

List materials needed to elicit routine and plan for varying stimuli with sufficient examples:	Four different sets of pajamas and daytime outfits; CD with motivational morning songs.
What is the plan for progressing from modeling to distributed practice?	Begin training with music on; pajama shirt off, and start training in the midst of Step 3 to establish concept. Demonstrate and isolate Step 3 and then begin training at Step 1. Use elastic and large clothes initially to minimize time and maximize number of trials. Once Steps 1–3 firmly established with clothes being handed to client, then increase time intervals and let him pick up clothes. When first three steps independent with 24-hour delay, begin chaining the last three steps.

WHO will help training outside of session?

☑ Support person identified to provide additional practice between sessions

☑ Sufficient variety of people identified to provide stimuli to allow generalization

Describe plan to train support person/people:	OT will conduct training and then have aide observe the last two sessions and follow scripted plan.

WHERE will I address this goal?

☑ There is a plan for generalization to different settings

☑ Measures of generalization across settings are incorporated into long-term goal

FIGURE 6.1. *(cont.)*

Consideration 3: Specifying the Desired Outcomes (Why?)

An important part of the planning process is to identify the desired outcome. The clinician must be clear about *Why* he or she is teaching this routine. At this juncture, the clinician specifies measurable goals and objectives and a plan for a multilevel evaluation.

Goal Writing

The planning process provides the ingredients necessary for writing clinical treatment goals and objectives. Treatment goals should specify the following components: *treatment approach, treatment target, objective performance measurement, criterion, level of independence,* and *conditions/context*. Table 6.4 provides examples of each of these components in the context of training multistep routines. Table 6.5 provides an example of incorporating the different goal components into specific written clinical goals.

TABLE 6.4. Sample Wording to Describe the Different Components of Therapy Goals for Multistep Routines

Who?	Will do what? (objective and operational)	In what context(s)?	To what criterion?	With how much assistance?
The client ...	... will complete a five-step laundry procedure given systematic instruction ... will complete a four-step showering procedure following SRT ... will complete a six-step lawn-mowing routing following a combination of systematic instruction and environmental modification	... immediately ... after a 5-second delay ... during therapy sessions with the clinician ... at home prior to cooking dinner ... at home at 1:00 P.M. ... in the lunchroom at work ... during recess at school ... when walking to his volunteer job ... while riding the bus to work ... when checking in at the recreation center	Sample session data Percent steps completed (with 100% accuracy over three consecutive sessions) Time interval client able to retain and demonstrate steps (following a 24-hour delay across 2 consecutive weeks) Time to complete all steps (within 10 minutes for three out of four opportunities)	... given clinician modeling ... with no more than two prompts from the clinician to look at the checklist ... following a prompt from the spouse to begin ... when the spouse sets watch alarm ... with the use of step-by-step audio instructions on voice memo ... independently
Nurse ... Care provider ... Spouse ...	... will provide cues to initiate a five-step morning routine and provide the client with checklist		Sample pre- and postimpact data Supervisor work evaluation (supervisor ratings will be ≤4 in all categories by the end of therapy). Caregiver burden index (spouse will complete caregiver index with a score of ≤10 3 weeks after goal mastery). Self-esteem rating (client will provide average rating ≥5; no scores <3 on a questionnaire). Improving total scores on Participation Objective Participation Subjective (Brown et al., 2009) (by 5 points or greater).	

TABLE 6.5. Sample Therapy Goals

Long-term goal with generalization to home

Following training using systematic instruction emphasizing errorless instruction, Mr. Bretz will independently complete his five-step cooking routine on three consecutive occasions at home after his wife sets out all the ingredients and the recipe. Mrs. Bretz will show a decrease of 3 points on the Caregiver Burden Index.

Short-term objective for initial acquisition during therapy

Using systematic instruction, Ms. Hill will independently demonstrate the five steps for filling her medication box and taking out the correct pills in response to the alarm, during therapy, for three consecutive sessions over a 2-week period.

Multilevel Evaluation

Chapter 4 detailed the importance of multilevel evaluation and discussed five distinct types of data that contribute to clinical decision making: (1) session data, (2) generalization probes, (3) maintenance probes, (4) pre- and postimpact data, and (5) pre- and postefficacy data. Session data are used to make daily clinical decisions about progress toward short-term objectives. Generalization and maintenance probes are taken periodically to assess durability and transfer of learning without prompting. These data allow measurement of progress toward long-term therapy goals. Pre- and postmeasures of impact and efficacy are taken as part of the baseline assessment—during planning—and after cessation of treatment. These data support clinical accountability.

The two therapy goals listed in Table 6.5 demonstrate the connections between goal writing and multilevel evaluation. The first example is a long-term goal. During the planning process, the clinician solicits input from the client and supports him or her to establish long-term goals and set expectations for progress. This process involves specifying the therapy approach (in this case, systematic instruction), the target routine (five-step cooking procedure), progress measurement (completion of all steps in the routine), a criterion for mastery (three consecutive sessions), the level of independence (independent), the context (at home) and the conditions for completing the target routine (when ingredients are set out).

Generalization probes taken in the client's own home will be most relevant to this outcome. This goal specifies the impact of training, with the expectation that the spouse's reported burden will be reduced when the client's goal is met, evidenced by a change in scores on a standardized scale. The choice of target outcomes and how they are measured direct the planning process. In this example, the clinician planned for the environmental modification of having the ingredients laid out for Mr. Bretz and incorporates that prompt into the task analysis. Such planning also alerts the clinician to take a baseline measure of burden from Mrs. Bretz.

In addition to specifying a long-term goal, the clinician identifies short-term objectives that reflect progress across therapy sessions. Many goals initially are addressed in clinical settings, so the short-term objective may be to establish the target routine prior to (or in some cases, simultaneously with) addressing it in the naturalistic context. An example of a short-term objective is shown in Table 6.5. The approach (systematic instruction), target (medication routine), objective performance measurement (completion of five steps), level of independence (independently), criterion (three sessions over a 2-week period), context (during therapy), and conditions (in response to an alarm) are all clearly specified and will be critical for guiding treatment conditions. The clinician may gradually introduce stimulus variation in the therapy session to promote generalization. In some cases, routines can be taught in the target context from the beginning of training. For example, service delivery models such as home health, telehealth, and school-based intervention, guarantee generalization. Regardless, it is important to determine how learning will be measured so that therapy can be directed by client performance. The clinician will be able to generate a data sheet in order to easily track this performance within and across sessions.

Consideration 4: Designing the Individualized Plan

The clinician incorporates the information gained during the needs assessment with the opportunities and constraints of the specific service delivery setting in order to design the best possible training plan. Form 6.1 in the Appendix (an enlarged version is on the book's page on The Guilford Press website) is a blank instructional planning worksheet, adapted from the version presented in Chapter 4 to accommodate the training of multistep routines. The task analysis generated during the planning process and the therapy goals incorporating multilevel outcome measurements are detailed on the plan. Figure 6.1 shows an example of a completed worksheet. Examples of completed worksheets are provided at the end of the chapter for two supplementary sample clients (see Figures 6.6–6.9).

PIE: IMPLEMENTING SYSTEMATIC INSTRUCTION
FOR MULTISTEP ROUTINES

The planning process reviewed in the above section sets up the clinician to provide effective and efficient training that will be carried out in the implementation phase. The planning process has generated (1) the task analysis listing the individualized, sequential steps for the routine and potential environmental triggers; (2) measurable goals and objectives to monitor performance; and (3) varied training stimuli to elicit practice of the routine. As a reminder, there may be prerequisite steps or knowledge that needs to be taught before training a multistep routine; these would be the first items addressed. For example, when training a swallowing routine, the clinician may first need to preteach the client what types of foods are allowed or how to execute a thickening process.

As outlined in Chapter 4, the implementation phase consists of three subphases of learning: initial acquisition, mastery and generalization, and maintenance. The specific instructional techniques vary with the learning phase. Before systematic instruction can begin for the targeted routine, the clinician first conducts an initial assessment probe to determine the client's ability to perform the multistep routine, and then chooses the training methods accordingly. This initial assessment establishes which steps the client can do and which steps need to be trained. The initial assessment is distinct from, and comes after, the *needs assessment*, which is the process used to identify the routine that should be targeted.

Initial Assessment

The purpose of the initial assessment is threefold: (1) identify steps that the client already knows, (2) determine where to begin in therapy, and (3) identify the most effective method of prompting. The initial assessment worksheet in Form 6.2 in the Appendix (an enlarged version is on the book's page on The Guilford Press website) is a generic example that can be used to list the steps of the target routine and types of prompts or supports needed.

In most cases, the process begins with a baseline assessment in which the clinician asks the client to demonstrate the routine at the level of independence indicated in the long-term goal (e.g., "without prompting"). If the client is unable to demonstrate a step, the clinician may model the previous step and ask the client to show what he or she would do next. The idea is facilitate completion of the whole routine, using whatever cues are necessary, in order to evaluate whether the client has the skills/knowledge for the procedure. These data provide a baseline against which outcome will be measured and allow the clinician to identify which steps the client may already know and where therapy should begin.

For the second part of the assessment, the clinician should determine what type of prompting (if any) should be provided as the clinician begins to fade prompts after the client demonstrates initial acquisition. This part of the initial assessment requires a *dynamic assessment* to determine what types of prompts or cues are most facilitative. The goal is to develop a cueing hierarchy by having the client try the routine with no cues and then start providing cues until he or she can do the step. For example, the clinician may model several sequential steps that the client did not know, then distract the client, and then assess the effects of different types of prompts. The effects of prompts, such as providing a keyword hint or a question (e.g., "What would you do next?"), to encourage self-monitoring can be informally probed to gather information for the cueing hierarchy. As reviewed in Chapter 3, direct modeling or physical demonstration usually provides the most facilitative cue; indirect prompts to self-monitor and opportunity cues (e.g., waiting for response) are the least facilitative. Table 6.6 provides examples of different cueing hierarchies.

In summary, most training begins with a one-session initial assessment that establishes baseline performance for the routine and identifies different levels of cueing. Figure 6.2 is a completed sample of the initial assessment worksheet.

TABLE 6.6. Examples of Cueing Hierarchies

Level of cue/prompt	Sample 1	Sample 2	Sample 3
I (most facilitative)	Model	Model	Model: Point to and read target step on checklist
II	Verbal: "Do X."	Verbal: Keyword for that step	Visual specific: Point to next step on checklist
III	Visual: Point to next item to be used.	Verbal: First letter of keyword	General: Remind client to look at checklist
IV	General: Recount previous step—"You just completed X."	General: Encouragement—"You're doing it. Try the next step."	General: Indirect cue to use checklist—"Where could you double-check the next step?"
V	General: Indirect hint to self-monitor—"How is it going?"	N/A	Opportunity Cue: Raised eyebrow; pregnant pause to encourage thinking

Initial Assessment		

Client: OS   Date: 5/23

Target Routine: Leaving house in A.M.

Antecedent to Start Routine: Alarm with verbal prompt—"Show me how you would get all your things gathered to leave for the bus in the morning"

LIST STEPS	ACCURACY (+/–/cued)	COMMENTS
1. Turn off alarm	+	Did automatically
2. Make sure backpack in spot on kitchen counter	–	Went to whiteboard
3. Go to kitchen whiteboard and take off marker	–	"Now I could look at board" but did not take off marker
4. Gather item #1 (lunch on second shelf in fridge) and place in backpack	–/cued	Clinician: "You just looked at board—what should you do?"
5. Check off on whiteboard	–	
6. Gather remaining items one at a time; put in backpack and check off on whiteboard	–/cued	Remembered to check off items when pen rolled on floor; put 2/3 items in backpack when prompted to get item
7. Erase whiteboard	–	
8. Leave for bus when second alarm goes off	+	Read alarm text "leave for bus" and went to the door

Baseline: 2 / 8

Dynamic Assessment to Establish Cue Hierarchy		
STEPS/ANTECEDENT	TYPE OF PROMPT/CUE	PERFORMANCE EFFECT
1. Modeled steps 1–3 and distracted client by having him count backward for 30 seconds. Then set off alarm.	a) Nodded toward backpack on hook b) Keyword prompt: backpack	a) Not helpful b) Elicited target. Got pack off hook, brought it to counter near whiteboard, and opened it.
2. Modeled steps 4–5 and distracted client by having him count backward for 30 seconds. Said "You've got your backpack ready now What should you do?"	a) Pointed to item on whiteboard b) Self-monitoring prompt "Think about the routine"	a) Elicited target b) Not helpful. Did not check off item or look at next item— asked me "What step is next?"

(cont.)

FIGURE 6.2. Sample completed initial assessment worksheet for morning routine.

Recommended Cue Hierarchy:	
Level I	Model
Level II	Point
Level III	Keyword
Level IV	Self-Monitor
Level V	Opportunity Cue

FIGURE 6.2. *(cont.)*

Initial Acquisition Phase of Training

The purpose of therapy at this phase is to establish the target action sequences that make up the routine. As noted in Chapter 4, fundamental to the initial acquisition phase is to *minimize the learner's errors, move from a massed to a distributed practice schedule,* and p*rovide sufficient practice or repetition* (Campbell et al., 2007; Cherry et al., 2009). Errors are minimized by the use of modeling and guided practice. The clinician initially provides intensive repetition and then allows longer time intervals between practice trials. Acquisition training should be systematic and sufficiently fast-paced to provide adequate learning opportunities and to keep the client engaged.

Each session begins with a probe to determine retention from previous sessions and indicate the step at which training should begin. Note that the session probe is different from the initial assessment. The initial assessment is a *one-time* evaluation to identify effective prompts and establish baseline performance, whereas the session probe occurs at the beginning of every training session and provides an opportunity for the clinician to observe the routine without prompts or supports and measures the client's retention from previous sessions so that the clinician will know where to start therapy. A progress monitoring form can be used to track performance on session probes and assess learning over time (see Form 6.3 in the Appendix; an enlarged version is on the book's page on The Guilford Press website). After the session probe, the training portion of the session begins. The clinician reviews the steps that were previously taught and models the next step in the routine, chained to the previous step. Depending on the client's retention of training from the previous session, the clinician models the two-step sequence (the previously learned step and the new step), and then has the client demonstrate the sequence. The clinician also incorporates strategies to increase client engagement (e.g., prediction of performance; self-recording of performance).

Below is an example of an elaborated clinician session script to illustrate the core components of training during initial skill acquisition for Days 2–4 of training. Note that the Initial Assessment was completed on Day 1. The "handwritten" font represents what the clinician would *say*, and the printed font below each script represents what the client would *do*.

Day 2 of Training (30-Minute Session)

"As you know, we're working on your laundry routine so that you can take care of your own laundry. Let's begin by figuring out what step in the routine we need to focus on. Here's the pile of clothes. Show me how you wash your clothes."

Clinician administers session probe and records performance on the progress monitoring form as shown in the Day 2 column of Figure 6.3 (client completes two steps).

"Nice. You have learned the first two steps. Let's add the next step. I measure the soap and dump it in. Measure and dump. Watch again, measure and dump. You do it and say 'measure and dump' as you complete these steps."

Clinician models and chains the new step to the previous step that was already learned, and emphasizes keywords during the demonstration. Client performs steps after clinician for several repetitions, with clinician prompting client to speak keywords.

Routine: Laundry Routine				
Long-Term Goal: ES will independently complete sorting and initiation of laundry with a verbal cue from his wife to begin the laundry on three out of four occasions.				
Initial Acquisition Short-Term Objective(s): Following systematic instruction, ES will independently complete the six-step laundry routine, in less than 6 minutes, with the therapist giving a prompt to get started.				
Steps	**Session Probe Data**			
	5/15 (Day 2)	5/16 (Day 3)	5/17 (Day 4)	5/18 (Day 5)
6. Add one pile and close lid	Cued: All set?	Cued: All set?	+	+
5. Turn water level to medium and pull knob to fill wash	−	−	−	+
4. Turn temp knob to warm	−	−	+	+
3. Dump soap in washer	Keyword cue: Dump	+	+	+
2. Measure soap	+	+	+	+
1. Sort clothes	+	+	+	+
Completion Time:	5 min	5 min 45 sec	6 min	5 min
Engagement Strategies:		(a) 4/5	(b) ✓	(a) None (b) ✓
Generalization Programming during Training:			Different pile of clothes	Moved soap
Comments: Trained using keywords: <u>sort</u>, <u>measure</u>, <u>dump</u>, <u>warm</u>, <u>medium</u>, <u>fill</u>, and <u>close</u>.				
Note: Graph the number of steps performed successfully each time the routine is probed.				

FIGURE 6.3. Sample completed progress monitoring form for laundry routine with daily session probe during initial acquisition phase of learning.

"Now I'm going to distract you for 2 minutes and see if you remember *measure* and *dump*." [Chats for 2 minutes.]

>Clinician distributes practice and repeats for three distributed trials.

"Good. Let's go back and add in these two steps. Show me the whole routine and say the keywords for each step."

>Clinician prompts with keywords for two repetitions, then fades cues. Client says keywords on own while repeating routine several times.

"Great—you have learned the first three steps. Let's add the fourth step. You dump the soap and then turn the temperature knob to warm. Watch me: *Dump and knob-to-warm*."

>Clinician models and chains new step to previous step that was already learned and emphasizes keywords during demonstration. Client performs steps several times, with clinician prompting using keywords.

"Now I'm going to distract you for 2 minutes and see if you remember *dump and knob-to-warm*." [Chats for 2 minutes.]

>Clinician distributes practice and repeats for three distributed trials.

"Good. Let's go back and add in these two steps. Show me the whole routine and say the keywords for each step."

>Clinician prompts with keywords on first trial, then fades cues. Client says keywords on own while completing all four steps for several trials.

Day 3 of Training

"Here's the laundry pile. You are going to show me how you sort and wash. What step do you think will be hard to remember?"

>Client responds that using the knobs is the most confusing. Clinician administers assessment probe and records performance on the progress monitoring form, as shown in the Day 3 column of Figure 6.3 (four steps).

"Nice. You have learned the first four steps. After dumping soap, you turn the temp knob to warm."

>Client has recognition memory and says, "Oh, yeah, *dump* and *warm*" and shows clinician without a model.

"Now I'm going to distract you for 2 minutes and see if you remember *dump* and *temp-to-warm*." [Chats for 2 minutes.]

>Clinician distributes practice and repeats for three trials, increasing time by 1 minute each time.

"Good. Let's go back and add in these two steps. Show me the whole routine and say the keywords for each step."

>Clinician prompts with keywords on first trial, then fades cues. Client says keywords with occasional cues while completing all four steps for several trials.

"OK, let's add the next step. Temp-to-warm and then water-to medium. *Temp-to-warm then water-to-medium.*"

Clinician demonstrates three times, and client follows with several practice repetitions while clinician speaks keywords.

"Now I'm going to distract you for 2 minutes and see if you remember *warm* and *medium*." [Chats for 2 minutes.]

Clinician distributes practice and repeats for three trials, increasing time by 1 minute each time.

"Good, let's go back and add in these two steps. Show me the whole routine and say the keywords for each step."

Clinician fades prompts. Client says keywords out loud and correctly demonstrates Steps 1–5.

Day 4 of Training

"Here's the laundry. Show me your routine."

Clinician administers session probe.

"Great—you've got almost all the steps! We'll finish learning the basic routine today. Before we begin, I'll have you keep track of where you are at. You see here the progress you made on learning the steps." [Shows client the progress monitoring form.] "Go ahead and put a '+' next to the first five steps you completed correctly. Then we'll add in the next one."

Clinician assists client in recording performance on progress monitoring form, as shown in the Day 4 column of Figure 6.3 (client completes four steps). Clinician teaches the last step in the sequence, following the same procedures above.

The above script and accompanying sample progress monitoring form (Figure 6.3) illustrate the following essential instructional components during the initial acquisition phase:

- Conducting session probe at the beginning of the session to determine where therapy should begin (data collected on the progress monitoring form [Form 6.3])
- Minimizing learner errors during practice (e.g., clinician demonstration, cues to say keywords)
- Providing high repetition with intensive massed practice to establish the skill
- Distributing or spacing practice as steps are learned
- Incorporating metacognitive strategies to increase learner engagement (e.g., anticipation of difficult steps, charting own data) and self-awareness

The clinician should have a method to record session data while steps are being taught. Figure 6.4 shows session data taken during Day 3 of therapy for the client described in the previous script. After the client completed the routine through Step 3,

Client: ES			Date: 5/16
Step	Number of Massed Practice Trials and Level of Cueing	Duration and Number of Distributed Practice Trials	Comments
1. Sort			
2. Measure			
3. Dump			
4. Warm		M+++ ++ @ 3 min ++ @ 6 min	Used keywords for 3 min trials only.
5. Medium			
6. Fill and Close			
Summary	Very secure at end of session for completing steps 1–4		
Recommendations for next session	If maintains _____ move to step 6		

Note: + correct; – incorrect; M = model; C = cued

FIGURE 6.4. Sample session data chart for day 3.

the clinician demonstrated Step 4, *selecting the water temperature*. The client practiced Step 4 three times in a row. The clinician then began distributing practice and had the client add Step 4 to the routine, increasing the delay between repetitions. The client was able to complete the routine without errors twice, after a 6-minute distracter task. As illustrated in the script, he maintained knowledge of this step during his session probe at the next session on Day 4. A blank session data form is provided in Form 6.4 in the Appendix (an enlarged version is on the book's page on The Guilford Press website).

What Happens When the Client Makes an Error or Does Not Demonstrate Learning?

If a client is not learning a particular step, it is important to *isolate that step* and provide intensive practice. For example, if the learner described in the laundry routine above made repeated errors on Step 4 when the clinician increased the time between repetitions from 1 to 2 minutes on Day 2, then the clinician would reduce the interval to 1 minute—the last interval at which the client was successful. The clinician also could isolate that step and provide additional massed practice of just turning the knob to warm, and then chaining it back to the routine at either a 1- or 2-minute interval. The following guidelines describe clinician actions when the client demonstrates errors.

- Guideline 1: When an error is demonstrated, interrupt any attempts by the client to "think through" the correct procedure; instead, provide the correct model and ask the client to repeat that step immediately.
- Guideline 2: If the client makes an error during the distributed practice sequence, return to the last time interval at which the client produced a correct response and begin training at that interval.
- Guideline 3: If a particular step is difficult to learn, isolate that step and chain it back to the routine by having the client practice the step multiple times, then having the client complete the preceding step and the troubling step together, and then moving to longer practice intervals.
- Guideline 4: If the client continues to make errors, reconsider the training target. The step may be confusing, too complex, too similar to other steps, or unnatural for the client to produce and may need to be modified.

By the end of each session, the client must have produced more correct responses than errors, or he or she risks learning the error responses rather than the correct procedures. In addition to the information provided in Chapter 5, these guidelines are outlined in the published manual for SR training (Brush & Camp, 1998), which also includes sheets for recording data on practice trials during the session. Additionally, training will emphasize generalization by extending the contexts and task parameters under which the client can perform the target task.

Mastery and Generalization Phase of Training

The next training phase begins when initial learning of the routine has occurred, but may not be consistent or firm. The emphasis at this stage is on mastery or increased fluency—the ability to complete steps in the routine faster and more automatically—and decreasing prompting or cueing. In general, once the client can demonstrate all the steps and accurately perform the probe administered at the start of each session, he or she will be in the mastery and generalization phase. Mastery and generalization of the target routine are accomplished by attending to three variables:

1. *Lengthening the distributed practice.* The clinician increases the interval between successive repetitions of the routine, until the learner can complete the steps independently after a long delay. For example, in traditional SR training (Brush & Camp, 1998), the routine is considered to be mastered if the client can produce it accurately and independently the following day.
2. *Incorporating or increasing stimulus variability.* The basic routine is established in the acquisition phase. During the mastery phase, the client practices initiating the routine under all relevant conditions, to facilitate generalization of learning to the contexts in which the routine will be used. This phase requires the clinician to provide more varied training stimuli and to involve people in the natural environments in the training process. Common factors to consider varying include the

training stimuli, times and events that will trigger the routine, people involved or present for the routine, and locations at which the routine is performed.

3. *Increasing metacognitive engagement.* The clinician identifies methods to enhance learner engagement and awareness and thereby facilitate mastery and generalization. The client is involved in selecting how to modify the target or environment as well as in goal setting and progress monitoring.

Table 6.7 provides examples of the above training components for the client learning to do the laundry routine described in the sample script.

The following is an overview of the components to be included in sessions addressing both initial acquisition and mastery of routines:

- Begin with a session probe (using the Progress Monitoring form [Form 6.3]) to determine retention from previous training.
- Review homework and other data on performance outside of therapy sessions.
- Review learned steps and model new step(s). Provide high amounts of practice with the new step (using the session data form [Form 6.4]).
- Increase the practice interval.
- Review the learned sequence.
- Assign home practice.

Maintenance Phase

As described in Chapter 4, therapy methods used in the maintenance phase are designed to increase the likelihood that a rehabilitation target will be retained beyond the cessation of therapy. A common problem for clinicians is that clients abandon learned routines once they are discharged from rehabilitation. Once a multistep routine has been learned fully, the best method to avoid relapse is to put it to ongoing use. The primary methods

TABLE 6.7. Examples of Training Elements That May Be Introduced in the Mastery Phase of Instruction for Sample Client Learning Laundry Routine

Lengthening distributed practice	Increasing stimulus variability[a]	Increasing metacognitive engagement
Clinician doubles the time between "Show me how you sort" and "Do the laundry" each time the client is correct, up to a 30-minute interval.	Invite different people (e.g., spouse, aide) to come into session and say, "OK, it's time to do the laundry." Different clothes are used for the practice sorting. Materials (soap, clothes basket) are put in different positions and places, so the client has to actively search for them and therefore be clear what step he is completing. Noise introduced (TV, phone, tape of traffic noise) to simulate the distracters in the home environment.	Client begins to time himself and tracks completion time. Client reflects on performance sheet about what went well. Client sets personal learning goals (e.g., date that he wants to be finished with learning the routine; move to a self-monitoring checklist with no input from therapist or spouse).

[a]The goal was to train this client to use his own laundry machine and not to teach a generalized laundry procedure, so he was trained only with his own machine.

for achieving this sustained application are *incorporating natural supports* and setting up the circumstances for *cumulative review*. The clinician identified natural supports during the planning phase and has considered training relevant people throughout the implementation phase. Training should help these individuals use cues or prompts to elicit the target routines, and to understand the need for repeated errorless practice if the client starts to relapse. The training of care providers in error-control techniques and the use of cueing hierarchies needs to be scheduled into the therapy process. Inviting care providers into the therapy session and demonstrating the techniques can be an efficient training method. Cumulative review, or periodic practice of previously mastered material, can be done either through ongoing training in the clinic or at the client's residence (provided by a care provider). Cumulative review is especially important for maintaining routines that are not practiced on a regular basis. Figure 6.5 shows a home practice log that the spouse of the sample client might use. This log sheet would ideally be designed in collaboration with the client, the spouse, and the therapist. The log data can provide useful information for ongoing problem solving as any new developments or challenges arise. Depending on the service delivery model and the complexity of the routine, follow-up visits or phone support may be provided to review the routine and identify any retraining needs.

PIE: EVALUATING LEARNING OF MULTISTEP ROUTINES

This manual emphasizes the importance of multilevel outcome evaluation. As noted, the planning process results in a long-term outcome goal and initial short-term acquisition objectives. Examples of these are shown at the top of Figure 6.3.

The clinician must measure progress toward the long-term goal and short-term objectives by measuring the *direct effects of instruction*. This is usually a measure of accuracy, fluency, or efficiency in completing the steps. In Chapter 4 these data were referred to as *session data*. In the laundry example, the clinician evaluated therapy progress with a session probe at the beginning of each session using the progress monitoring form (see Figure 6.3). These data allowed the clinician to assess retention of previously taught target steps by measuring the number of steps recalled—as a measure of accuracy—and the total time to complete the laundry routine—as a measure of efficiency. Session data were used to evaluate the client's learning of individual routines during the practice instruction. Figure 6.4 shows data from a therapy session focused on training Step 4. The number of trials and duration of the practice trial were recorded.

A clinician also measures *global effects of therapy*, including generalization, long-term maintenance, and the impact of training. These data are likely to contain measures of client performance in target contexts (accuracy, efficiency, and frequency), level of support needed in specified environments and conditions, and caregivers' reports of functional impact in everyday contexts. In the laundry example, these data were collected using the home log shown in Figure 6.5. In this case, one desired outcome of training was to increase the client's sense of independence and productivity, as measured on a rating scale developed with the client. In addition to the amount of support, the number of steps completed independently and qualitative notes on performance were logged by the spouse. Pre- and postimpact data from the standardized measure of caregiver burden could potentially demonstrate the impact of training, if the spouse reported reduced burden at the conclusion of the training. It is challenging to collect

Date	How laundry was initiated (verbal cue OK)	Number of steps completed independently	Cues or prompts	Issues/solutions	Client self-rating (1–3 scale)?
5/23	"It'd be a good time to do laundry."	7/7	A hint to use the keywords	Slow—talked aloud to keep himself on track.	2 = "I did OK"
5/30	"Can you start the laundry?"	7/7	None needed		2 = "I did OK"
6/6	"Thanks for doing the laundry."	6/7—forgot to put in soap	Soap was put away in cupboard	Will leave soap out on shelf.	1 = "I didn't like needing reminders"
6/13	Left a note	0	Didn't initiate	Seems like he needs someone to directly tell him to get started.	1 = "I didn't like needing reminders"
6/20	"Will you do the laundry?"	7/7	None	Seemed irritated that I came into room to monitor. Probably try to just periodically check.	1 = "I didn't like needing reminders"

FIGURE 6.5. Home log for laundry routine, kept by client's spouse to encourage maintenance and measure impact.

efficacy or control data for multistep routines, given that they are highly structured, domain-specific targets. It may be useful to compare performance on the target routine with performance on other routines that have a similar number of steps and difficulty. For example, a comparison to the laundry task could be the client's independence in cleaning the bathroom—which, like laundry, might be done once or twice per week. The type of outcome data needed to measure progress in therapy and the ultimate impact of intervention must be individualized for each client.

SUPPLEMENTARY EXAMPLES

This section provides additional examples of performance sheets from clients at an assisted living center for adults with ABI. Residents participated in a group where they set up a weekly coffee bar. Group members volunteered for different multistep routines necessary to host the coffee bar and were taught using the procedures outlined in this chapter. Tasks included making coffee, baking, making crafts to sell, and operating the cash register. Residents were matched to each of the target routines and were trained during individual sessions held at the facility. Examples are provided for training two residents on the same task: operating the cash register: The *instructional planning worksheet* shows task analyses for operating the cash register (Figures 6.6 and 6.9); the *initial assessment worksheet* was used to determine where to begin training and identify prompts (Figures 6.7 and 6.10); the *progress monitoring form* was used to measure therapy progress (Figures 6.8 and 6.11); and a *staff log* helped to evaluate and encourage generalization and maintenance (Figures 6.12 and 6.13).

(text resumes on page 139)

Long-Term Goal:	John will independently take money and make change during coffee hour 2 weeks after training completed.

Initial Acquisition Objectives:	John will independently demonstrate all eight "cash machine" steps with 100% accuracy and no cueing for 3 consecutive days during therapy.

(Specify target, approach, objective performance, independence, criterion, and context/conditions.)

Prerequisite Skills:	(1) counting money (bills and change) to be taught prior to initiating routine, and (2) refreshing skills on calculator—especially putting in numerical values for money sums

WHAT will I teach the client to do?

Task Analysis (List Steps)

1. When you start, count existing money in drawer using calculator to add it up
2. Write amount on sheet
3. Say the price for the coffee looking at the menu and put in calculator ("The single espresso is two dollars")
4. Take amount from customer and say amount out loud (e.g., "You gave me a five")
5. Subtract that amount on calculator
6. Give the change on calculator to the client
7. At end of hour total amount in drawer
8. Write on sheet

☑ It is a functional target
☑ It is customized to client
☑ Context/antecedent specified
☑ Progress measurement specified in long-term goal and/or acquisition objectives

Plan to enhance client motivation/engagement:	Client chose this volunteer task and is social, so likes the interaction; saying money amounts aloud helps w/staying on task.

WHEN and HOW will I teach the instructional target?

Therapy Frequency:	3	/ week
Session Duration:	5	min
Therapy Duration:	6	Sessions, Weeks, (Months)

☑ There is opportunity for sufficient practice within sessions
☑ There is opportunity for sufficient practice across sessions

(cont.)

FIGURE 6.6. Sample completed instructional planning worksheet for Client 1.

List materials needed to elicit routine and plan for varying stimuli with sufficient examples:	Bills, coins, calculator, record sheet. Start with only two espresso drinks and two calculations. Increase different amounts given by consumer and then increase different drink options.
What is the plan for progressing from modeling to distributed practice?	Will teach routine in distinct phases before linking together: (1) counting money; (2) making correct change. When steps in each phase can be done with verbal prompting using keywords, will fade verbal prompts and move to distributed practice. When two phases are mastered, will put sequence together.

WHO will help training outside of session?

☑ Support person identified to provide additional practice between sessions

☑ Sufficient variety of people identified to provide stimuli to allow generalization

Describe plan to train support person/people:	Residential staff will attend one therapy session a week. Starting the third week of training; they will make the coffee menu and supply the bills/coins for training in order to invest them in the process.

WHERE will I address this goal?

☑ There is a plan for generalization to different settings

☑ Measures of generalization across settings are incorporated into long-term goal

FIGURE 6.6. *(cont.)*

Initial Assessment		
Client: Client 1		Date:
Target Routine: Taking cash from customers		
Antecedent to Start Routine:		

LIST STEPS	ACCURACY (+/–/cued)	COMMENTS
1. Count money using calculator	–	
2. Write amount on sheet	Cued "Record amount"	Read sheet and figured out where to put sum
3. Say price; input calculator	–	When told to input the amount, he input the correct numbers
4. Say client amount	Cued "Say amount aloud"	
5. Subtact client amount on calculator	Cued "Subtract"	Used calculator correctly
6. Give change	Cued "Give amount on calculator"	
7. At end, total amount in drawer	Cued "Total amount in drawer"	Needed model to get started
8. Write amount on sheet	Cued "Record amount"	

Baseline: 0 / 8

Dynamic Assessment to Establish Cue Hierarchy		
STEPS/ANTECEDENT	TYPE OF PROMPT/CUE	PERFORMANCE EFFECT
Step 1	Point plus verbal cue "Count amount"	Step completed correctly—knows how to count the money and use calculator
Step 3	"How will you remember the price after reading it on the menu?"	"Say it aloud" (primed from previous demonstration)
Step 6	"Coffee costs $1.50; I gave you $2.00. Show me what you do to make sure you give me correct change."	Used calculator
Step 7	"It's the end of the hour. What do you do?"	Guessed wrong
Step 7	Point/keyword	"Count"

(cont.)

FIGURE 6.7. Sample completed initial assessment worksheet for Client 1.

Recommended Cue Hierarchy:	

If he doesn't know step, simple word and pointing provide cue; if he has recognition, can use a specific question cue.

Level I	Point plus keyword
Level II	Keyword
Level III	Specific question cue (ask question, the answer to which is the target step)
Level IV	Opportunity cue (clinician pause; raised eyebrow)

FIGURE 6.7. *(cont.)*

Routine: Client 1

Long-Term Goal: John will independently take money and make change during coffee hour 2 weeks after training completed

Initial Acquisition Short-Term Objective(s): John will independently demonstrate all eight "cash machine" steps with 100% accuracy and no cueing for 3 consecutive days during therapy

Steps	Session Probe Data				
	7/3	7/4	7/5	7/6	7/7
7. Write on sheet	–	–	–	–	–
6. At end of hour, total amount in drawer	–	–	–	–	–
5. Give the change on calculator to the client	–	–	–	–	+
4. Subtract that amount on calculator	+	–	+	+	+
3. Take amount from customer and say amount out loud (e.g., "You gave me a five")	+	–	+	+	+
2. Say the price for the coffee looking at the menu and put in calculator ("The single espresso is two dollars")	+	+	+	+	+
1. When you start, count existing money in drawer using calculator to add it up	+	+	+	+	+
Completion Time:	Not measuring—just working on recall				
Engagement Strategies:	Looked at list of steps first and circled hard ones				
Generalization Programming during Training:			Played background tape with café noise		
Comments:	Retained training over weekend!	Having an off day— feeling sad	More confident		More confident

Note: Graph the number of steps performed successfully each time the routine is probed.

FIGURE 6.8. Sample completed progress monitoring form for Client 1.

Long-Term Goal:	SR and whiteboard visual organizer will be used to teach Laura to take money and make change during coffee hour. Two weeks after training Laura will complete transactions with no more than two staff cues to look at list for every two customers.

Initial Acquisition Objectives:	Laura will complete cash register procedure in clinic with nonspecific cues to "Look at next step."

(Specify target, approach, objective performance, independence, criterion, and context/conditions.)

Prerequisite Skills:	Counting change backward

WHAT will I teach the client to do?

Task Analysis (List Steps)

1. Put customer money in drawer section labeled "customer"
2. Write customer amount on right column of small whiteboard in front of drawer
3. Write coffee price on left column of small whiteboard in front of drawer
4. Count backward from price to how much customer gave you and give money to client
5. Look customer in eye and say "Thank you."

☑ It is a functional target
☑ It is customized to client
☑ Context/antecedent specified
☑ Progress measurement specified in long-term goal and/or acquisition objectives

Plan to enhance client motivation/engagement: Verbal reinforcement as client completes steps. Have client predict hardest/easiest steps looking at task analysis during training sessions and review progress sheet.

WHEN and HOW will I teach the instructional target?

Therapy Frequency:	3	/ week
Session Duration:	50	min
Therapy Duration:	6	Sessions, Weeks, (Months)

☑ There is opportunity for sufficient practice within sessions
☑ There is opportunity for sufficient practice across sessions

(cont.)

FIGURE 6.9. Sample completed instructional planning worksheet for Client 2.

List materials needed to elicit routine and plan for varying stimuli with sufficient examples:	Money box w/sections labeled; cash, menu, whiteboard with task steps and columns for recording customer amount and coffee price. Start with only one coffee amount and calculations. Increase different amounts given by consumer and then increase different drink options.
What is the plan for progressing from modeling to distributed practice?	Increase time delay and add new step after client can retain step with verbal cue "Look at list" for 3 minutes.

WHO will help training outside of session?

☑ Support person identified to provide additional practice between sessions

☑ Sufficient variety of people identified to provide stimuli to allow generalization

Describe plan to train support person/people:	Residential staff involved in needs assessment and helped develop task analysis and whiteboard format. They will attend two sessions to observe SR technique.

WHERE will I address this goal?

☑ There is a plan for generalization to different settings

☑ Measures of generalization across settings are incorporated into long-term goal

FIGURE 6.9. *(cont.)*

Initial Assessment		
Client: Client 2		Date:
Target Routine: Cash register		
Antecedent to Start Routine: "Pretend you are working the cash register for coffee hour. Here's your materials. Show me what you would do if I ordered a coffee that cost $1.50 and gave you $2.00."		

LIST STEPS	ACCURACY (+/–/cued)	COMMENTS
1. Put customer money in drawer section labeled "customer"	–	Unable to complete any steps without complete verbal instruction and monitoring
2. Write customer amount on right column of small whiteboard in front of drawer	–	
3. Write coffee price on left column of small whiteboard in front of drawer	–	
4. Count backward from price to how much customer gave you and give money to customer	–	
5. Look customer in eye and say thank you.	–	

Baseline: __0__ / __5__

Dynamic Assessment to Establish Cue Hierarchy		
STEPS/ANTECEDENT	TYPE OF PROMPT/CUE	PERFORMANCE EFFECT
Step 1	Verbal instruction plus modeling	Step completed correctly
Step 2	How will you remember the amount the customer gave you?	"I could find a piece of paper?"
Step 2	"Show me how could you use this whiteboard to help you remember that I gave you $2 for the coffee?"	Wrote whole sentence "She gave me $2 for coffee"
Step 2	Model ... then "You try it"	Did it correctly

Recommended Cue Hierarchy:		
(Will need modeling and instruction before being able to fade cueing)		
Level I	Model plus verbal instruction	
Level II	Model only	
Level III	Verbal instruction	
Level IV	keyword	

FIGURE 6.10. Sample completed initial assessment worksheet for Client 2.

Routine: Taking cash from customer

Long-Term Goal: SR and whiteboard visual organizer will be used to teach Laura to take money and make change during coffee hour. Two weeks after training Laura will complete transactions with no more than two staff cues to look at list for every two customers

Initial Acquisition Short-Term Objective(s): Laura will complete cash register procedure in clinic with nonspecific cues to "look at next step"

Steps	Session Probe Data				
	8/23	8/24	8/25	8/26	8/27
5. Look customer in eye and say thank you	−	−	−	C model	C keyword
4. Give money to client	−	C model	+	+	+
3. Count backward from price to how much customer gave you	C model	C keyword	+	+	+
2. Write coffee price on left column of small whiteboard in front of drawer	+	+	+	+	+
1. Put customer money in drawer section labeled "customer"	+	+	+	+	+
Completion Time:	NA	NA	8 min	7'50"	7'
Engagement Strategies:	I role-played being "customer" she knew at residence, which she thought was fun				
Generalization Programming during Training:	Before I started, I had her "visualize coffee bar with customer line"		Brought in other residents to help role play		
Comments: C = cued		"Oh, yeah" when given keyword	Seems to really like learning task		

Note: Graph the number of steps performed successfully each time the routine is probed.

FIGURE 6.11. Sample completed progress monitoring form for Client 2.

Date	Staff initial	Performance log	Comments
6/10	AT	Helped four customers and remembered the steps for all of them. Got confused once, but customer retold him the price of the coffee and he fixed the error.	
6/18	MF	Helped five customers. Needed a reminder the first time through, so got out old checklist with steps and then after the first customer he was independent.	Might be good to have steps listed and have him review at the beginning of each time, especially if it's been a few days.

FIGURE 6.12. Staff log showing maintenance and generalization data for Client 1.

Date	Staff initial	# customers	# prompts to look at list	Comments
Monday	OS	4	3	With practice, feel she will become more independent
Wednesday	ES	4	2	
Friday	ST	3	3	
Monday	OS	4	2	
Wednesday	ES	2	2	Made the task list in red pen, and he looked at it more independently

FIGURE 6.13. Staff log showing maintenance and generalization data for Client 2.

Client 1 sustained a brain injury 4 years prior to intervention in a motor vehicle accident. He had worked in retail and had some preserved knowledge about handling money. He had mild impairments in attention and executive functions and moderate impairments in memory, particularly new declarative learning. Training materials with performance data for Client 1 are shown in Figures 6.6–6.8 and Figure 6.12. Client 2 had a middle cerebral artery stroke 3 years prior to intervention, with severe residual cognitive impairments most notably in executive functions and working memory. Interview with family members revealed relatively preserved procedural memory for automatic sequences. The routines for Client 2 involved more prompting and more environmental supports to accommodate the severity of her impairments. Most significant was her inability to hold on to information when performing an activity; therefore her supports included a way to record needed information during the transaction. Training materials with performance data for Client 2 are shown in Figures 6.9–6.11 and Figure 6.13. Customization and specificity of routines are evident when comparing the two clients' routines. The first client was able to use a calculator, whereas the second client required steps to be listed and a graphic organizer to help her record the information as needed.

SUMMARY

This chapter applied the PIE framework training components to teaching individuals with significant cognitive impairments to complete functional multistep routines. The *planning* process emphasizes task analysis, in which the clinician deconstructs the target routine into a series of sequential steps, with careful consideration of the client profile, environment, and relevant task conditions. The *implementation* process begins with an initial assessment to determine baseline performance and identify a prompting hierarchy. The *intervention* phase begins with consideration of instruction practices that are important to the initial acquisition phase of treatment. At this stage, the clinician provides (1) high levels of correct practice, minimizing errors, with (2) sufficient repetition of the steps while (3) chaining the steps together as they are learned—all are critical to laying down the steps. Learner engagement is facilitated by using collaborative goal setting and involving the client in progress monitoring. As the learner progresses to mastery, the clinician increases stimulus variability, lengthens intervals between practice repetitions of the target, and incorporates more metacognitive, client-directed activities into the training. In the maintenance phase, the clinician works to incorporate natural supports to enhance generalization and long-term retention of the routine. The steps in this process are summarized in Figure 6.14.

APPLICATION EXERCISES

1. Look at the sample multistep routines listed in Table 6.1. Select one that you might teach in your practice, or generate your own routine in a relevant functional domain. Write the task analysis or steps for the routine on a blank initial assessment worksheet. Create a client profile, then generate hypothetical assessment data and fill in the form for that client.

2. Using the sample wording in Table 6.4, generate two different long-term therapy goals for the routine you selected in the first exercise (a) for a patient with severe memory impairments who will be living in a supported environment; and (b) for a patient who currently is living alone or will be discharged to an independent living situation.

3. Using the sample data shown in the progress monitoring form in Figure 6.3, rewrite the data for the session on 5/18, showing no retention of information learned during the 5/17 session. Generate a session data sheet based on the new probe data you just generated for 5/18. The session data sheet should show the step you created, the results from massed and distributed practice trials, and any cueing or prompting you provided.

4. Generate two examples for measuring generalization and maintenance of the target routine.

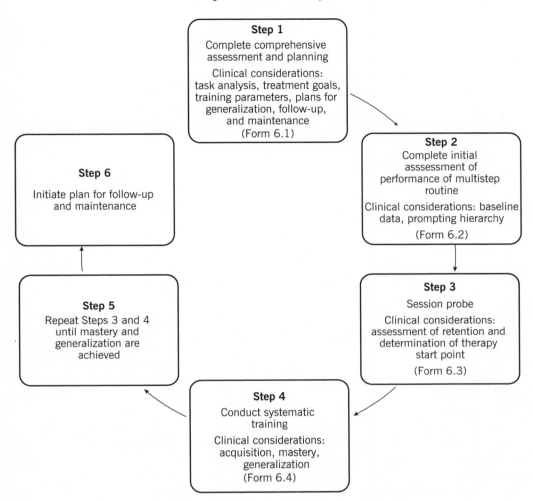

FIGURE 6.14. Illustration of training sequence.

CHAPTER 7

Training the Use of External Cognitive Aids

External cognitive aids provide people with cognitive impairments a method for carrying out desired or intended actions. These tools or devices compensate for cognitive impairments by either limiting demands on a person's impaired ability or by modifying the task or environment to match the client's abilities. The purpose of an external aid is to reinforce a person's residual abilities, substitute alternative methods for activity completion, or provide external support to complete a desired task (LoPresti, Mihailidis, & Kirsch, 2004).

The benefits of external cognitive aids are self-evident. They can support the completion of functional activities in naturalistic settings. Further, they can reduce caregiver burden and stress by helping individuals with cognitive impairment function more independently. A less-obvious benefit from the use of technological aids is that they can decrease the "digital divide" for clients with cognitive impairments, who have often been denied the advantages provided by technology (Sohlberg et al., 2005).

A number of different labels have been used to refer to external aids, including *cognitive orthoses*, *cognitive prosthetics*, and *assistive technology* (Cole, 1999; Kirsch, Levine, Fallon-Kreuger, & Jaros, 1987). More recently, the term *assistive technology for cognition* (ATC; LoPresti et al., 2004) has been adopted as a collective term to describe the range of aids that has been developed to address the needs of individuals with information-processing impairments.

Although some researchers in ATC limit their definition of cognitive prosthetics to tools that use computer technology and are specifically designed to help people compensate for cognitive impairments, this chapter uses the term to refer to a wide range of tools that includes low-tech and mainstream devices as well as specialized technology. That said, the increasing use of technology to help individuals compensate for cognitive impairments is one of the most notable advances in neuropsychological rehabilitation in recent years (Wilson, 2009). Despite the rehabilitative potential afforded by technological devices, however, and the growing number of affordable, accessible devices, clinicians do not implement them as often as one might expect, in part because many clinicians are uncomfortable or inexperienced with technology (Hart, Buchhofer, &

Vaccaro, 2004). Clinicians treating patients with cognitive impairments have a responsibility to reverse this trend and become familiar with the range of technology potentially useful to their patients.

An additional barrier to effective use of cognitive aids is the lack of systematic training provided to clients to teach device use. As discussed in the section on Research Support, the lack of details about training methods is a major gap in the research literature. Furthermore, clinicians, clients, and other stakeholders commonly report that aids are forgotten at home and generally not used in everyday life. This chapter aims to bridge this gap by reviewing instructional methods to train the use of external aids that help people with cognitive impairments function more independently. Although we focus on tools used to help manage deficits in attention, memory, and executive functions, we recognize that people with cognitive disabilities often have other limitations, including impairments in physical functions (e.g., reduced fine motor control and speech intelligibility), sensory abilities (visual, auditory, or tactile), language (reading, writing), and psychosocial functions (e.g., depression). This chapter does not cover the use of devices that address these other impairment areas; however, the principles and procedures for device selection and instruction are broadly applicable. For example, clinicians supporting the use of augmentative and alternative communication devices or training the use of environmental controls may be able to adapt the assessment and training sequences in this chapter for these applications.

The heterogeneity of cognitive impairments and accompanying limitations among individuals with ABI necessitates an individualized aid selection process. The P or planning phase of the PIE framework encourages careful attention to the range of domains that comprises an individual's user profile when considering appropriate options for devices. For example, certain devices may require adequate fine motor control to press buttons, sufficient motivation and executive functions to initiate device use, and sufficient visual acuity to read text displays. Features of a device that make it more "user-friendly" for one group may make it less so for another (LoPresti et al., 2004); hence clinicians need to implement a careful needs assessment.

TYPES OF EXTERNAL COGNITIVE AIDS

The most important predictor of successful long-term external aid use is careful selection. The aid needs to be well matched to the user and the environment. Hence, the process of selecting an aid is a critical clinical skill and begins with a clinician's becoming familiar with the range of assistive options with which to help clients compensate for their impairments.

The assistive technology literature describes a wide variety of aids, ranging from highly technical devices that compensate for cognitive impairments across environments and task domains, to low-technology tools designed for single task guidance. Figure 7.1 summarizes five key characteristics that can be used to discriminate among different aids: device complexity, target task, area of cognitive compensation, target population, and availability. *Device complexity* primarily refers to the cognitive demands involved in using a device. High-tech devices that require more steps and more technical knowledge would be considered to have greater complexity. An example of a complex device would be the iPhone manufactured by Apple. It requires some familiarity with Macin-

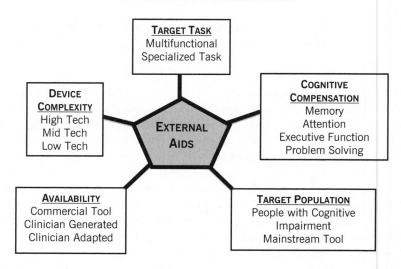

FIGURE 7.1. Key characteristics of external aids.

tosh computer interfaces or training to use this type of interface, although applications have been developed for use by individuals with cognitive and communication impairments (e.g., Locabulary, a communication application downloadable from iTunes). The nature of the *target task* is another important feature that defines an external aid. Tools may be multifunctional and designed to be used across tasks and contexts, or they may have one specific purpose. For example, an electronic calendar system in a personal digital assistant (PDA) or smart phone may be used for scheduling appointments, keeping a "to-do" list, and recording medication schedules. By contrast, a key-finder tool could be used solely for a specialized location task. Table 7.1 lists a range of tools categorized by complexity and target task.

Tools might also be selected based on the *type of cognitive impairment for which they compensate*. For example, an hourly watch chime can be used as an orientation/alerting signal for someone with an attention deficit, whereas a person with a prospective memory impairment would use an appointment reminder. Many tools assist with a variety of cognitive impairments. The *target population* for which a tool is designed is also a key feature. Some tools, such as the specialized task guidance systems listed in Table 7.1, are designed specifically for people with cognitive impairments, whereas other tools, such as cell phones, are designed as mainstream aids. As such, some aids may be commercially available at conventional stores, whereas others may need to be ordered from a manufacturer. Commercially available aids may also be adapted by a clinician to make them more usable; for example, the clinician may write simplified instructions for using a PDA or cover buttons that won't be used by, or are too complex for, a particular client. A few sophisticated high-tech aids are designed to be flexible in this regard (e.g., the Planning and Execution Assistant and Trainer [PEAT] available at *www.brainaid.com*), allowing users progressively more control and access as their cognitive skills improve. Alternatively, clinicians may generate a tool that matches a client and the target task. For example, the clinician and client might collaborate to develop a specialized checklist linked with an alarm.

TABLE 7.1. Examples of Tools Categorized by Complexity and Type of Target Task

Low-tech/specific task

- Calculator
- Phone dialer
- Electronic speller, thesaurus, dictionary
- Watch/clock
- Key finder
- Mail sorter baskets
- Financial planner
- Posted instructions on appliance (e.g., operating instructions for washer) or vocational activity (e.g., filing instructions)

- Pill box reminder
- Alarm clock
- Oven timer
- Labeler
- Color coding files, instructions, baskets
- Map; posted directional signs

Mid-tech/specific task

- Camera

High-tech/specific task

- Specialized or adapted software programs to facilitate writing (SeeWord), reading (e.g., *www.kurzweiledu.com*), e-mail (e.g., *www.coglink.com*)
- Global positioning system

Low-tech/multifunction

- Post-it notes
- Checklists
- Appointment calendars
- Car memo pads

- Voice mail
- Answering machine
- Watch beeps

Mid-tech/multifunction

- Data watches (e.g., Timex data watch; Fossil Wrist Palm, Casio Databank)
- Voice recorder/digital recorder
- Cell phone
- Pagers

High-tech/multifunction

- Smart phone (e.g., iPhone; Blackberry)
- Specialized task guidance systems (Planning and Executive Assistant and Trainer—PEAT; ISAAC, Pocket Coach)

- Personal digital assistants (PDAs)

Table 7.2 provides examples of external aids that have demonstrated utility for individuals with ABI. The domains of complexity, type of task, target population, and availability are listed for each aid. With the electronic and digital revolution, options for external aids are vast and proliferating. The clinician's challenge is to keep current on the range of options and be familiar with the characteristics of useful external aids.

RESEARCH SUPPORT

A large body of literature supports the efficacy and effectiveness of external aids for improving independence and life participation for people with cognitive impairments. A review of the literature in assistive technology for cognition spanning 20 years concluded that technological solutions are available and can be effective in helping people with ABI participate in many activities that would not otherwise be possible

TABLE 7.2. Examples of Assistive Tools Used to Compensate for Different Types of Cognitive Impairments

Cognitive impairment	Common behavioral manifestation	External aid option	Description of aid
Memory domain: *decreased recall*	Unable to access desired verbal or visual information	Voice recorder (Van den Broek et al., 2000)	Mid-tech, multifunction, commercially available, mainstream design
Memory domain: *decreased prospective memory*	Inability to initiate intended actions at target time	Alphanumeric pager (Wilson et al., 2001)	Mid-tech, multifunction, commercially available, mainstream design
Memory domain: *multiple processes (prospective and retrospective memory)*	Forgetting to make phone calls, arrive at appointments	Commercial smart phone (Svoboda et al., 2009)	Mid-tech, multifunction, commercially available, mainstream design
Attention domain: *decreased sustained attention*	Poor task persistence; increasing errors over time	Task guidance system (LoPresti et al., 2008)	High-tech, multifunction, commercial, designed for CI population
Attention domain: *decreased selective attention*	Difficulty focusing when distractions present; poor performance at school or work	Use of desk screen (Sohlberg & Mateer, 2001b)	Low-tech, specialized task, clinician adapted, designed CI population
Attention domain: *alternating attention*	Unable to switch between tasks or find place when interrupted	Checklist paired with alarm (Sohlberg & Mateer, 2001b)	Low-tech, multifunction, clinician generated, developed for person with CI
Executive function domain: *decreased initiation*	Does not begin goal activities	Reminder card with self-monitoring checklist (Sohlberg, Sprunk, & Metzelaar, 1988)	Low-tech, specialized task, clinician generated, developed for person with CI
Executive function domain: *decreased organization*	Begins multiple tasks without finishing	PDA (Gentry et al., 2008)	Mid-tech, multifunction, commercially available, mainstream design
Executive function domain: *decreased self-regulation*	Acts before thinking, resulting in performance errors	Use of a posted "stop sign" in work space (Sohlberg & Mateer, 2001b)	Low-tech, specialized task, clinician generated, developed for person with CI
Problem-solving domain: *decreased sequential processing*	Unable to carry out multistep tasks	Memory notebook with task sequences (Donaghy & Williams, 1998)	Low-tech, multifunction, clinician adapted, developed for person with CI
Problem-solving domain: *decreased reasoning*	Poor repair and strategy generation, resulting in difficulty completing task after making error or dealing with novel situation	Planning and Execution Assistant and Training System (PEAT; Levinson, 1997)	High-tech, multifunction, commercial, designed for CI population

Note. CI = cognitive impairment; PDA = personal digital assistant.

(LoPresti et al., 2004). A practice guidelines paper synthesized the findings from 21 studies containing a total of 270 participants and concluded that training the use of external aids should be a practice standard in ABI (Sohlberg et al., 2007). The authors noted, however, that although the basic outcome question "Are external aids helpful?" can be answered affirmatively, critical questions related to candidacy, device selection, user evaluation, and specific training protocols have yet to be answered.

A recent study illustrates the need for careful planning and systematic instruction to train people with acquired cognitive impairments to use external aids (Bowman et al., 2010). Fourteen patients with ABI received training from an occupational therapist to learn how to use electronic memory aids (e.g., a computerized daily schedule; reminders to check the stove and doors) while living in a training apartment for 5 days. During the first day, patients received up to 3 hours of standard introduction on using the aids. For the second and third days patients received training, as needed, based on their learning. Training ranged from 1 to 3 hours per day and used errorless techniques to show sequences of steps to use the aids, with scripted instructions to ensure clarity. The level of reminders and cueing was adjusted according to each participant's learning ability. Results showed that three participants were able to learn to use the aids independently in the time frame, eight advanced in their learning and required fewer reminders, and three were unable to learn to use the aids. The authors interpreted their findings as support for the use of systematic instruction, including error control during the acquisition phase, recognizing that for some patients training will need to be even more individualized and allow more time and support during the learning process. The authors also noted the importance of patient motivation and of choosing devices that meet patients' needs.

While there continues to be a need for research on factors that contribute to ease of device adoption and methods to promote generalization and maintenance, the existing literature suggests the following general predictors of successful aid use (Wilson, 2009):

- *Age.* Younger people tend to compensate better.
- *Severity of impairment.* People with very severe impairments tend to compensate less well.
- *Specificity of deficit.* Those with focal deficits appear to compensate more successfully than those with widespread cognitive impairments.
- *Premorbid use of strategies.* People who used compensatory aids premorbidly appear to compensate better after ABI.

Clinicians must be mindful of factors influencing candidacy for aid use, and they must be systematic in their needs assessments, their training of device use, and in their measurement of use and impact. The remainder of this chapter describes methods to promote effective practices in these areas.

PIE: PLANNING TRAINING FOR EXTERNAL COGNITIVE AIDS

As reviewed in detail in previous chapters, the planning portion of the PIE framework encompasses four considerations:

1. Identifying key learner characteristics (Who?)
2. Selecting the treatment target (What? Where? When?)
3. Specifying the desired outcomes (Why?)
4. Designing the individualized plan

Established assessment protocols in the assistive technology field address the first three considerations and lead to the fourth, development of the training plan. Typically, these protocols are part of a needs assessment that matches an individual to an appropriate device or technology. Central to all models of ATC selection is the concept that selection of a device or tool must be a team-based decision that includes the user's preferences and takes into consideration contextual factors that are likely to contribute to ultimate success. Below we review four different protocols designed to facilitate selection of a device that matches the abilities, needs, and environment of the device user.

External Aids Needs Assessment

Matching Person and Technology Assessment

Perhaps the most comprehensive and formalized tool currently available for facilitating device selection is the Matching Person and Technology assessment (MPT; Scherer et al., 2007). The MPT is commercially available and consists of a collection of forms designed to facilitate clinical recommendations for assistive technology. The goal is to identify a tool *for a specific user, for a specific purpose, in a specific environment*. The MPT assessment framework is a collaborative process beginning with consideration of technology relevance (e.g., the client's needs, preferences, and history), moving to specific technology and person matching, and concluding with follow-up and assessment of the "match quality" after the client has implemented the recommended technology. The client can complete the forms or a clinician can use them as interview guides.

The MPT assesses limitations, strengths, goals, and potential interventions relevant to (1) body functions (speech/communication, mobility, dexterity, seeing, hearing, reading/writing), and (2) activities (household, health maintenance, recreation/leisure, self-care, employment, thinking/understanding/remembering). Within these areas, it surveys the client's history of support and technology use and current perspectives on technologies. A critical part of the assessment process is psychosocial questions related to areas such as self-determination, personal view of capabilities, motivation, and reliance on the therapist for tool use. A quick screen can be completed in 15 minutes, and comprehensive assessment can be completed in 45 minutes.

Compensation Techniques Inventory

The Compensation Techniques Inventory (CTI; Appendix 7.1; an enlarged version, Form 7.1, is on The Guilford Press website) is a survey instrument used in Sohlberg's clinic that is designed to efficiently collect information in order to establish (1) primary areas of need, (2) past successes or challenges with using strategies/devices, and (3) current strategy use. It is an elaboration of the Compensation Techniques Questionnaire developed at the Mayo Clinic. A strength of the CTI is that it facilitates a systematic review of usage for a range of scheduling tools and their subfunctions to determine if the client can independently use a scheduling aid (e.g., entering scheduled events, entering "things to do," referring to entries, setting alarm, checking off entries, and rescheduling when needed). This gives the CTI an advantage over many protocols, which typically ask about device use in a unitary fashion rather than delineating the different functions and subfunctions that comprise the domain the device is designed to help.

The CTI can be completed independently or as part of an interview during a needs assessment. It helps the clinician survey device use and thus select tools that will both build on familiar or previously successful device use and also establish a baseline frequency of occurrence for cognitive problems for which the device can compensate. It assumes that the clinician will have information about the client's cognitive, physical, sensory, and psychosocial functioning. It also assumes that the clinician will investigate the client's preferences and environmental supports.

Needs Assessment for Selection of External Aids

The Needs Assessment (NA) protocol (Sohlberg & Mateer, 2001b; see Appendix 7.2) is an interview guide designed to help the clinician conduct a comprehensive needs assessment in order to identify the external aid most likely to be adopted. This protocol facilitates the collection of information in three broad areas: (1) organic factors (cognitive/learning profile and physical profiles); (2) personal factors (spontaneous use of personal preference for compensation strategies; self-awareness, acceptance of disability, and goals); and (3) situational factors (financial resources, available support, context for using the device).

TechMatch

The TechMatch website (*www.coglink.com/techmatch*; see Appendix 7.3) contains a computer survey designed to help clinicians and care providers match people with cognitive impairments to computer tools that will help them perform desired activities. The care provider completes a survey, in collaboration with the client, and the program generates a response profile and algorithms that lead to technology recommendations. The survey shown in Appendix 7.3 asks questions related to device use in five domains: (1) technology (experience, interest, abilities), (2) environment (public computing options, available assistance, transportation needs), (3) user needs (motoric, reading, writing), (4) cognitive ability, and (5) personal situation (financial, attitudinal). The TechMatch assessment is limited, however, as it evaluates client usage for a restricted range of technology options: a desktop computer, laptop, netbook, PACK drive (portable adapted computer key—a USB drive loaded with specialized programs that can be used in public computers), and cell phone (smart phone). The survey responses can be summarized in a report that a clinician can use to request insurance or other funding for a device.

A review of available assessment protocols reveals the wide range of factors that needs to be considered when matching a client to a tool. Table 7.3 summarizes the primary factors. It is important to recognize that no single instrument or interview will identify *the* right tool. The clinician will need to integrate information from different sources and creatively anticipate what functions the tool will need to serve. In other words, the needs assessment should not only facilitate a good match for a tool, but it should define *how* the tool will meet the identified needs of the client. Usually the clini-

TABLE 7.3. Summary of Critical Factors to Consider in Needs Assessment

Assessment domain	Instrument(s) addressing this area	Options for obtaining information
Client cognitive/learning profile	MPT, CQI, NA, TechMatch	Neuropsychological testing; collaborative interview (including corroborative source)
Physical abilities related to device usage	MPT, NA, TechMatch	Occupational and/or physical therapy assessment; collaborative interview
Goal/target activities	MPT, CQI, NA, TechMatch	Collaborative interview
History of tool use	MPT, CQI, NA, TechMatch	Collaborative interview
Preferences for tools	MPT, CQI, NA, TechMatch	Collaborative interview
Client resources (e.g., financial)	MPT, NA, TechMatch	Collaborative interview
Client awareness/motivation	MPT, NA	Neuropsychological testing; collaborative interview
Client self-determination/expectation	MPT	Neuropsychological testing; collaborative interview
Environmental supports	MPT, CQI, NA, TechMatch	Home observation; collaborative interview
Consideration of specific devices	CQI, TechMatch	Collaborative interview (helpful to have sample tools to demonstrate)

Note. CTI, Compensation Techniques Inventory; MPT, Matching Person and Technology; NA, Needs Assessment.

cian and client need to make decisions or engage in problem solving beyond the initial assessment. This need is illustrated by the following clinical examples:

- The assessment results suggest that a client will need an alarm function. The clinician must consider what interval(s) need to be available (e.g., hourly, pre-alarm warning, annual setting, repeated alarms). Not all devices have variable alarm functions; hence this function needs to be incorporated into the selection process.
- The assessment process suggests that a client needs a salient prompt to compensate for an impairment in initiation. The client might benefit from distinctive ring tones for specific callers or custom alarms that can serve an alerting function.
- The assessment process has led to the selection of a portable global positioning system (GPS) that the client can use for community transportation; it also has identified declarative memory impairment as a primary challenge. The clinician will need to think through how to remind the client to recharge the GPS system, since these tools quickly drain battery power and the client may not remember to recharge it without a reminder.
- The assessment process suggests that a voice-messaging system would be a preferred scheduling tool given a client's limited writing ability. The clinician should

anticipate how the client will archive or delete old messages, because that consideration may affect which model of voice recorder is selected.

The need to match a user to a device via a comprehensive assessment process is emphasized in the ATC literature and in clinical practice. It is also important to recognize that the alignment of each client's needs and abilities with device features *changes over time*, not only at critical transition points (e.g., discharge from hospital to home or from rehabilitation to community living, beginning new employment, returning to school), but also with ongoing changes such as developmental improvements in executive functions and improvements in awareness or acceptance of disability. One of the biggest challenges is that these transitions are typically accompanied by a change in service providers, and new providers will have to be explicitly trained to support ATC use. Anticipating these junctures is important in the selection process.

In summary, the burden is on the clinician to (1) synthesize the information from the needs assessment, (2) be knowledgeable about options for external aids (including methods to adapt or generate custom tools), and (3) anticipate how the aid can be adapted to meet currently identified needs as well as anticipated future needs.

Designing the Individualized Plan

After conducting the needs assessment, the clinician will have gathered the information necessary to design an individualized training plan, including a specific tool, goal, and context. The next step is to construct a task analysis for teaching the steps to use a device, with consideration of contextual variables that may support or impede this use. From the very beginning of the planning process, the clinician must consider how to evaluate impact of the device. Sometimes a client may be successfully taught to use a device, but the tool does not have the desired influence on everyday functioning. Data evaluating effectiveness are necessary so that the therapy plan can be adjusted as needed.

The instructional planning worksheet shown in Form 7.2 in the Appendix (an enlarged version is on the book's page on The Guilford Press website) and Figure 7.2 (completed example) will facilitate planning of device training, promoting generalized use, and achieving the desired impact. The instructional planning worksheets reviewed in Chapters 4, 6, and 8 are customized in this chapter for the training of external aids. The table in the top portion of the planning sheet can be used to specify prerequisite skills. Sometimes the goal is for the client to use all components of a particular device function, whereas other times it may be that the client only uses one component. For example, someone other than the client might enter information on the client's calendar system, and the client learns only to check and carry out what is listed in each entry.

In the completed client example shown in Figure 7.2, a training plan is outlined to teach a client, Maria, to use the scheduling function in her cell phone. Maria, a 62-year-old woman who had a right CVA, went through initial inpatient rehabilitation and then transitioned home. She was receiving weekly outpatient speech and occupational therapy. The following key factors were identified in the needs assessment that led to the selection of the particular aid and the generation of Maria's individual training plan:

External Aid: _Schedule function on cell phone_

Primary Function	Requisite Skills	Impact/Goal	
		Short-term	Long-term
Make and follow scheduled agenda	• Enter events on calendar • Set alarm • Complete activities with alarm prompt • Check off completed events	Maria will respond to alarmed activities and initiate them as indicated	Maria will independently set and follow daily schedule

Long-Term Goal: _Maria will independently enter daily agenda from morning planning with her husband into her phone calendar and initiate and complete 90% of alarmed events for 1 week_

Initial Acquisition Objectives: _Maria will independently demonstrate steps for entering events and alarms in phone calendar in clinic for two to three trials with 10-minute delay_

(Specify target, approach, objective performance, independence, criterion, and context/conditions.)

WHAT will I teach the client to do? (Use of Tool)

Task Analysis (List Steps)

1. _Locate calendar screen when given agenda_
2. _Identify correct date and time_
3. _Enter event from planning agenda_
4. _Locate alarm screen_
5. _Select correct alarm options_

6. _Take phone out of purse when alarm goes off_
7. _Turn off alarm_
8. _Initiate activity (pantomime in clinic)_
9. _Type "X" next to activity_

☑ Plan is customized to client

☑ Context/antecedent specified

☑ Progress measurement specified in long-term goal and/or acquisition objectives

Plan to enhance client motivation/engagement: _Initially schedule preferred activities (TV shows, grandchildren calls)_

(cont.)

FIGURE 7.2. Sample completed instructional planning worksheet.

Plan to involve environmental supports:	• Collaborate with husband and Maria to establish mutual daily planning time at home • Husband to attend last 15 minutes of each session

WHEN and HOW will I teach the instructional target?

Therapy Frequency: _____2_____ / week
Session Duration: _____50_____ min
Therapy Duration: _____4_____ Sessions, (Weeks,) Months

☑ There is opportunity for sufficient practice within sessions
☑ There is opportunity for sufficient practice across sessions

List materials needed to practice using tool and plan for varying stimuli with sufficient examples:	Phone; home planning sheet; list of typical events organized by preferred and less preferred; data sheet
What is the plan for progressing from modeling to distributed practice?	High repetition; chaining steps and then insert delay. Steps 6–9 will be practiced first in the clinic with simple tasks in order to establish need for using phone. Then scheduling mechanics in Steps 1–5 will be taught.
WHERE will the tool ultimately be used?	home
WHO will support training and tool use?	husband
Describe context:	Couple will plan day over morning coffee and husband will complete planning sheet during this time. As he tidies up, Maria will transfer information to phone. Daily events will be carried out at home or in walking distance to house.
Describe plan to train support people:	Husband will participate in the last 15 minutes of treatment to collaborate on training plan.

FIGURE 7.2. *(cont.)*

• *Client's primary need*: The priority for Maria and her husband was for Maria to be able to stay alone at home and initiate productive activity. Her husband was concerned that she would sit and watch television the entire time he was at work.

• *Client's history of aid use*: Premorbidly, Maria used a paper-and-pencil planner that she brought with her to therapy. She had a well-developed sense of following a timed agenda, suggesting a good foundation for learning to refer to a schedule in her current condition.

• *Key cognitive challenges*: Interview and cognitive testing revealed that impairments in declarative memory, initiation, and awareness were critical considerations for selecting a device and planning therapy. Maria would need a detailed written schedule and a method for marking what she did, to compensate for her memory limitations. Her awareness deficits suggested that a salient auditory prompt might be needed to remind her to check the schedule. Initiation deficits also suggested that she might benefit from a concrete demonstration of the advantage of using her scheduling system. It was thus decided to train the second half of her routine by first training her to acknowledge the alarm and then act on it for preferred activities. Her limitations in insight and awareness suggested that a support person would need to generate the schedule with Maria's input and that she would not be independent in creating the schedule items.

• *Environmental factors*: An interview and home visit revealed that breakfast and morning coffee was a time that was already ritualized in the couple's day and could be utilized for the planning time. The clinician worked with the couple to generate a list of "preferred" activities (e.g., leisure and social activities such as neighborhood walks, family phone conversations, gardening, and tracking the stock market) and household chores that were still well established in her repertoire and that she valued (e.g., vacuuming, dusting, sweeping porches), and these were incorporated into the training plan.

When the clinician takes time to explicitly consider the above factors, the resulting training plan is customized to the client and is more likely to lead to achievement of the desired goals.

PIE: IMPLEMENTING SYSTEMATIC INSTRUCTION FOR THE USE OF EXTERNAL COGNITIVE AIDS

The planning process leads to the selection of an external aid and the generation of a training plan; this section outlines factors important for implementing that training plan. Teaching the use of an external aid is often best conceptualized as two sets of activities: (1) teaching the *mechanics* of using the aid, and (2) organizing the *supports and reinforcements* necessary for the client to use an aid in the *target contexts*. Whereas the planning process ensures that key factors relevant to addressing both sets of activities will have been considered, the initial therapy plan is largely determined by whether a person needs extensive instruction in the implementation or procedures for using the selected tool as a prerequisite to being able to implement the tool in his or her setting. For example, if a client has a significant declarative memory impairment that affects the ability to learn new information, he or she may need very structured, errorless practice using SR to learn procedures related to device use (see SR worksheets in Chapter 5). This type of training follows the procedures outlined in Chapter 6, training the use of multistep routines.

The task analysis for using the external aid is generated on the planning sheet (Form 7.3 in the Appendix; an enlarged version is on the book's page on The Guilford Press website). The clinician then determines whether there is a need for structured training to use the tool *or* whether the client already knows the mechanics for tool use and needs training to establish the habit of using the aid. Figure 7.2 shows that the client, Maria, needs training in both sets of activities. The clinician generated a plan to teach Maria the steps for using her iPhone scheduler *and* to ensure that use was supported and established in her home environment, so that she could achieve her goal of independently following an agenda when her husband was away. Figure 7.3 provides a flowchart emphasizing the notion that different clients will begin the training process with different instructional objectives.

As discussed throughout this text, it is useful to think of instruction for people with cognitive impairments as having three phases: acquisition, mastery/generalization, and maintenance. *Acquisition* refers to the initial phase of laying down a concept, behavior, or procedure; it comprises the processes needed to establish new learning or relearning.

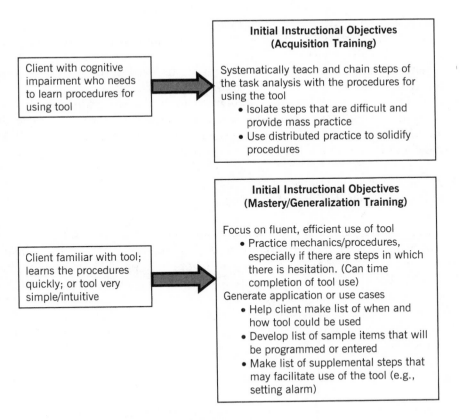

FIGURE 7.3. Initial instructional objectives differ depending on the client profile.

Mastery is the phase in which the client learns to use the tool more fluently. It includes *generalization* training to extend learning to new contexts or tasks. *Maintenance* is the continued use or demonstration of the learning in the target contexts. The following sections describe the procedures used in each phase when training ATC use.

Initial Acquisition Phase of Training

The purpose of therapy at this phase is to establish the motivation and procedures for using the selected external aid. It is critical from the outset to ensure that there is buy-in from the client. Researchers have suggested that a vital predictor of the adoption of ATC and determiner of long-term use is a person's *initial reaction*, including perceptions of the relative advantages or disadvantages of the device in terms of usability and impact on the client's quality of life (Lenker & Paquet, 2004). Hence, a person's introductory experience using the tool is important. If the client has an initial positive experience and sees advantages to using the device, his or her intention to use the device is reinforced.

Five important clinical actions will maximize the likelihood of initial positive experiences and continued use of the ATC:

1. Selection of the tool is based on a comprehensive needs assessment with attention to key contextual and client factors.
2. The selection process is collaborative; the client participated in for choosing and customizing the device.
3. The tool and the procedures for using it are tailored to the individual and his or her environment.
4. Initial training of device use (for clients who need instruction in the procedures) is set up to ensure success: Systematic instruction is used to teach procedures in an efficient manner, tailored to the client's learning strengths and challenges, so the client is able to use the device as quickly as possible.
5. Training examples are relevant to and valued by the client and thus reinforce device use from the outset. The examples help clients to understand the benefits of the tool from the start of training.

The first two training considerations are met during the selection process, as previously reviewed. The next three are ensured by following the systematic instruction process for the acquisition phase reviewed in Chapter 6 (pp. 122–127) and Chapter 8 (pp. 205–208). The decision tree in Figure 5.1 and the SR worksheets, also in Chapter 5, can be used to plan training. A recap within the context of external aids is provided below for clients who need to learn the actual procedures. To illustrate the implementation of the training procedures described in this section, we provide the following three case examples.

Case 1

Tyrone was a 60-year-old male who had an anoxic event when he suffered a heart attack 10 months prior to his ATC assessment. He received intensive inpatient and outpatient cognitive and cardiac rehabilitation. Testing revealed a severe declarative memory impairment: Tyrone was amnesic for daily events. He displayed limited self-awareness and was stimulus bound (i.e., required concrete "here-and-now" instructions and could not think in abstract terms). His procedural memory was intact, and he could learn routines and procedures, although because of his declarative memory impairment he could not recall the learning episode or recall learned content when asked. However, if Tyrone got started on a task, he would continue the task sequence if it was in his premorbid procedural repertoire or had been systematically taught as a new routine. Although easily fatigued, Tyrone had no significant motor or sensory limitations. Prior to his heart attack, Tyrone was an auto mechanic, owner of a repair shop, and avid jazz music enthusiast. Tyrone lived with his wife of 40 years and had two grown children who lived out of state. After Tyrone's hospitalization, the family sold the auto repair shop to Tyrone's brother, Wayne.

The needs assessment revealed that restoring Tyrone's ability to work at the shop was a priority. A goal was established for him to be able to complete inventory tasks while at the shop. His basic data entry skills were intact, and he had retained procedural learning for the basic inventory system. Tyrone indicated that he would enjoy the sense of productivity from completing the daily inventory task.

Case 2

Laurine was a 43-year-old woman who experienced a hemorrhagic stroke that resulted in severe impairments in cognition and swallowing. At the time of her evaluation, she had been moved to inpatient rehabilitation. A neuropsychological evaluation showed severe impairments across cognitive areas, most notably in declarative memory and problem solving. The immediate needs identified by staff were to advance her diet by improving her swallowing and increase her initiation of goal-directed activity. These goals were in preparation for Laurine's transition to a skilled nursing facility in which scheduled events would be listed on wall calendars and posted reminders.

A needs assessment revealed that prior to her illness Laurine had worn a watch with an alarm and used a multifunctional written planner to track both work and home tasks. Although she was compliant when asked to engage in a task and she verbally indicated an interest in following an agenda, she did not initiate tasks and required prompting with task materials in view in order to begin an activity. The staff's priority was to train Laurine to use a reminder system that would cue her to start specific activities, including swallowing exercises. The team designed a data-watch linked to a large wall calendar with agenda items posted. The goal was for Laurine to learn the routine of looking at her watch when she heard the alarm, then using the time cue to find a particular time on the posted agenda, where there would be visual prompts to do her swallowing exercises, fill out a meal request, or press the call button to ask for her medications. The diagram of the swallowing exercise, the meal form, and the call button were all displayed next to the wall agenda.

Case 3

Emma was a 17-year-old senior in high school who had suffered a mild TBI while playing soccer 3 months prior to her assessment. As a result of the injury, Emma experienced attention deficits, intermittent headaches, and cognitive fatigue, all of which interfered with her school performance. She was unable to focus more than 30 minutes without getting a headache. Before her injury, Emma had been an average student and had used a written planner to manage her academic and extracurricular tasks. She carried a cell phone and was adept at using it for calls, texting, and accessing the Internet. Her priorities were to implement a headache management program recommended by her physician and use attention facilitation behaviors that would help her focus on schoolwork. Emma and the clinician decided to program the scheduling function of her cell phone with reminders to engage in her target headache management and attention behaviors on a set schedule. The schedule also cued Emma to text pain and attention ratings to her mother, who would enter them on a data collection sheet to bring to the therapist. This aspect of the program provided needed progress data for the therapist and, at the same time, encouraged Emma to engage in self-monitoring.

Initial Assessment (before the First Training Session)

In most cases, the assessment process begins with a baseline assessment, in which the client is asked to demonstrate how to use the device with the amount of prompting specified in the long-term goal. The clinician should use an initial assessment form listing the steps for using the external aid. Generic forms are shown in Figures 7.4–7.6, or the clinician can design a customized form. The purpose of this evaluation is to obtain baseline performance data and identify any steps the client may already have mastered. The results indicate where therapy should begin. Conducting this evaluation may take only a few minutes, depending on the device and the length of the dynamic assessment.

If the initial assessment reveals that the client is unable to demonstrate the sequence of steps to be used in accessing the device, the clinician might then model an individual step and have the client "show me what you would do next" to determine if he or she knows individual steps. Now the clinician knows if steps can be bundled together and the amount of practice that might be needed. After determining what steps the client does or does not know, the clinician should conduct a dynamic assessment to determine the type of prompting (if any) that should be provided during the training process. Because the clinician will fade prompts as the client acquires the steps, it is important to know what type of prompting is most facilitative.

Figures 7.4–7.6 show examples of completed initial assessment forms for the three case examples: Tyrone, Laurine, and Emma. Tyrone knew how to turn on the computer and access the inventory program, so those two steps were combined into one step for the task analysis. For Laurine, initial assessment revealed that she heard and attended to the watch beep and looked at the text on the watch face, but did not follow the directions stated in the text. Because she would initiate action if the therapist pointed to the text, the plan was to use pointing as a prompt, then fade it once that step became automatic. Emma was independent in using her phone reminder system to initiate her symptom management protocol. She and the therapist had designed the system collaboratively to fit with her school schedule and needs. She did not need help learning the system but would need support to implement it in her everyday life.

(text resumes on page 162)

Initial Assessment		

Client: _Tyrone_   Date: _10/28_

External Aid: _Inventory Task_

Antecedent to Use Aid: _Brother will set up work space with forms, computer, pen, timer, and radio_

LIST STEPS	ACCURACY (+/–/cued)	COMMENTS
1. Set timer for 45 minutes	cued	"How long will you work?"
2. Turn on computer and open parts inventory program	+	
3. Take first customer receipt in stack and put on paper stand	+	
4. Find parts section and enter in number of part on line 1	−	
5. Cross off corresponding parts line with red line when entered	−	
6. Repeat Steps 3 and 4 for all lines with parts listed	−	
7. When all parts on receipt are entered, put receipt in outbox	−	
8. Start with next receipt and repeat Steps 3–7	−	
9. When timer goes off, finish the current receipt and take break, listening to jazz station while you wait for your brother to come review progress and set next goals	−	

Baseline: _2 / 9_

Dynamic Assessment to Establish Cue Hierarchy		
STEPS/ANTECEDENT	TYPE OF PROMPT/CUE	PERFORMANCE EFFECT
"Find parts section"	Direct verbal	+
Point to parts section	Pointing	+ Correct when there was not too much of a delay; otherwise he forgot task
"What do you do first?"	Question cue	+ Turned on computer

Recommended Cue Hierarchy:		

Level I   _Direct verbal cue_

Level II   _Pointing_

Level III _Question cue_

Level IV   _____

FIGURE 7.4. Sample completed initial assessment worksheet for Case 1, Tyrone.

Initial Assessment		

Client: Laurine   Date: 6/4

External Aid: Agenda

Antecedent to Use Aid: Watch beep

LIST STEPS	ACCURACY (+/–/cued)	COMMENTS
1. Notice watch beep	+	
2. Read text on watch	–	With direct verbal cue
3. Walk to wall agenda	–	
4. Look at watch and find corresponding agenda item	–	
5. Find material for agenda item (form, exercise illustration, or call button)	–	
6. Initiate action	–	
7. Press red button on watch	–	
	–	

Baseline: 1 / 9

Dynamic Assessment to Establish Cue Hierarchy		
STEPS/ANTECEDENT	TYPE OF PROMPT/CUE	PERFORMANCE EFFECT
1. Watch beeped	Direct verbal cue "Read text"	+
2. Watch beeped	Pointing to watch	+
3. Watch beeped	Question cue "What next?"	+
4. "Read the text and follow instructions"	Direct verbal cue	+ "Walk to agenda"
5. "Read the text, now what?"	Question cue	– (When pointed to agenda, she walked to it)

Recommended Cue Hierarchy:		

Level I   Direct verbal cue

Level II   Pointing

Level III   Question cue

Level IV

FIGURE 7.5. Sample completed initial assessment worksheet for Case 2, Laurine.

Initial Assessment

Client: Emma   Date: 8/23

External Aid: Phone

Antecedent to Use Aid: Watch chime

LIST STEPS	ACCURACY (+/–/cued)	COMMENTS
1. Press silence when watch chimes	+	
2. Look at schedule screen	+	
3. Initiate breathing and neck/shoulder stretches	+	
4. Text Mom current activity (e.g., listening to lecture; reading) and rating on attention and headache scales	c	Remember to look at "notes"
5. If rating on either scale above 2, take break	+	

Baseline: 4 / 5

Dynamic Assessment to Establish Cue Hierarchy

STEPS/ANTECEDENT	TYPE OF PROMPT/CUE	PERFORMANCE EFFECT

Not necessary

Recommended Cue Hierarchy:

Level I _____

Level II _____

Level III _____

Level IV _____

FIGURE 7.6. Sample completed initial assessment worksheet for Case 3, Emma.

Session Activities

If the initial assessment reveals that the client needs to be taught the procedures for using a device, the clinician moves to the acquisition phase. If the client already knows how to use the device, the clinician moves to the mastery/generalization phase. In our case examples, both Tyrone and Laurine would require training to learn the steps to use their external aids, whereas Emma could move directly to the mastery phase.

To recap: There are three fundamental components of the initial acquisition phase—*minimize the learner's errors, move from a massed to a distributed practice schedule,* and *provide sufficient practice or repetition.* Each session begins with a session probe to determine retention from previous sessions and indicate the step where training in the current session should begin. Note that the session probe differs from the initial assessment. The initial assessment, as described above, is a *one-time* evaluation to identify effective prompts and establish baseline performance, whereas the session probe occurs at the beginning of *every* training session and is an observation of the client's device use without prompting or support. The aim of session probes is to show retention and direct where to start therapy that session. A progress monitoring form (see Form 7.4 in the Appendix; an enlarged version is on the book's page on The Guilford Press website) can be used to track session probe data as an indication of learning over time and to inform the therapist about where to begin training during each session.

Figures 7.7 and 7.8 show progress monitoring forms for Tyrone and Laurine. The data for Tyrone show that he was learning and retaining one to two steps each session. The data for Laurine suggested that she was not initiating the steps with the watch beep and corresponding text after four sessions of practice.

The session probe is followed by a review of steps that were taught in previous sessions and a model of the next step identified in the task analysis, chained to the previous step. Depending on the client's retention, the clinician models the two-step sequence (learned step and new step) and then has the client demonstrate the sequence. The clinician also incorporates strategies to increase client engagement (e.g., prediction of performance, self-recording of performance), as needed. The clinician keeps session data in order to know how to proceed in therapy (see Form 7.5 in the Appendix; an enlarged version is on the book's page on The Guilford Press website).

Figures 7.9 and 7.10 provide examples of session data for Tyrone and Laurine. For Tyrone's session, the clinician was chaining the new Step 5 to the previously learned and retained Step 4. The initial trial was modeled and then cued, using the cueing hierarchy, starting with an explicit verbal cue. The clinician then isolated Step 5 and provided mass practice. One more trial was completed with chaining of Step 5 to Step 4, then the client completed the whole sequence, beginning with Step 1 and using distributed practice at 1-, 5-, and 10-minute intervals. Laurine's training was less successful. Session data showed an attempt to teach Step 2. Laurine could do it with a model, but as soon as the model was withdrawn, she required a direct verbal cue to complete that step. This led the clinician to decide to try a talking watch or voice organizer to determine if auditory speech prompts would be more effective.

(text resumes on page 167)

External Aid: Inventory task

Long-Term Goal: Tyrone will independently work on inventory for 45 minutes in duration completing at least 10 receipts with no more than one error

Initial Acquisition Short-Term Objective(s): With verbal prompts to get started and to continue, Tyrone will be able to independently enter in parts data for three sheets with 100% accuracy in the clinic

Strategy Steps/Component	Session Probe Data				
	11/1	11/2	11/3	11/4	
9. When timer goes off, finish the current receipt and take break, listening to jazz station while you wait for your brother to come review progress and set next goals	–	–	–	–	
8. Start with next receipt and repeat Steps 3–7	–	–	–	–	
7. When all parts on receipt are entered, put receipt in outbox	–	–	–	+	
6. Repeat steps 3 and 4 for all lines with parts listed	–	–	–	+	
5. Cross off corresponding parts line with red line when entered	–	c (point)	+	+	
4. Find parts section and enter in number of part on line 1	+	+	+	+	
3. Take first customer receipt in stack and put on paper stand	+	+	+	+	
2. Turn on computer and open parts inventory program	+	+	+	+	
1. Set timer for 45 minutes	c	c	+	+	
Completion Time:	N/A	N/A	5 min 3 receipts	8 min 6 receipts	
Supports:	• Computer booted to program • Pen and receipts in sight on table • Written cue card to "double-check entries"				
Motivational/Engagement Strategies	• Tyrone keeping track on number of days till he gets to go back to shop to work • Timing self on tasks • Listens to jazz station during breaks				
Generalization Programming:	Use receipts and computer from shop				
Comments:	Need to put timer in view with "45 min" sticker				

Note: Graph the number of steps performed successfully each time the routine is probed.

FIGURE 7.7. Sample completed progress monitoring form for Case 1, Tyrone.

External Aid: Watch and agenda

Long-Term Goal: Laurine will respond to watch beep when no one is in room, look at corresponding agenda item, and complete it at least three times daily for 3 consecutive days

Initial Acquisition Short-Term Objective(s): With therapist pointing to wall agenda, Laurine will read and initiate corresponding item in response to watch beep for three consecutive trials

Strategy Steps/Component	Session Probe Data				
	6/7	6/8	6/9	6/10	
7. Press red button on watch	–	–	–	–	
6. Initiate action	–	–	–	–	
5. Find material for agenda item (form, exercise illustration, or call button)	–	–	–	–	
4. Look at watch and find corresponding agenda item	–	–	–	–	
3. Walk to wall agenda	–	–	–	–	
2. Read text on watch	–	dv	dv	dv	
1. Notice watch beep	⊢——⊢——⊢——⊣				
Completion Time:	N/A	N/A	N/A	N/A	
Supports:	Pointing cues (agenda and materials) Reminded her of goal prior to beginning				
Motivational/Engagement Strategies:	Verbal reinforcement				
Generalization Programming:	Modeled agenda after one in d/c SNF				
Comments: dv—direct verbal prompt				Limited to no retention	

Note: Graph the number of steps performed successfully each time the routine is probed.

FIGURE 7.8. Sample completed progress monitoring form for Case 2, Laurine.

Step	Number of Massed Practice Trials and Level of Cueing	Duration and Number of Distributed Practice Trials	Comments
Client: Tyrone		**Date:** 11/2	
1. Set timer for 45 minutes		1 min 5 min 10 min + + +	
2. Turn on computer and open parts inventory program		+ + +	
3. Take first customer receipt in stack and put on paper stand		+ + +	
4. Find parts section and enter in number of part on line 1	C C + + + +	+ + +	
5. Cross off corresponding parts line with red line when entered	M C + + + + + +	+ + +	
6. Repeat steps 3 and 4 for all lines with parts listed			
Summary	Helped to isolate and provide mass practice Client charted progress data on progress monitoring form, which appeared to be reinforcing		
Recommendations for next session	Step 5 seems firm. If retains 1–5 on session probe tomorrow, move to Step 6		

Note: + correct; − incorrect; M = model; C = cued

FIGURE 7.9. Sample completed session data form for Case 1, Tyrone.

Client: Laurine			Date: 6/10
Step	**Number of Massed Practice Trials and Level of Cueing**	**Duration and Number of Distributed Practice Trials**	**Comments**
1. Notice watch beep	+ + + + + + + + + + +		With model or direct verbal prompt, Laurine reads text. If there is any delay, she does not initiate reading
2. Read text on watch	M M M M M M C M M C M M C		
3. Walk to wall agenda			
4. Look at watch and find corresponding agenda item			
5.			
6.			
Summary	Unable to reduce prompting Initiation deficit very severe		
Recommendations for next session	Abandon text and try with audio-talking watch		

Note: + correct; – incorrect; M = model; C = cued

FIGURE 7.10. Sample completed session data form for Case 2, Laurine.

The following provides an overview of the training sequence:

1. A probe is taken at the beginning of each session and recorded on the progress monitoring form. This session probe tells the clinician where to begin in therapy.
2. Training during the session focuses on:
   - Minimizing learner errors during practice (clinician demonstration, fading of prompts)
   - High rates of repetition with intensive massed practice in the acquisition phase to establish the skill, if needed
   - Chaining newly learned steps with previously learned steps
   - Distributing or spacing practice once the steps are learned
   - Incorporating metacognitive strategies to increase learner engagement (e.g., anticipation of difficult steps, charting own data, reinforcement)

Mastery and Generalization Phase of Training

The phrase *mastery and generalization of training* refers both to strengthening the client's skill in using the external aid and also to broadening the contexts and increasing the independence with which the aid is used. For clients who already know how to use their aids, such as Emma in the above case example, training would start with encouraging generalized use outside of the clinic. Often this involves a combination of counseling, education, and establishing self-monitoring routines.

For clients who need to learn the actual steps or procedures for aid use, illustrated by Tyrone and Laurine in the above case examples, the mastery phase of training begins as soon as the basic steps have been taught. Therapy focuses on increasing the consistency and fluency with which the aid is used, which is accomplished by varying the factors (e.g., practice distribution) and reducing prompts. The client's goal may be to implement the steps faster or more automatically with an increasing level of independence. In a randomized, controlled trial evaluating SR training (Bourgeois et al., 2007), much of the researchers' efforts were devoted to training people to use previously prescribed devices consistently and appropriately. This fluency aspect of training is critical and often not built into therapy programs.

To promote mastery and generalization of external aid use for clients learning the actual steps or mechanics of their device, clinicians need to attend to the following instructional characteristics described in earlier chapters (e.g., see SR worksheets in Chapter 5):

1. *Lengthening the distributed practice.* The clinician increases the interval between practice trials to reinforce independent tool use over increasingly longer periods of time. When the session probe administered at the beginning of the session indicates sufficient fluency with the steps, the clinician can start varying training contexts to promote generalization.
2. *Quickly correcting any errors and providing additional repeated practice on that step or sequence, before fading prompts.* When an error is made, the clinician:

- Interrupts and provides correct practice on that step.
- Returns to the last time interval that resulted in a correct response and begins training at that interval.
- Isolates a step that the client is not performing accurately and provides intensive practice until that step is mastered, then chains it back to the routine (i.e., have the client practice the step multiple times and then complete the preceding step and the difficult-to-learn step together before moving to longer practice intervals).

When clients such as Tyrone and Laurine become more fluent with the basic use of their external aids, therapy will focus more on generalization. Clients such as Emma will begin therapy by working on generalization because they already know how to use their external aids. The following two instructional techniques help to promote generalization.

Introducing Natural Supports and Context Variability into the Training

To encourage use of the external aid in natural contexts, it is important to define everyday antecedents or triggers that prompt the client to employ the aid, and also to use varied training stimuli to promote use in different situations. Examples of these methods include:

- Varying the prompts that alert the need to use the aid
- Involving the support people who will be present in the target environment
- Providing training in the target context

Facilitating Natural Reinforcement for Using the External Aid

For clients to become consistent in their use of assistive tools, they need to have sufficient opportunities and reinforcement. A clinician can assist by:

- *Ensuring that there are opportunities for using the aid.* For example, if a client is using a calendar to track appointments and dates, he or she will need events to schedule and attend so that there are natural consequences to aid use or nonuse. The clinician should check with care providers to ensure that there are such dates to provide the client with practice using the aid. Occasionally, a clinician may need to develop opportunities by scheduling contrived events (e.g., call our office on Tuesday at 3:00 to get the results of our testing"). This type of approach may provide interim practice, keeping in mind that the client's performance in this context will not be the final measure of training success, while community integration activities are being established.

- *Building in reinforcers.* The clinician should identify external or internal cues that will encourage aid use. For example, if a client is learning to use a PDA for tracking "things to do," generalization might be facilitated by scheduling preferred tasks in addition to chores. Involving the client in goal setting to specify how the aid will help achieve desired goals may also reinforce its use. Similarly, tracking the beneficial impact of aid use (e.g., measuring memory successes when using a PDA) will be reinforcing to the client.

The therapy target for our third case example was for Emma to use her cell phone to promote self-monitoring and management of somatic symptoms (headache and fatigue). She was instructed to follow a programmed schedule for breathing and stretching when prompted by her watch chime. She was then to document her current activity, rate the severity of her symptoms, and text this information to her mother. This sequence had been developed collaboratively with Emma, her mother, and the psychologist. A memo was sent from the psychologist to her teachers explaining the plan and asking for permission to have Emma sit near the door and quietly leave for her stretching break if alerted by her watch. Emma's psychologist worked to facilitate generalized use of the strategy by using the following techniques:

- Involving natural supports (Emma's teachers) in the plan. The teachers came up with an idea to have a chair outside the classroom door so that Emma would have a place to sit to do her stretches.
- Reinforcing Emma's initiation of her strategy by having her mother immediately respond to the text with supportive statements.
- Reviewing Emma's self-ratings showing gradual improvement in attention and decrease in headache pain, which showed that her stretching, breathing exercises, and pacing were effective.

Maintenance Phase

Many devices end up in a closet gathering dust. The best insurance against device abandonment has been detailed in the preceding sections: (1) selecting a device that meets the needs of the client, (2) effectively training the use of the device, and (3) setting up ongoing reinforcement and support for device implementation. If it is an option, it may be helpful to increase the time interval between therapy sessions or schedule follow-up visits to promote generalization and make any needed adjustments to the plan for using the device.

Measuring therapy outcomes ultimately requires probes of device use over time. Some clinics or practices have mechanisms for following up with patients to gather such information. One method for encouraging maintenance when there is no funding for follow-up is to provide clients with data charts or feedback surveys that can be mailed back to the clinician, thereby reinforcing use of the device and offering an opportunity to reflect on any needed updates. Figure 7.11 shows an example of a questionnaire that was sent to the client's brother to gather maintenance data for case example 1. The clinician should establish the follow-up system and schedule of visits prior to the client's discharge from therapy. A blank follow-up questionnaire is provided in Form 7.6 in the Appendix (an enlarged version is on the book's page on The Guilford Press website). Encouraging clients and families to provide this maintenance data can support ongoing device use.

Date: _February 9_____

___4_____ week follow-up

Dear _Wayne_____,

This purpose of this letter is to check in and see how _Tyrone's computer invoice system_____
is working. Please use the rating scales to indicate how much help is currently required to use the tool(s) learned
in rehabilitation in comparison to how much you anticipated needing to assist, in addition to rating the frequency
of use. Thank you for completing the information and returning this follow-up letter so that we can track recovery
and outcomes.

Level of Independence	Expected Level of Independence	Frequency of Use	Comments

Independence Rating:

1 = Unable

2 = Lots of help

3 = Occasional help

4 = Reminders only

5 = Independent

Frequency of Use:

0 = Never

1 = One time a week

2 = A few times a week

3 = Most days

Please call _Sarah at 223-4444_____ if you have any questions
or would like reminders about training or would like to schedule a follow-up visit.

FIGURE 7.11. Sample completed follow-up form to collect maintenance data.

PIE: EVALUATING OUTCOMES WHEN TRAINING EXTERNAL COGNITIVE AIDS

Previous chapters in this manual have emphasized the importance of multilevel outcome
evaluation. The clinician will need methods to measure (1) whether the client learns *how
to use* the device, (2) whether the client *initiates using the device in the target contexts*,
and (3) the *effect or impact of using the device*. The first area is an important measurement domain for clients who need acquisition training, such as Tyrone and Laurine.
In these cases, the clinician initially measures progress toward the long-term goal and
short-term objectives by measuring the client's accuracy, fluency, or efficiency in using
the external aid. Data measuring these outcomes are the training data shown in the
progress-monitoring examples in Figures 7.7 and 7.8.

A clinician also should measure use of the external aid in functional contexts as well as determine overall outcome or impact of having learned to use the aid. We can look to the literature evaluating the efficacy of external aids for examples of different types of outcome measurement. The review by Sohlberg et al. (2007) identified seven different outcome measures that were used as dependent variables in research studies:

1. *Frequency of use* (Ownsworth & McFarland, 1999; Schmitter-Edgecombe et al., 1995; Wilson, Emslie, Quirk, & Evans, 2001; Wright et al., 2001; Yasuda et al., 2002). Some external aids display usage data. For example, if a client is being trained to use a medication chart to record time, date, and dose, the clinician can document the number of recordings. Similarly, a clinician may count the number of entries in a diary or journal for a client using this aid for psychosocial or memory goals.

2. *Performance on structured tasks designed to capture the demands of the target function* (van den Broek, Downes, Johnson, Dayus, & Hilton, 2000). A clinician can structure an assessment to determine if the aid is used successfully. For example, to measure outcome of training a client to use the scheduler function in a cell phone, the clinician might set up a probe and give the client different events that would need to be scheduled, and then record whether the client initiated scheduling them and whether they were scheduled accurately. Ideally, the clinician has taken baseline and posttreatment data to evaluate treatment effects.

3. *Retrospective questionnaires assessing performance in the domain facilitated by the external aid* (Donaghy & Williams, 1998; Hart, Hawkey, & Whyte, 2002; Ownsworth & McFarland, 1999; Quemada et al., 2003; Schmitter-Edgecombe et al., 1995; Wilson et al., 2001). The clinician can design or use an existing tool that queries the client on the aspect of everyday functioning with which the target aid was selected to assist. A common example of this type of measurement is the use of everyday memory questionnaires to determine if the frequency of forgetting has decreased with the introduction of an external aid.

4. *Performance on the tasks cued by the aid* (Kim, Burke, Dowds, & George, 1999; Kerns & Thomson, 1998; Kirsch, Levine, Lajiness-O'Neill, & Schnyder, 1992; Kirsch et al., 2004a, Kirsch et al., 2004b; Squires et al., 1996; Wade & Troy, 2001; Wilson, Evans, Emslie, & Malinek, 1997; Wilson et al., 2001; Yasuda et al., 2002; Zencius, Wesolowski, & Burke, 1990). A useful way to measure outcome is to determine whether the client is carrying out the target tasks the aid is designed to prompt. For example, if a client is using a navigation device such as a GPS system, an outcome measurement strategy might be to document the number of trips completed successfully in a 1-week period. Similarly, to measure outcomes for a client learning to use a checklist system for completing vocational tasks, the clinician may ask the client's employer to record the number of tasks completed without cueing.

5. *Ratings of participant preference, satisfaction, or perception of improved performance* (Kim, Burke, Dowds, Boone, & Park, 2000; Ownsworth & McFarland, 1999; Schmitter-Edgecombe et al., 1995; Wilson et al., 2001; Wright et al., 2001). Rating systems can be established to solicit and measure a client's perceptions of factors related to usability and impact.

6. *Anecdotal reports of effectiveness of the aid* (Burke, Danick, Bemis, & Durgin, 1994; Fluharty & Priddy, 1993). Narrative accounts of client use of an aid are often reported as outcome data in the literature. These reports typically come in the form of diary entries or data from semistructured interviews.

7. *Objective tests of impairments* (e.g., Donaghy & Williams, 1998; Kerns & Thomson, 1998; Quemada et al., 2003; Schmittter-Edgcombe et al., 1995; Wilson et al., 2001; Wright et al., 2001). Performance on standardized tests could be used as an outcome measure if there was an assumption that the use of the external aid would lead to improved functioning in the area being assessed (e.g., if Emma's increased use of relaxation strategies improved her performance on an attention test, or if an aid that prompted a patient to exercise improved measures of physical function). In most cases, external aids are introduced as compensatory techniques without an expectation that use of the aid will lead to improved cognitive or physical functioning or changes in the underlying impairment.

The above measures offer options for documenting generalization and the impact of training the use of external aids. Depending on the type of training and the aid, and the specific type of outcome to be measured, the clinician can select the measures most appropriate to the client.

Maintenance or long-term use of trained devices is the ultimate measure of success. The Assistive Technology Outcomes Measurement System project (Lauer, 2004; Rust, & Smith, 2006) surveyed donors of assistive technology and asked why their devices were no longer being used. Respondents used terms such as *abandonment, refusal, avoidance*, and *noncompliance* as negative reasons for ceasing to use their aids, but there were positive reasons as well. Most notably was advancement to a less restrictive device or improvement in function so that a device was no longer needed. They suggested that the more neutral term *discontinuance* be used when evaluating outcomes. Their results remind clinicians that multiple factors may contribute to the decision to discontinue use of a device, and that there must be a mechanism in place to assess changes in a client's environment or abilities that may warrant the need for a new system or adaptations to the way an external aid is used. Follow-up visits with professionals or enlisting care providers to conduct ongoing monitoring and needs assessments are important aspects of outcomes measurement. Figure 7.11 shows an example of an attempt to gather these data. The data could be gathered via phone call, e-mail or postal mail.

PUTTING IT ALL TOGETHER:
A CASE APPLICATION FROM THE LITERATURE

A recent single-case experiment evaluated the outcome of training a client with severe anterograde amnesia to use a smartphone to compensate for a declarative memory impairment that limited the client's ability to perform prospective tasks and recall recent events (Svoboda, Richards, Polsinelli, & Guger, 2009). The training was consistent with the principles of the PIE framework described in this chapter. Smartphone training consisted of two phases: basic skill acquisition and real-life generalization. The first phase used principles of errorless learning to teach content and procedures required for use of target applications on the smart phone. Each application was broken into its component steps. Performance on each component step was measured using a cueing hierarchy. The criterion for moving to the next stage of training was 98% correct on all steps within a single training session. The client successfully acquired all three calendar functions that were targeted in eight 1-hour training sessions.

In the generalization stage, the clinician introduced novel applications using the same errorless learning approach, and gave take-home assignments to use the phone for increasingly complex tasks. The client successfully and rapidly acquired the skills for using the address book, camera, camcorder, voice recorder, and other functions of the phone. In addition to session data measuring number of trials to criterion, outcome was measured as the percent of five assigned phone calls successfully completed by the client each week. Impact was measured by a standardized memory questionnaire filled out by the caregiver that involved rating the frequency of occurrence of common memory mistakes and an assessment of smartphone use.

Results showed that the client demonstrated consistent and novel generalization of smartphone skills across a broad range of real-life memory-demanding circumstances. The authors suggested that theory-driven, systematic, hierarchically organized training can allow individuals with severe memory impairment to exploit commercially available tools to successfully support memory.

SUMMARY

Technology advances over the past several years have created virtually endless options for external aids that can help clients with cognitive impairments live more fully and independently. However, the array of choices and opportunities to adapt devices to people's individual circumstances can be overwhelming for clinicians. The process of developing goals and implementing training can be streamlined by the use of (1) a comprehensive needs assessment to identify a tool that is well matched to a client and his or her ecology, and (2) systematic planning and therapy implementation that adheres to the instruction principles shown to be effective for people with cognitive impairments. The use of multilevel evaluation can guide therapy efforts by revealing which aspects of the external aid have been learned and which require further instruction to ensure that the client masters use of the aid. Identifying methods to measure generalization and impact and monitor long-term needs maximizes the possibility that an external aid will be used consistently over the long term and that it makes a difference in the life of the individual client. We conclude with a summary of the clinical sequence for selecting and training the use of an external aid. This sequence is shown in Figure 7.12.

1. Complete a needs assessment to identify appropriate aid and instructional needs (see Appendices 7.1–7.3).
2. Design an individualized training plan outlining methods for meeting training needs, task analysis, and supports to be implemented (see Instructional Planning Worksheet for External Cognitive Aids, Form 7.2).
3. Administer an initial assessment, a one-time probe to determine the performance baseline and prompting hierarchy (see Initial Assessment Worksheet for External Cognitive Aids, Form 7.3).

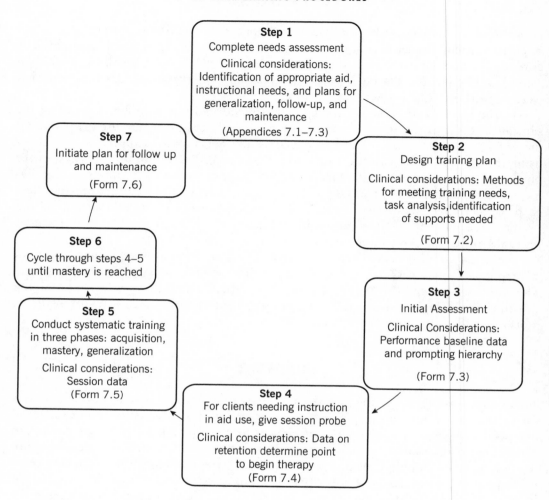

FIGURE 7.12. Clinical sequence for selecting and training use of an external aid.

4. For clients needing instruction to learn the steps for using the aid, begin each session with a probe to determine retention and where to begin in therapy (see Progress Monitoring Form for External Cognitive Aids, Form 7.4).

5. Conduct systematic training, adhering to guidelines for learning phases of acquisition, mastery, and generalization (see Session Data Form for External Cognitive Aids, Form 7.5).

6. Cycle through Steps 4 and 5 until mastery is reached.

7. Initiate the plan for follow-up and maintenance (see Follow-Up Form to Collect Maintenance Data, Form 7.6).

APPLICATION EXERCISES

1. Pair up with a peer and practice conducting a needs assessment using the CTI in Appendix A as an interview guide. Your peer should assume the role of a person who has difficulty managing some daily tasks due to memory impairment and who has insight into his or her problems. Think about expanding on questions that would help you identify an appropriate external aid. Then switch roles.

2. Look at the external aids listed in Table 7.1. Select one that is familiar to you and develop a task analysis, listing the steps for training a hypothetical patient to use the aid. Use your results to Steps 3–5.

3. For the tool you selected in exercise 2, write a hypothetical long-term goal and short-term objective for training use of the aid. Be sure to make the goal and objective measurable and specify the target context and amount of support needed.

4. Generate two possible ways to measure your client's progress for each of the following: (a) learning to use the external aid (session data), (b) using the aid in the target context (generalization data), and (c) the effect of using the aid in everyday life (impact data).

5. Generate an example of how you, as the clinician, might facilitate generalized use of the external aid you are teaching your client.

6. Using the Progress Monitoring Form (Form 7.4), generate session data for Case 1 for 11/4 based on the probe taken that day, as shown in the column for 11/4. Which step would you begin training? Based on progress to date, what would you anticipate accomplishing in that session?

7. Again using Form 7.4, generate two sets of hypothetical probe data that could be entered into the progress monitoring for case 1 during the next session on 11/5. Have the first set of probe data show that the client retained what was taught, based on your session data from 11/4, and the second set of probe data show that the client had not retained what you taught and that you need to back up and review.

APPENDIX 7.1. Compensation Techniques Inventory

Client Name:			Date:		
I. Independence Screen					
Life Tasks	**How much help needed? (see rating scale)**	**Comments (check any that are important goal areas)**			✓
Making appointments					
Financial management					
Social arrangements					
Shopping					
Meal planning and preparation					
Cleaning					
Laundry					
Driving					
Personal care					
1 = unable; 2 = lots of help; 3 = occasional help; 4 = reminders only; 5 = independent					
II. Functional Cognition Screen					
Cognitive Issue	**Frequency of Problem (see rating scale)**	**Comments (check any that really bother you)**			✓
Don't know the date					
Miss appointments					
Lose keys					
Double schedule					
Forget to complete tasks at home or work					
Don't know what appointments are coming up next week					
Have trouble organizing days and tasks that need to be completed					
Start but don't finish tasks					
Lose track of time					
Cannot stay focused and return to task when interrupted					
Forget what I did yesterday					
1 = happens constantly; 2 = happens frequently; 3 = happens occasionally; 4 = rarely happens; 5 = not an issue					

APPENDIX 7.1. *(cont.)*

Type of Aid	Frequency of Use PRIOR	How Useful PRIOR	Frequency of Use NOW	How Useful NOW
Past and Current Compensation Use				
EXTERNAL SCHEDULING AIDS				
Wall Calendar *Location* _____				
• Enter scheduled events				
• Enter "things to do"				
• Refer to entries				
• Check off entries				
• Reschedule as needed				
Planner *Type* _____				
• Enter scheduled events				
• Enter "things to do"				
• Refer to entries				
• Set alarm				
• Check off entries				
• Reschedule as needed				
Electronic Scheduler *Type* _____				
• Enter scheduled events				
• Enter "things to do"				
• Refer to entries				
• Set alarm				
• Check off entries				
• Reschedule as needed				
OTHER EXTERNAL AIDS				
Voice recorder				
Car memo pad				
Digital stopwatch				
Wristwatch				
Bulletin board with notes				
Home filing system				
Post-it notes				
Reminders on fridge				
Pill reminder system				
Voice mail				
Calculator				
Camera				
Others:				

APPENDIX 7.1. *(cont.)*

Type of Aid	Frequency of Use PRIOR	How Useful PRIOR	Frequency of Use NOW	How Useful NOW
STRATEGIES				
Use cue card of compensation techniques				
Stop and think				
Slow down to work carefully				
Recheck work for accuracy				
Ask direct questions if needed				
Follow written directions				
Ask for help if unsure				
Self-talk (talk through a plan)				
Repetition (repeat to self or review information repeatedly)				
Write down and repeat information to self				
Others:				
ENVIRONMENTAL ADAPTATIONS				
• Label house or work drawers/cupboards				
• Organized filing system				
• Keep space neat				
• Sit in a quiet place to work				
• Remove irrelevant or distracting items				
Others:				

Frequency of Use Scale: 0 = never; 1 = 1X/week; 2 = a few times/week; 3 = most days
Helpfulness Scale: 0 = N/A or not useful; 1 = rarely helps; 2 = pretty helpful; 3 = very helpful

APPENDIX 7.2. Needs Assessment

Client Name:	Date:

I. Cognitive Profile

Check the areas that are of concern.	For those areas that are checked, describe the nature of the impairment.
☐ Episodic memory (ability to remember daily events and personal experiences)	
☐ Semantic memory (ability to remember facts and knowledge-based information)	
☐ Prospective memory (ability to remember to initiate a planned future action at a specific time)	
☐ Procedural memory (ability to learn procedures or steps—may be learning without awareness)	
☐ Retrograde amnesia (pattern of loss of memory for events prior to injury)	
☐ New learning (ability/rate of learning new information)	
☐ Decreased attention	
☐ Limitation in executive functions (e.g., initiation, planning, organization)	
☐ Reduced reasoning/problem solving	
☐ Language problems (affecting ability to read, write, or type entries)	

II. Physical Profile

Check the areas that are of concern.	For those areas that are checked, describe the nature of the impairment.
☐ Visuoperceptual problems (affecting ability to read, write, or type entries)	
☐ Motoric difficulties (affecting ability to write in, manipulate, or carry a tool)	
☐ Auditory problems (affecting ability to hear alarms or watch beeps)	

APPENDIX 7.2. *(cont.)*

III. Personal Factors

A. Current or Past Use of Memory/Organizational Aids (Check all that apply)

☐ No systems used   ☐ Notes to self

☐ Calendar in the home   ☐ Wore a watch

☐ Datebook system   ☐ Electronic system

☐ Spouse/partner keeps track of things   ☐ Other

Comments:

B. Level of Acceptance/Awareness of Memory Impairment (Check best description)

☐ Has limited understanding or awareness of impairment (awareness deficit due to organic brain damage)

☐ Exhibits significant psychological denial (difficulty accepting disability)

☐ Can state knowledge of impairment but does not think aids are necessary

☐ Openly discusses memory problem but inconsistent in using compensation strategies

☐ Appears willing to learn and use aids

C. Client Preference for a Memory System

Appearance (color, style, size)	
Types of functions (e.g., calendar, things to do list, budget planner)	
Mode (electronic, written, auditory, pictoral)	

D. Financial Resources

☐ Insurance (or third-party willing to pay)

☐ Personal funds available to purchase system of choice

☐ Funds available for system up to _____ dollars

☐ No funds available

E. Available Support

☐ Patient would need to be able to utilize systems independently due to lack of available support

☐ Family/staff/significant others able and willing to be trained but will require structured program

☐ Persons to be involved with patient will vary; will need to provide description of system, procedures for using it, and methods for providing assistance

APPENDIX 7.2. *(cont.)*

IV. Situational Factors

Context: Describe goal of external aid _____

When and where would it be used: _____

Functions of systems—external aid system will need to provide the following functions:

☐ Autobiographical information (personal history, orientation sheets, photos, fact sheets, etc)

☐ Daily schedule

☐ Calendar

☐ Things to do

☐ Daily diary/events log

☐ Specific journal (e.g., anger log)

☐ Therapy goals

☐ Other

Recommendations: _____

APPENDIX 7.3. TechMatch Survey

Technology

1. Check all of the items below that describe common technologies your (or your client) has successfully used on a regular basis since experiencing a cognitive change:
   - ☐ A remote control for electronic devices such as TV
   - ☐ A game console (xBox, Nintendo, Wii) hooked to TV
   - ☐ An electronic calendar or PDA
   - ☐ An answering machine to record and later recall phone calls
   - ☐ A DVD player
   - ☐ A watch with a programmable alarm
   - ☐ A portable music player (iPod, MP3)
   - ☐ None

2. Check all of the computer technologies below that you (or your client) has successfully used since experiencing a cognitive change:
   - ☐ Laptop computer
   - ☐ Desktop computer
   - ☐ An electronic calendar or PDA
   - ☐ Cell phone
   - ☐ BlackBerry
   - ☐ Flash/USB drive
   - ☐ Other _____
   - ☐ None

3. Check all of the following devices you (or your client) tried to use, but found too complex or didn't work:
   - ☐ Laptop computer
   - ☐ Desktop computer
   - ☐ An electronic calendar or PDA
   - ☐ Cell phone
   - ☐ BlackBerry
   - ☐ Flash/USB drive
   - ☐ Other _____
   - ☐ None

4. Check all of the items below that describe activities you (or your client) now does on a computer:
   - ☐ Sends and receives e-mail
   - ☐ Plays games by self
   - ☐ Plays challenging games with other people
   - ☐ Looks at different Internet sites for fun or to get information
   - ☐ Uses a calendar or address book
   - ☐ Listens to music on the Internet
   - ☐ Buys music on the Internet and saves it on computer
   - ☐ Writes letters or other short documents
   - ☐ Does lots of writing and saves it on a computer
   - ☐ Searches for a map or driving directions
   - ☐ Stores and edits photographs
   - ☐ Other _____
   - ☐ None

APPENDIX 7.3. *(cont.)*

5. Check all of the items below that describe activities you (or your client) aren't now doing but wants to do on a computer:
   - ☐ Send and receive e-mail
   - ☐ Play games alone
   - ☐ Play challenging games with other people
   - ☐ Look at different Internet sites for fun or to get information
   - ☐ Use a calendar or address book
   - ☐ Listen to music on the Internet
   - ☐ Buy music on the Internet and save it on a computer
   - ☐ Write letters or other short documents
   - ☐ Do lots of writing and save it on a computer
   - ☐ Search for a map or driving directions
   - ☐ Store and edit photographs
   - ☐ Other _____
   - ☐ None

6. Check one item below that describes your (or your client's) current level of knowledge about using the Internet:
   - ☐ Can use almost any computer to find what is needed on the Internet
   - ☐ Can find what is needed on the Internet using a computer that is familiar
   - ☐ Can find what is needed on the Internet if steps are written down and using a familiar computer
   - ☐ Can find what is needed on the Internet if someone is nearby to help when needed
   - ☐ Hasn't yet successfully used the Internet

Environment

1. Check all of the settings below that you (or your client) currently visits:
   - ☐ Public space in a group home, assisted living facility, or apartment building
   - ☐ Public library
   - ☐ Disability center
   - ☐ Community center
   - ☐ Community college or university computing lab
   - ☐ Assistive technology center
   - ☐ Work setting, work readiness, or career center
   - ☐ Brain injury rehabilitation center
   - ☐ Other _____
   - ☐ None of the above

2. Check all of the people that you (or your client) would be comfortable around when using a computer:
   - ☐ Only a therapist or care provider
   - ☐ Family
   - ☐ Friends
   - ☐ People at work or school
   - ☐ Strangers in a public setting

3. Check all of the places where you (or your client) would feel comfortable using a computer:
   - ☐ Public space in a group home, assisted living facility, or apartment building
   - ☐ Public library

- ☐ Disability center
- ☐ Community center
- ☐ Community college or university computing lab
- ☐ Assistive technology center
- ☐ Work, work readiness, or career center
- ☐ Brain injury rehabilitation center
- ☐ Own home or apartment
- ☐ Other _____

4. Check all items below that describe the type of support you (or your client) has for using technology:
   - ☐ A support person available at home who knows how to use electronic devices
   - ☐ A support person who can visit at home to help
   - ☐ Someone to call who will answer questions over the phone
   - ☐ A personal assistant who could help outside of the home
   - ☐ No support for using technology

5. Does your client's living environment have Internet access now?
   - ☐ Yes
   - ☐ No
   - ☐ I'm not sure

6. Check all items below that describe the methods your client uses to get around town:
   - ☐ Can walk to nearby businesses
   - ☐ Can ride a bike to businesses in town
   - ☐ Can ride the bus to businesses in town
   - ☐ Drives own car
   - ☐ Is not able to get around town without assistance

7. Check all items below that describe the type of assistance your client has when traveling to distant locations around town:
   - ☐ Does not need assistance
   - ☐ Has someone who drives when leaving home
   - ☐ Uses a disability transit service
   - ☐ Does not leave home

8. Does your client currently have a desktop computer at home that is available for use?
   - ☐ Yes
   - ☐ No

User Needs

1. Check all items below that describe how your (or your client's) hands work when picking up something thin, like a piece of paper:
   - ☐ Could pick up a piece of paper with either hand
   - ☐ Could pick up a piece of paper with one hand, but not the other
   - ☐ Hands would probably shake or tremble
   - ☐ Would be very slow but could do it
   - ☐ Would probably wrinkle the paper
   - ☐ Could not pick up or hold a piece of paper

APPENDIX 7.3. *(cont.)*

2. Check all items below that describe things you (or your client) can do with your (or his or her) hands:
   - ☐ Use a joystick to play video games
   - ☐ Open a doorknob
   - ☐ Open a toothpaste tube
   - ☐ Use tweezers to remove a splinter
   - ☐ Can't do any of these things

3. Check all items below that describe how you (or your client) would read a story:
   - ☐ Reads whole books, such as paperback or library books
   - ☐ Reads shorter stories, like those in the newspaper or magazines
   - ☐ Reads books that have a lot of pictures with words, like graphic novels
   - ☐ Reads simple books with a lot of pictures and little or no writing, like comic books
   - ☐ Listens to books on tape
   - ☐ Does not read

4. Check one item below to show the smallest writing you (or your client) can comfortably read:
   - ☐ Smallest Font
   - ☐ Small Font
   - ☐ Medium Font
   - ☐ Big Font
   - ☐ Can't read any of it

5. Check all items below that describe your (or your client's) spelling and writing:
   - ☐ Never misspells words
   - ☐ Misspells words not used a lot
   - ☐ Is often unsure about spelling
   - ☐ Makes quite a few spelling mistakes
   - ☐ Does not write

6. Check one item that describes your (or your client's) ability to carry objects that are quite heavy, for example, a few large books:
   - ☐ Can put them in and take them out of a backpack or other case
   - ☐ Would not be able to carry heavy items without help

7. Check one item that describes your (or your client's) ability to carry objects that are slightly heavy, such as just one large book:
   - ☐ Would be able to put it in and take it out of a backpack or other case
   - ☐ Would not be able to carry a large book without help

8. Check all statements that describe your (or your client's) ability to carry and use a small object like a key:
   - ☐ Can remove/replace the key from around his or her neck on a string
   - ☐ Can insert and turn a key to unlock a door
   - ☐ Would need help to use a key

APPENDIX 7.3. *(cont.)*

Cognitive Ability

1. Check all statements that describe how you (or your client) plans and organizes daily activities:
   - ☐ Is spontaneous with little planning
   - ☐ Plans each day's activities ahead of time
   - ☐ Plans activities, but has trouble following through
   - ☐ Needs someone else to help with daily planning
   - ☐ Follows a routine each day

2. Check all statements below that describe what happens when you (or your client) needs to learn the steps to use a new type of machine or technology:
   - ☐ Learns independently by reading an instruction manual
   - ☐ Benefits from having written instructions attached to the equipment
   - ☐ Prefers if someone gives verbal instructions and then stands by to help
   - ☐ Requires an experienced instructor to teach each step
   - ☐ Other _____

3. Check all statements below that describe your (or your client's) ability to remember a secret name or number, for example, a combination number used for a locker:
   - ☐ Can remember a secret name or number
   - ☐ Would write a secret name or number in a safe place and keep it to use when needed
   - ☐ Needs help to remember a secret name or number
   - ☐ I'm not sure how well my client would do this

4. Check all statements that describe your (or your client's) ability to remember to take something small, like a library card, when leaving home:
   - ☐ Would probably forget the library card
   - ☐ Would always remember to take the library card
   - ☐ Would use a checklist to remember to take the card
   - ☐ Would store the library card in the same place to help remember it
   - ☐ Would need help from someone else to remember to take the library card

5. Check all statements that describe your (or your client's) ability to remember to bring an overdue book when going to the library:
   - ☐ Would always remember to take the book
   - ☐ Would add the book to a checklist to remember to bring it
   - ☐ Would place the book in a spot it could be seen when leaving home
   - ☐ Would need someone's help to remember the book
   - ☐ Would probably forget to take the book
   - ☐ Other _____

6. Check one statement that describes how you (or your client) would use a machine for the first time, like a grocery store self-check-out scanner:
   - ☐ Would read and follow the instructions without any difficulty
   - ☐ Would read the instructions, and would ask for help if necessary
   - ☐ Would ask for help instead of trying to follow instructions independently
   - ☐ Would never use a machine like the scanner; would always go to the aisle where a clerk checks out customers
   - ☐ Other _____

APPENDIX 7.3. *(cont.)*

7. Check one statement that describes what you (or your client) would do on a rainy day if carrying something delicate outside like a wrapped birthday present:

   ☐ Would pay attention to the weather forecast, and would be sure to protect the gift so it would stay dry

   ☐ May not listen in advance to a weather forecast, but would always carefully protect a nice gift if it might rain

   ☐ Would need reminders from someone to protect the gift before leaving home

8. Check one statement that describes your (or your client's) ability to pay attention in a distracting environment:

   ☐ Can concentrate to start and finish a task even if there is a lot of noise and activity

   ☐ Can start a task, but if people are talking or moving around nearby, the distraction can reduce accuracy or slow performance

   ☐ Can start a task, but if people are talking or moving around nearby, will lose concentration and have to start over again

   ☐ Needs to be in a quiet room to start and finish a task when concentrating

   ☐ Has difficulty with concentration even in a quiet room

Personal Situation

1. Check one statement that describes how flexible you (or your client) is financially for buying new devices or services:

   ☐ Able to purchase whatever technology is needed

   ☐ Could spend a few hundred dollars to get a device if it was really useful

   ☐ Has a very limited budget with less than one hundred dollars to spend on technology

   ☐ Would only like to use technology that is free

2. Check one statement that describes your (or your client's) attitude toward doing new things:

   ☐ Will stick with a new task until it is figured out

   ☐ Easily tries new tasks but has trouble sticking with them if not successful right away

   ☐ Not much of a risk taker so needs a lot of support to try new things

   ☐ Only likes to do what is comfortable and familiar. Does not like to branch out with new tasks

3. Check one statement that describes how motivated you (or your client) is for tasks that are challenging:

   ☐ Motivated and stimulated by difficult challenges

   ☐ Likes a slight challenge

   ☐ Is easily discouraged

   ☐ Won't try if something will be hard

4. Check one statement that describes how you (or your client) feels about change and variety in life:

   ☐ Is happiest if able to do different things and go different places often

   ☐ Likes a moderate amount of variety in life

   ☐ Likes to have only a little variety in life

   ☐ Likes to go to the same places and do the same things most days

   ☐ Is most comfortable with a lot of structure in life—variety just complicates things

TechMatch is a service of Personal Technologies, LLC. Copyright 2009 by Lynn E. Fox, McKay Moore Sohlberg, Stephen Fickas, Jason Prideaux, and Anthony Wittig. Reprinted by permission. The online survey generates recommendations based on survey responses. Development was funded by Grant No. H133S070096 from the National Institute on Disability and Rehabilitation Research.

CHAPTER 8

Training the Use of Metacognitive Strategies

Metacognition is our ability to think about thinking. This includes knowing when and how to use a strategy that will help us understand, learn, and remember. The development of metacognitive ability begins early in life and continues into late adolescence, when we can effectively judge whether we need to study in advance for a test or can cram the night before, or know that when we have a lot to do, it is helpful to write things down on a list. Metacognition has two components: being able to monitor our own thoughts, and being able to use that information to make changes that improve our thinking and behavior (Dunlosky & Metcalfe, 2009). People with TBI often have problems in both aspects of metacognition: They are unaware or less aware of deficits (i.e., poor monitoring), and they do not easily make changes in their thinking in response to changing demands (i.e., impaired executive functions) (Kennedy & Turkstra, 2006). As a result, they often need formal training in strategies that will help them use their residual cognitive abilities effectively.

In this chapter, we discuss instructional procedures for training individuals to regulate their behavior or thinking. Strategies can be simple, such as teaching a person with an executive function impairment to say each step in a recipe out loud in order to stay focused on completing the steps in order. Most types of instruction have a strategy component. For example, elaboration and association, discussed in Chapter 5, are strategies that can be used by the clinician to help clients learn facts and concepts. The current chapter, however, focuses on training clients to use strategies independently to improve their thinking or learning.

For the clinician, the first step in providing effective metacognitive strategy instruction is to know the range of strategy options. Strategies can be divided into two basic categories: (1) *task-specific* strategies, such as using a reading comprehension strategy to improve the understanding and retention of text; and (2) *general* strategies that can assist with the completion of a wide variety of target tasks, such as a self-monitoring strategy that can be used to teach any multistep routine. We begin by describing these two types of strategies and the research evidence in support of each. After delineating the different options for teaching strategies and the supporting the evidence, the PIE framework is used to explain and organize the key instructional components important for training clients to use any type of strategy.

STRATEGY OPTIONS:
GENERAL VERSUS TASK-SPECIFIC STRATEGIES

What Are General Metacognitive Strategies?

The field of neuropsychological rehabilitation provides strong evidence supporting the training of metacognitive strategies to assist people with cognitive impairments in achieving their goals. Most studies have focused on strategy use for managing impairments in three cognitive domains: attention (e.g., sustaining and shifting attention), executive functions (e.g., organization, inhibition/impulse control, self-correction), and memory (e.g., recall, remembering to carry out intentions). At the core of metacognitive strategy training is teaching an individual to self-regulate thoughts and actions—that is, to "think about his or her own thinking"—and to self-monitor performance during an activity (Kennedy & Coelho, 2005). The goal is for the learner to use methods that provide some control over his or her own learning and behavior.

Strategies to Manage Impairments in Attention and Executive Functions

Most of the evidence supporting strategy instruction for improving attention and executive functions comes from studies of metacognitive strategy instruction (MSI; Kennedy et al., 2008). MSI uses direct instruction to teach individuals to regulate their own behavior and deliberately monitor how they are performing a target task, then change their behavior if performance is not optimal (Sohlberg et al., 2005). To self-regulate, individuals need to (1) identify an appropriate goal, (2) anticipate what they need to do to reach that goal, (3) identify possible solutions to challenges, (4) self-monitor and evaluate progress, and (5) modify their behavior or strategy use if they are not making adequate progress. MSI thus can be used to address difficulties with problem solving, planning, initiation, organization, and task persistence—all of which are commonly impaired in individuals with TBI and other acquired cognitive disorders. Table 8.1 lists examples of MSI techniques that have been evaluated in the literature and shown to produce positive clinical results.

There is substantial evidence to support the use of MSI with young to middle-age adults with brain injury when improvement in everyday functional problems is the goal, as shown by an evidence review and meta-analysis (Kennedy et al., 2008). Most participants maintained gains from therapy, but there was variability in the extent to which participants generalized strategy use beyond the targets trained in therapy. Further support for MSI can be found in the extensive literature on teaching students with learning disabilities, who often have attention and executive function impairments that resemble those seen in TBI (Ylvisaker et al., 2002). Teaching students with learning disabilities to self-monitor thoughts and actions during academic tasks has been shown to be highly effective for improving accuracy and productivity and for promoting on-task behavior (Hughes, Ruhl, Schumaker, & Deshler, 2002; Reid, Trout, & Schartz, 2005). Effective MSI approaches from the learning disabilities field include teaching students to self-monitor their level of attention or engagement, and teaching them to chart or rate their perceptions of their performance. There is growing evidence to support the use of step-by-step self-regulation sequences for helping students to complete school-related goals, similar to those discussed in the adult neurogenic literature. An extensive review (Reid et al., 2005) demonstrated large effect sizes for teaching self-monitoring to students

TABLE 8.1. Description of Metacognitive Strategies

Metacognitive strategy	Description	Supporting research evidence
Problem-solving therapy (PST)	*Problem-solving process:* Participants taught steps for sequences such as: "Problem Identification and Analysis"; "Generation of Hypotheses and Decision Making"; "Evaluation of a Solution."	von Cramon et al. (1991)* von Cramon & Matthes-von Cramon (1994)
Time pressure management (TPM)	*Problem-solving process:* Intervention first helps with increasing self-awareness and acceptance of disability, then participants taught step-by-step problem-solving approach rehearsed under increasing distractions.	Fasotti et al. (2000)*
Problem solving with impulse control	*Problem-solving process:* Participants taught to document impulsive reactions to problem situations and identify strategies to avoid reactions.	Rath, Simon, Langenbahn, Sherr, & Diller (2003)*
Verbal mediation	*Self-instruction process for problem solving and goal completion:* Participants taught to verbalize steps of multistep tasks and fade talking to whispering and then inner speech.	Cicerone & Wood (1987) Cicerone & Giacino (1992)
Goal attainment	*Goal-setting process:* Participants taught steps to set goals and actively monitor progress toward goals.	Webb & Gluecauf (1994)
Goal management training (GMT)	*Goal-completion process:* Participants taught six steps: Stop, define main task, list steps, learn steps, execute task, check results.	Levine et al. (2000)*
Self-monitoring	*Self-monitoring process:* Participants taught to make predictions and monitor performance via anticipating their own performance and/or recording task progress.	Cicerone & Giacino (1992) Suzman, Morris, Morris, & Milan (1997)
Self-monitoring (WSTC)	*Self-monitoring process:* Participants taught self-monitoring steps associated with acronym WSTC: What am I supposed to be doing? Select a strategy. Try the strategy. Check the strategy.	Lawson & Rice (1989)
Self-monitoring (Error self-regulation)	*Self-monitoring process:* Participant taught to self-evaluate previous performance, anticipate future difficulties, and consider possible corrective strategies. Predictions were compared to therapist evaluations.	Ownsworth, Quinn, Fleming, Kendall, & Shum (2010)

Note. * indicates that research provided a high level of supporting evidence using a randomized controlled trial.

with learning challenges, to reduce inappropriate behavior, and increase academic accuracy and productivity. Similarly, a review by Mooney, Ryan, Uhing, Reid, and Epstein (2005) reported large effect sizes for studies that used self-management strategies for students with disabilities to increase engagement and academic productivity.

Strategies can also be used to assist clients with sequencing the different steps involved in a task. For example, Butler and colleagues (2008) developed a package of cognitive strategies designed to be used in "task preparation," "during a task," and "posttask" (see Table 8.2). The strategies were evaluated with school-age children and adolescents who had attention and executive function impairments from the effects of radiation and chemotherapy for cancer treatment (Butler et al., 2008). As shown in Table 8.2, strategies were designed to address impairments that interfered with academic performance. The overall results were positive; however, training of these cognitive strategies was part of a larger intervention package that also targeted affective state, motivation, and confidence, making it difficult to discern the extent to which positive effects were due to cognitive strategy instruction alone.

Strategies to Enhance Learning New Declarative Information

Memory strategies, commonly called mnemonic strategies, are techniques or methods that are employed to enhance or improve learning and/or recall of target information. These are called *internal* strategies, because they rely on conscious thought by the user, as contrasted with *external* strategies such as notebooks and planners that compensate for changes within the learner and attempt to lessen cognitive demands (see Chapter 7). In general, internal memory strategies require individuals to carefully attend to the information to be learned, which by itself can enhance learning. These strategies include elaboration, visualization, and creating mnemonics, which were reviewed in Chapter 5

TABLE 8.2. Sample of Metacognitive Strategies Used at Different Times during a Task for Students with Attention and Executive Function Impairments

Task preparation strategies	During-task strategies	Posttask strategies
"Magic words" Selected to increase confidence or assist with affective state	"Talk to myself" Verbal mediation	"Check my work" Increase self-monitoring
"Soup breath" Relaxation technique	"Mark my place" Assist with sustained attention	"Ask for feedback" Increase self-monitoring
"Game face" Approach task with confidence and minimize distraction	"Start at top" or "Row by row" Assist with organization and attention	"Reward myself" Increase engagement
"World record" Increase engagement	"Time out" Pacing strategy	
"Warm up my brain" Increase readiness	"Look at floor" Increase focus during public speaking or reading tasks	
	"Ask for a hint" Solicit support	

Note. Based on Butler et al. (2008).

as methods to teach facts and concepts. In this chapter, we focus on the independent use of internal strategies by the learner, who must have sufficient metacognitive ability to recognize when the strategy will be helpful. Internal memory strategies aim to facilitate access to stored semantic networks of information and to use these networks to assist with storage and retrieval processes (West, 1995). They are useful for helping clients learn a specific body of new information—particularly, for learning disparate items and coalescing them into one memory. According to Wilson (1995), use of internal memory strategies can be effective because of the following:

- Strategies encourage a deeper level of processing, which improves recall.
- Strategies often integrate isolated information.
- Strategies often provide built-in retrieval cues.

Table 8.3 lists examples of internal memory strategies and supporting research.

There are major caveats to using internal memory strategies, however, and not all research results are positive. Kaschel et al. (2002) summarize some of the reasons that researchers and clinicians may be reticent to employ internal memory strategies:

TABLE 8.3. Description of Memory Strategies

Memory strategy	Description	Supporting research
Visual imagery Structured imagery training	Using hierarchical exercises and specific generalization and transfer training in three-staged training process involving acquisition of imagery technique.	Kaschel et al. (2002)
Visual imagery Method of loci	Memorizing known series of locations and creating a visual image of information to be remembered in each location.	West (1995)
Verbal elaboration First-letter mnemonics and rhymes	Generating expression or rhymes to help remember target information.	Wilson (1995)
Verbal elaboration Elaborative encoding	Transforming information held in short-term memory in ways that facilitate storage in long-term memory by creating associations with other semantically or acoustically related information.	Oberg & Turkstra (1998); O'Neil-Pirozzi et al. (2010)
Visual imagery and verbal elaboration Story method	Creating a story and generating visual images incorporating information to be remembered.	O'Neil-Pirozzi et al. (2010); Wilson (1995)
Retrieval techniques Mental retracing	Systematically reviewing previous actions to trigger target information.	Wilson (1991)
Retrieval techniques Alphabetic searching	Searching through alphabet in hopes letter will act as cue for word or name	Moffat (1984)
Retrieval techniques Alphabetic searching	Systematically proceeding through the alphabet in attempt to get phonetic trigger of target information.	Wilson (1991)

- Strategies can be too complex for people with cognitive impairments.
- Strategies can be unnatural and difficult to apply to everyday life activities.
- Generalized use of memory strategies rarely occurs in people with cognitive impairments, particularly impairments in executive functions.

These limitations make sense when we consider that metacognitive impairments are common among individuals with acquired memory disorders. Kaschel and colleagues (2002) discuss the factors important for addressing these potential barriers. The results from their rigorous, controlled evaluation suggest that imagery training can enhance recall, providing it incorporates specific training components. (See the Example from the Literature on page 211.) They demonstrated improved delayed recall of everyday relevant verbal materials (stories and appointments) when their training used systematic instruction. This training included a hierarchy of exercises that gave the participants practice in using the strategies and then helped them transfer the use of strategies to their everyday lives.

O'Neil-Pirozzi and colleagues (2010) also conducted a controlled study evaluating the effects of teaching internal memory strategies to people with brain injury. Researchers administered a 16-week small-group memory therapy program to 54 adults with TBI who were more than 1 year postinjury, and compared their memory test scores to those of a group that received no training. Training methods included semantic association (e.g., categorization and clustering items according to meaning), elaboration, and visual/auditory imagery. There was a significant benefit of training, and gains were maintained after 1 month with no treatment. Consistent with our earlier discussion about cognitive prerequisites for internal strategies, benefits were seen primarily in participants with mild–moderate TBI. As discussed in Chapter 5, individuals with more severe cognitive impairments may not be candidates for training in strategies that require insight and independent use.

Metacognitive strategies vary greatly in terms of complexity. Many interventions are multidimensional and address a range of behaviors or processes important for completing any goal or retaining different sets of information. For example, both goal management training (GMT) (Levine et al., 2000) and WSTC (What am I supposed to be doing? Select a strategy. Try the strategy. Check the strategy; Lawson & Rice, 1989) train ordered sequences of self-questioning that are designed to help with planning, organization, self-monitoring, and problem solving. In personal metaphor training, developed by Ylvisaker and Feeney (2000), clients learn to perform complex constellations of positive behaviors by first identifying a role model who embodies qualities they admire, and then learning to internalize those qualities and "act" like that person. These authors argued that although personal metaphors might seem too abstract for persons with cognitive impairments, in fact, they are a way to make complex information simple and accessible to these individuals. In support of this premise, they noted that metaphors can be effective even for very young children (e.g., telling a child to act "like a big girl") before metacognition has developed.

Researchers (e.g., Spikman, Boelen, Lamberts, Brouwer, & Fasottie, 2010) also have trained cognitive strategies to improve lifestyle (e.g., following healthy diet and exercise regimen), organization and planning (building daily routines to target individual goals), and attention (e.g., mindfulness exercises). By contrast, other interventions target a single strategy designed to teach a specific behavior or method that will increase task accuracy. For example, an individual can be taught to use alphabet searching when he or she has word-finding problems (Wilson, 1991), or to simply record perception of accuracy on tasks in order to increase self-monitoring (Butler et al., 2008; Cicerone & Giacino, 1992). A focused strategy can thereby be used to address a discrete aspect of executive function or memory that is a barrier to successful performance. Alternatively, a more general strategy can be used to address multiple impairments.

This section has reviewed a wide range of metacognitive strategies, each with its own unique characteristics. Taken together, there is substantial evidence to support the use of metacognitive strategy instruction for people with attention, memory, and executive function impairments (Ehlhardt et al., 2008).

The following are a few examples of activity-level measures that might be used to assess outcomes of strategy-based training:

- Number of errors when using the strategy to perform a target task or activity
- Number of accurate solutions generated when using a particular problem-solving strategy
- Number of completed steps for complex tasks
- Frequency of occurrence of memory failures or other problems targeted by the strategy
- Perception of stress or burden following strategy training
- Perceived cognitive symptom severity

Restorative or Compensatory?

It is not clear whether metacognitive strategy training is restorative (i.e., remediating the cognitive impairment so that the person can complete the task the same way as before the injury) versus compensatory (i.e., completing the activity successfully, often by doing the same task in a different way than before the injury). In general, the benefits of strategy instruction are more likely to be observed in performance of activities rather than in scores on standardized tests of memory, attention, and executive function. These benefits suggest that strategy instruction is compensatory. However, investigations have shown impairment-based improvements following MSI, suggesting that it might be restorative. For example, von Cramon, Matthes-von Cramon, and Mai (1991) demonstrated that participants who received treatment that involved teaching them a problem-solving strategy improved on three of five intelligence subtests. Similarly, in their study of time pressure management, Fasotti, Kovacs, Eling, and Brouwer (2000) reported significant improvements on two out of three standardized memory tests and on all three attention tests. It becomes blurrier when the efficacy measures closely resemble the training tasks. For example, Kaschel et al. (2002) showed that patients with mild memory impairments who were taught to generate distinct images rapidly and to use them for retrieval of information they had read or to carry out intended actions showed improvements on standardized memory tests that contained items similar to the training stimuli. One of the target memory tests required recall of stories and appointment information; these were the same stimuli domains used in the training. In any case the brain is changing in response to experience, so the distinction of restorative versus compensatory might not be that meaningful to the individual client.

Regardless of the underlying mechanisms of improvement, a general principle is that strategy use will generalize to the extent that the target processes are similar across domains. For example, a strategy for focusing attention would not be expected to help with learning new facts in a person with a declarative memory impairment; however, if impairments in focused attention were responsible for why the person could not retain new facts, then an attention strategy would be helpful. For this reason, strategies targeting self-monitoring and self-regulation often have a broad impact, as these processes are common to many tasks in daily living. It is important for clinicians to be familiar with a range of evidence-based metacognitive strategies as options for their clients.

What Are Task-Specific Metacognitive Strategies?

The strategies just discussed are linked to specific cognitive domains, such as attention or memory. In this section, we discuss strategies that are used when the goal is to be able to perform a specific task or activity, such as reading a book, cooking a meal, or getting from one place to another. A task-specific strategy can be generated for virtually any type of activity and customized to the profile of the individual client. As such, the training of these strategies shares many characteristics with approaches to training multistep routines (Chapter 6), which are everyday routines in which a sequential set of steps is completed in a chronological order (e.g., steps to do the laundry). As discussed in Chapter 6, the client learns the routine by performing it step by step, often with training procedures such as errorless learning, and practices until the steps become automatic. Task-specific strategies are also focused on *how* to complete a target activity (e.g., *take notes* when reading a book, *check and recheck a recipe* when cooking a meal, *look up at signs* when getting from one place to another but they consists of unique task sequences). Thus, task-specific strategies are metacognitive strategies in which the focus is on completing a specific activity, often within a specific context (Sohlberg & Mateer, 2001b). The strategy is generated by first defining the task and context, then identifying a process that effectively reduces performance barriers caused by the cognitive impairment. Table 8.4 provides five examples of different task-specific strategies.

The first three strategies listed in Table 8.4 pertain to academic or school-related activities. This is the domain that has received the most research attention and thus serves as an evidenced-based example of this approach. Reading comprehension strategies have been evaluated with readers with a variety of cognitive impairments, including people with ABI, older adults, and people with developmental cognitive and language disorders. These strategies are particularly useful for people with acquired cognitive–communication disorders such as TBI, because they compensate for impairments in self-regulation and memory. For example, if a student with TBI does not have good judgment about how well he or she has learned new information, these approaches can provide structured steps that foster full understanding of the material.

In general, most reading strategies include methods to facilitate (1) previewing, (2) active reading, and (3) reviewing content. The reading comprehension strategy that has been subjected to the most evaluation in children is reciprocal teaching (RT). This strategy is designed to teach readers four strategies to improve reading comprehension for narrative text: predicting, clarifying, questioning, and summarizing (Palincsar & Brown, 1984). A meta-analysis by Rosenshine and Meister (1994) showed positive

TABLE 8.4. Description of Activity-Specific Strategies

Activity specific strategy	Description	Supporting research

Reading comprehension strategies
  Reciprocal teaching
    PQRST (preview, question,
      review, state, test),
    SQ3R (survey, question,
      read, recite, and review)
	Techniques to increase contextual understanding, encoding, and reviewing	Bussman et al. (2000); Rosenshine & Meister (1994); West et al. (1995); Wilson (1992)

Writing strategy
  Graphic organizer to structure
    content
	Use of graphic organizer with flowcharts to guide writer to indicate topic sentences and supporting details	Ylivsaker & Feeney (1998)

Study agenda	Time-ordered agenda with instructions for listing homework goals and anticipated completion time	Sohlberg & Mateer (2001b)

Traveling to novel places	Destination arrival protocol for going to public places with steps for identifying:
	  (1) handicapped parking and ramps
	  (2) restroom
	  (3) seating to rest
	  (4) "helper" person
		Case examples from Sohlberg's clinic

Image–name match	Sequence for remembering names	McCarty (1980)

effects of RT on reading comprehension—findings that have been confirmed by many subsequent studies (e.g., Souvignier & Mokhlesgerami, 2006).

A different example of a task-specific strategy is the image–name match method, a strategy designed solely for the purpose of remembering people's names. As outlined by Wilson (2009) there are four strategy stages:

1. Identifying a distinguishing feature on the target individual (e.g., frizzy hair).
2. Generating a keyword that represents a concrete object for the name (e.g., Coleman is Coal-Man).
3. Converting the keyword to a mental image (e.g., a lump of coal sitting on a man's head).
4. Visualizing the face with the prominent feature enlarged with the name's image superimposed on top of the enlarged feature (Coal-Man on top of a mass of the individual's frizzy hair).

This method has been used with older adults who have cognitive decline (Yesavage, 1984) and with people with brain injury (Wilson, 1992), for whom remembering names is an important goal. However, as noted above, the independent use of strategies such as the image–name match often is not feasible for people with acquired cognitive impairments, and the process of generating the images might need to be directed by the clinician, as described in Chapter 5. In summary, a task- or activity-specific strategies have been evaluated in the research literature. Taken together, the results suggest that training individuals to implement a strategy to complete a target task or skill will enhance performance on that activity.

PIE: PLANNING FOR METACOGNITIVE STRATEGY INSTRUCTION

By now you are familiar with the four considerations critical to the therapy planning process. In this section, we review the key planning considerations specific to the training of general and task-specific metacognitive strategies.

Consideration 1: Who Is the Learner?

The clinician first considers the abilities and potential vulnerabilities of the individual client. Assessing the client's cognitive–linguistic, physical, and sensory abilities in addition to relevant affective and social support parameters provides critical information for selecting an appropriate strategy and planning how best to train the client to use that strategy. Generating a profile of essential learner characteristics often occurs simultaneously with planning Consideration 2, as the learner profile informs the selection of the strategy. Assessment of learner characteristics may require some combination of standardized testing, observation on functional measures, and interviews with the client and relevant support persons.

In terms of candidacy for strategy training, as discussed above, the client must have sufficient motivation and awareness to recognize the benefits of the strategy and consider using it. Strategy use requires an internally generated cognitive-behavioral response. In contrast, facts and concepts (Chapter 5), highly structured procedural routines (Chapter 6), and the use of external aids (Chapter 7) *can* be trained as automatic behavioral sequences that tap into procedural memory without significant client insight. However, the initial use of a metacognitive strategy requires the user to understand when to implement it and how it will be helpful (Sohlberg & Mateer, 2001b). Ideally, strategy use will become automatic over time with practice.

Consideration 2: Selecting the Strategy (What? Where? When?)

In conjunction with generating a learner profile, the clinician needs to identify the specific strategy to be trained and delineate the subcomponents. The following three planning questions help to guide this process:

1. *What* is the specific need?
2. *Where* is the target environment?
3. *When* will the client implement the strategy?

The clinician begins the planning process by *specifying the need* that the strategy will address. Selecting a best-fit strategy requires conducting a systematic needs assessment. Depending on the client, the needs assessment may consist of an interview with him or her or with a relevant support person. Alternatively, the assessment may involve a home or community visit to evaluate the target environment. These visits are critical when the clinician cannot otherwise obtain information about environmental factors that will influence strategy use. For example, training the client to use a study agenda is unlikely to be effective if there is no reliable workspace at home and assignments are easily lost. The clinician's task is to determine which assessments are necessary and feasible.

A needs assessment is the process by which *the clinician identifies factors unique to the client and environment that will determine the best strategy for the client's needs.* Essentially, the clinician is conducting an ecological assessment, integrating relevant client characteristics (cognitive–linguistic, psychosocial, physical, and sensory) with environmental considerations, then generating possible strategy options that will address the need and be usable by the client in his or her environment. Figure 8.1 depicts the clinical decision-making process necessary for identifying a good match. In some cases it might be necessary to conduct a dynamic assessment to determine which strategy will be most useful. For example, a clinician may assist the client in using two different strategies to complete a task, and then compare their effectiveness in helping the client achieve the target. The client also provides input about preferences for different types of strategies (particularly if a clinician-proposed strategy looks conspicuous in public or is something he or she never would have used premorbidly). The adoption of a strategy is more likely if a client is involved in the selection, has endorsed its utility, and perceives it to be useful (Borkowski, Carr, & Pressley, 1987). The two clinical case applications at the end of this chapter illustrate the systematic strategy selection process. Figures 8.2 and 8.3 provide a summary of the strategy selection process for these cases.

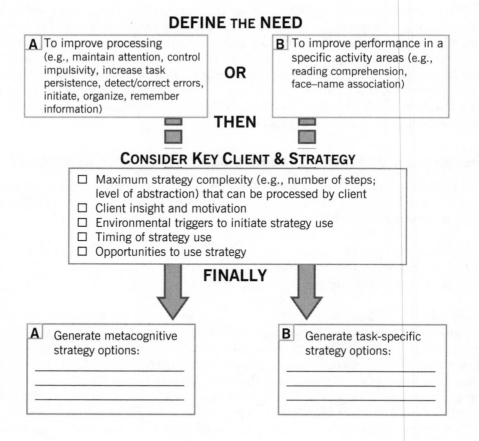

FIGURE 8.1. Matching strategy, need, and client.

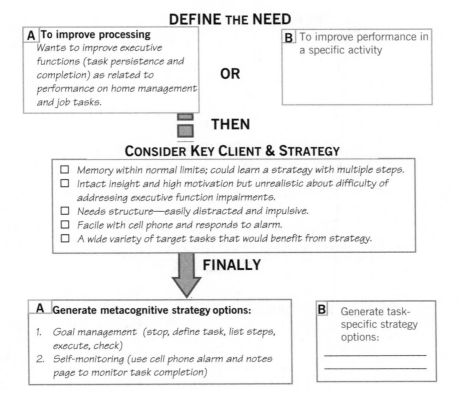

DEFINE THE NEED

A To improve processing

Wants to improve executive functions (task persistence and completion) as related to performance on home management and job tasks.

OR

B To improve performance in a specific activity

THEN

CONSIDER KEY CLIENT & STRATEGY

☐ *Memory within normal limits; could learn a strategy with multiple steps.*
☐ *Intact insight and high motivation but unrealistic about difficulty of addressing executive function impairments.*
☐ *Needs structure—easily distracted and impulsive.*
☐ *Facile with cell phone and responds to alarm.*
☐ *A wide variety of target tasks that would benefit from strategy.*

FINALLY

A Generate metacognitive strategy options:

1. *Goal management (stop, define task, list steps, execute, check)*
2. *Self-monitoring (use cell phone alarm and notes page to monitor task completion)*

B Generate task-specific strategy options:

_____
_____

FIGURE 8.2. Strategy selection process for case 1.

Consideration 3: Specifying the Desired Outcomes (Why?)

An important part of the planning process is to identify the desired outcome. The clinician must have a clear to the question *Why am I teaching this strategy?* Expectations for learning should be identified as part of the planning process. At this juncture, the clinician specifies measurable goals and objectives and plans for multilevel evaluation.

Goal Writing

Chapter 6 outlined the components necessary for writing treatment goals and objectives, including *treatment approach, treatment target, objective performance measurement, criterion, level of independence,* and *conditions/context.* The case applications at the end of this chapter have corresponding instructional planning worksheets (Figures 8.4 and 8.5). These worksheets provide examples of two long-term goals and two initial acquisition objectives and illustrate how goal components may be addressed.

Multilevel Evaluation

The clinician first needs to evaluate the client's understanding of, and ability to use, the strategy or demonstrate the steps in the strategy that have been taught. In addition, the

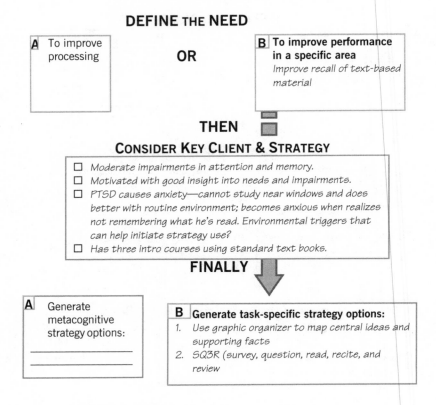

DEFINE THE **NEED**

A | To improve processing

OR

B | To improve performance in a specific area
Improve recall of text-based material

THEN

CONSIDER KEY CLIENT & STRATEGY

☐ *Moderate impairments in attention and memory.*
☐ *Motivated with good insight into needs and impairments.*
☐ *PTSD causes anxiety—cannot study near windows and does better with routine environment; becomes anxious when realizes not remembering what he's read. Environmental triggers that can help initiate strategy use?*
☐ *Has three intro courses using standard text books.*

FINALLY

A | Generate metacognitive strategy options:
_____
_____

B | Generate task-specific strategy options:
1. *Use graphic organizer to map central ideas and supporting facts*
2. *SQ3R (survey, question, read, recite, and review*

FIGURE 8.3. Strategy selection process for case 2.

clinician needs to measure whether strategy use is being generalized and maintained in the target environments and, if so, whether the strategy is addressing the identified need. Previous chapters have detailed the importance of multilevel evaluation for measuring these different types of outcomes. Five distinct types of clinical data have been defined: session data, generalization probes, maintenance probes, impact data, and efficacy data. When training clients to use strategies, these different data sources are necessary to (1) monitor the learning of strategy use and guide instruction decisions, (2) evaluate the client's implementation of the strategy in the intended context, and (3) measure the impact of strategy use. Table 8.5 (p. 203) provides examples of the different types of data and how they may be used to support instruction and the attainment of long-term goals.

Consideration 4: Designing the Individualized Plan (How)

By now the clinician has gathered the information necessary to design an individualized instructional plan. Form 8.1 in the Appendix (an enlarged version is on the book's page on The Guilford Press website) provides a worksheet to help the clinician design a plan that incorporates information collected during the evaluation. Figures 8.4 and 8.5 show completed instructional plans for the two case examples.

Long-Term Goal:	Improve task completion for home and work activities by implementing self-monitoring strategy independently at least four times a day with a "temptation to stray" rating of 1 or 0 for 1 full week.
Initial Acquisition Objectives:	Note in journal examples at home and work of how strategy could have helped or prevented identified task completion problems; verbalize and demonstrate all steps of the self-monitoring strategy in the clinic with no prompts.

(Specify target, approach, objective performance, independence, criterion, and context/conditions.)

WHAT will I teach the client to do?
Strategy (List Steps)

1. Identify target activity for 45-minute period and estimate time needed/desired using "Notes" application on cell phone

2. Set alarm on cell phone for 15-minute intervals

3. When alarm goes off, notice what's been completed during the interval

4. If you stayed on task, (a) take a moment to compliment self; (b) rate "temptation to stray" scale on Notes page and then continue on goal activity

OR

4. If you strayed from target task, (a) put away distracter task; (b) rate "5" on "temptation to stray" scale and return to goal activity

5. Repeat steps 3 and 4

6. Repeat steps 3 and 4

Strategy (Checklist)

☑ Strategy addresses identified need(s)
☑ Client has sufficient insight/awareness
☑ Strategy is customized to client
☑ Context/antecedent specified
☑ Progress measurement specified in long-term goal and/or acquisition objectives

Plan to enhance client motivation/engagement:	• Logging performance on cell phone using application familiar to client • In clinic check-ins will graph the ratings, show performance, and set weekly goals

WHEN and HOW will I teach the strategy?

Therapy Frequency:	1	/ week
Session Duration:	45	min
Therapy Duration:	6	Sessions, (Weeks,) Months

☑ There is opportunity for sufficient practice within sessions
☑ There is opportunity for sufficient practice across sessions

List materials needed to elicit strategy use and plan for varying stimuli with sufficient examples:	Cell phone; list of common home and work activities; journal for logging baseline information

What is the plan for progressing:	Practice in clinic session using items from journal and progress to reporting on actual performance. If generalization slow, provide reminders on cell phone during the week.

FIGURE 8.4. Sample completed instructional planning worksheet for case example 1.

Long-Term Goal:	Will use SQ3R strategy when reading assignments for history and literature for 3 weeks, as evidenced by homework agenda sheets; will improve performance on history and literature quizzes with no grades lower than a B.
Initial Acquisition Objectives:	Independently verbalize and demonstrate SQ3R strategy using class textbooks in clinic session

(Specify target, approach, objective performance, independence, criterion, and context/conditions.)

WHAT will I teach the client to do?
Strategy (List Steps)

1. SET YOUR HOMEWORK SPACE and REVIEW PREVIOUS READING: (a) Make sure you are in one of your routine spots; (b) do your breathing; (c) take out your homework agenda sheet and fill out the top and review any earlier entries.
2. SURVEY: Look through the chapter or reading section and read all the headings and subheadings and side text boxes.
3. QUESTION: List three main concepts you think you will learn from the reading and list two questions you have about the topic.
4. READ: Read the selected text that you identified on the agenda based on how much time you have.
5. RECITE: Every time you come to a new heading, go back and say in your head the main points and ideas from the previous section—mark on your sheet.
6. REVIEW: When you finish your selected section, review your questions, markings on the text and your homework agenda.

Strategy (Checklist)
☑ Strategy addresses identified need(s)
☑ Client has sufficient insight/awareness
☑ Strategy is customized to client
☑ Context/antecedent specified
☑ Progress measurement specified in long-term goal and/or acquisition objectives

Plan to enhance client motivation/engagement:	Keep graph of % recall of probe questions during strategy practice in clinic to show how strategy increases recall; verbally reinforce use of strategy as shown on homework agenda.

WHEN and HOW will I teach the strategy?

Therapy Frequency: _____2_____ / week
Session Duration: _____30_____ min   (Fall term)
Therapy Duration: _____8_____ Sessions, (Weeks,) Months

☑ There is opportunity for sufficient practice within sessions
☑ There is opportunity for sufficient practice across sessions

List materials needed to elicit strategy use and plan for varying stimuli with sufficient examples:	Textbooks and copies of homework agenda

What is the plan for progressing:	Progress from shorter to longer and more complex reading passages as strategy is mastered.

FIGURE 8.5. Sample completed instructional planning worksheet for case example 2.

TABLE 8.5. Examples of Strategy Measurement

Type of data	Examples	Purpose
Session data	• Number of strategy steps demonstrated in clinic with no prompting • Longest time interval client retained and demonstrated the entire strategy • Ability to independently list and describe each step in the strategy • Ability to independently state purpose and benefit of strategy • Number of possible applications client able to generate for using strategy during week	• Measure knowledge and ability to carry out strategy • Guide decisions about progress toward short-term objectives and indicate when to move on or provide more review
Generalization probes	• Number of entries in strategy diary • Number of teacher observations of independent strategy use • Number of strategy checklists completed during the week • Spouse/significant other's ratings in strategy log • Number of times lost place during reading session • Number of reminders to return to task	• Measure use of strategy in intended context
Maintenance probes	• Number of times strategy used weekly according to entries in the strategy log for initial 2 months following cessation of treatment • Number of strategy checklists turned in to teacher during weeks 2 and 3 after therapy	• Measure implementation of strategy over time
Impact data	• Grades on weekly history quizzes • Number of items on "to-do" list completed independently • Ability to greet church group members by name, as reported by spouse/significant other • Caregiver burden rating for spouse/significant other reminders • Improvements on the Inattention Rating Scale	• Measure whether implementation of strategy is meeting identified need
Efficacy data	• Changes on Behavioral Assessment of Dysexecutive Syndrome • Improvements on Paragraph Recall subtest; stable performance on Design Fluency subtest (control data)	• Primarily measure impairment-based changes

PIE: IMPLEMENTING SYSTEMATIC INSTRUCTION FOR METACOGNITIVE STRATEGY TRAINING

The planning process reviewed in the above section lays the groundwork for training that will be carried out in the implementation phase. The planning process has generated (1) the target strategy with its individual steps or behaviors, (2) measurable goals and objectives to monitor performance, and (3) training stimuli to facilitate learning the strategy components. The next phase is to *implement* the strategy training. The following section details the different training phases. The therapy dose needed to train a person with cognitive impairments to use strategies varies greatly depending on the client and strategy; separate training phases may not even be necessary. A review of compensatory memory strategy interventions reported a wide array of therapy doses, ranging from a single hour of training to programs that required 30 treatment hours over several weeks (West, 1995). There are no set guidelines for treatment dosage, and, unfortunately, these decisions are often driven by funding constraints. Careful documentation and measurement of client performance can help the clinician determine the optimal amount and schedule of therapy.

The following knowledge and skills are important for independent and effective strategy use and transfer to everyday life.

Knowledge
- The client must know the goals of the strategy and the specific procedures or steps involved.
- The client must recognize tasks or environments that will benefit from strategy use.
- The client must know how strategy use will meet his or her needs.

Affective and Motivational States
- The client should believe that the strategy will be useful, the level of effort to use the strategy will be worthwhile, and that he or she is capable of implementing the strategy.
- The client should feel motivated to use the strategy and be engaged in the process of strategy development and training.

Skills
- The client must have the requisite cognitive, sensory, and motor skills to make decisions about *how* and *when* to use the strategy.

The sequence of steps in the training program depends on the extent to which the client meets the above prerequisites. The clinician will begin the implementation phase by assessing the client's knowledge, emotional disposition, and relevant skills. The strategy has been selected with input from the client using the PIE planning process. The clinician can interview the client to ascertain the depth and strength of knowledge and skills surrounding the selected strategy in order to identify where to begin in therapy. Specifically, using the above list as an assessment guide, the clinician can generate questions and ask the client to demonstrate knowledge. Sample questions are listed below.

Sample Questions Assessing Requisite Knowledge
- "If you implement [the target strategy], how do you think it will help you?"
- "What are the specific steps you would follow to apply [the target strategy]?"
- "When do you think you would use [the target strategy]?"

Sample Questions Assessing Requisite Affective and Motivational States
- "If our therapy time is successful in teaching you to use [the target strategy] in your everyday life, do you think it will be valuable? Why or why not?"
- "How hard do you think it will be to do [the target strategy]?"
- "Do you think it will be worth it?"

Requisite Skills (Cognitive, Physical/Sensory, Metacognitive)

- "Show me how you might use our strategy to do [the goal activity]."
- "Show me what you would do if [a given circumstance or event] occurred?" (Provide scenarios for client to demonstrate ability to use, not use, and adapt strategy appropriately.)

If the client lacks requisite knowledge and beliefs, the acquisition phase of training will need to address teaching these concepts and information (see Chapter 5). Clients with milder cognitive impairments, particularly those with good executive function, may be able to see a demonstration of the strategy, use it in their home environment, and quickly become independent in applying it to a variety of situations; others will require formal training and planning for generalization and maintenance. Below we outline training phases with the understanding that the clinician will identify which areas need to be addressed for any given client.

Initial Acquisition Phase of Training

The purpose of therapy in this phase is to establish the client's conceptual knowledge about how and when to use the target strategy and to have him or her demonstrate the basic components. For some clients, the clinician may need to teach this information as a set of concrete facts. For example:

- "The goals of this strategy are to help me _____."
- "I use this strategy when _____."
- "These are the steps of the strategy _____."

The clinician can write down the information and have the client assist in generating the answers, and then review the information using the errorless and distributed practice regimen discussed in Chapter 5 for training facts and concepts. Form 8.2 in the Appendix (an enlarged version is on the book's page on The Guilford Press website) is a sample data collection sheet monitoring a client's learning of basic strategy information. Four questions are asked at the beginning and end of the therapy session. The question wording should be varied to avoid a stimulus-bound response. As explained in Chapters 1 and 5, clients with severe memory impairments may learn a hyperspecific response, so that the same words trigger an automatic response that is not processed consciously. For example, the clinician may vary the phrasing of the question "How can your strategy be useful to you?" to "Why would you want to use your strategy?" or "Share some benefits you might get from using this strategy." This variation helps train the concept and prevent hyperspecificity. Figure 8.6 is a sample completed data sheet.

A second goal of the initial acquisition phase is to ensure that the client can perform the strategy correctly in an optimal context (e.g., with maximum support and structure and no distractions). The clinician teaches the client the individual steps or components of the strategy, typically using the errorless learning and distributed practice methods described in Chapter 5. Readers should review the information in that chapter, particularly the principles for establishing a new behavior when a client has cognitive impairments.

Knowledge Questions	DATE					
	10/5 (beginning of session)	10/7 (end of session)	10/12 (beginning of session)	10/14 (end of session)	10/19 (beginning of session)	10/21 (end of session)
What is the name of your strategy?	M	A	A	I	I	I
Describe the steps in your strategy	M	A	A	I	I	I
What are examples of when you would use your strategy?	M	M	A	A	I	I
How can your strategy be useful to you?	M	M	M	A	A	I

M = Modeled—presented entire answer
A = Assisted—gave partial response
I = Independent, no cues

FIGURE 8.6. Sample completed data sheet for measuring strategy knowledge.

Acquisition of the strategy often requires providing explicit cues to prompt steps or components. The clinician begins by modeling strategy use, then may introduce one of the following learning supports as the strategy is being practiced:

- Checklist of the strategy steps
- Written cue cards prompting strategy steps
- Environmental cue (e.g., alarm) to initiate strategy
- Client states each step or a keyword representing that step as it is implemented

Ideally, the client internalizes the steps of the strategy, and these supports are withdrawn during the mastery phase—although some clients may benefit from or require an ongoing reference such as a checklist or auditory prompt. The clinician demonstrates the different components of the strategy and then has the client implement it. With practice, the client should be able to retain the target strategy steps over increasing time intervals. This retention may be achieved through the use of distributed practice, using the aforementioned learning supports as determined by the clinician. Figure 8.7 shows a completed data sheet for recording client performance for a client learning to use a self-talk strategy. The data were taken early in the acquisition phase. This sample client has already demonstrated knowledge of the strategy, understanding of the benefits and how to use it, and has moved on to actually practicing the strategy during a structured therapy session. Once the client can independently demonstrate the use of the strategy

Strategy: Verbal mediation

Long-Term Goal: Complete all household tasks (cooking and cleaning) on chore list within scheduled time frame with no prompting from husband

Initial Acquisition Short-Term Objective(s): Independently use the self-talk strategy, up to the "say aloud" step for home chores, that is practiced during the clinic session

Strategy Steps/Component	Session Probe Data				
	1/25	1/27	1/30	2/1	
5. When completed, fill out chore performance sheet					
4b. Say step in your head as you complete it					
4a. Say each step/action aloud as you do it	Model	I X2 (2 steps done indep)	I X3	+	
3. Begin task	+			+	
2. Gather needed materials	+	+	+	+	
1. Select chore from list and state chore and target time aloud	+	+	+	+	
Supports (e.g., written cues, checklist, say aloud, auditory prompts):	Index card with steps listed	Index card with steps listed	Faded index card	Faded index card	
Motivational/Engagement Strategies:	Records own progress on performance sheet	Records own progress on performance sheet	Records own progress on performance sheet	Records own progress on performance sheet	
Generalization Programming during Training:					
Comments:		Understands concept of saying steps aloud—needs reminder to do it	Understands concept of saying steps aloud—needs reminder to do it	Ready to move to inner speech step (4b)	

Note: Graph the number of steps performed successfully each time the routine is probed.

FIGURE 8.7. Sample completed progress monitoring form.

on target tasks in the clinic, training will move on to the generalization phase. There may be instances when the strategy can be trained directly on the actual target from the beginning. For example, people with mild impairments may be able to learn the strategy and take it home for use immediately. For people with more severe impairments, practice in the actual context is optimal, as generalization is then automatic.

Mastery and Generalization Phase of Training

The mastery phase occurs when knowledge about the strategy purpose and procedures has been acquired but strategy implementation is not consistent and has not been generalized to the natural environment. For clients who have executive function impairments but relatively intact declarative memory, moving to the mastery and generalization phases may occur after a single session. Clients with moderate-to-severe declarative learning impairments may require more practice and review to learn the basic strategy steps. Information about when to implement the strategy also may need to be taught formally. Failure to generalize treatment gains to everyday life is the hallmark of executive function impairments, so these patients will require specific attention to generalization as a part of their training process, as discussed in Chapter 2 and below.

The goal of the mastery and generalization phase of training is to increase the fluency and automaticity with which the client implements the strategy in everyday life. These goals are achieved by attending to the following three aspects of training.

Fading Learning Supports

To fade learning supports is to progressively withdraw supports such as clinician prompts and cues. The client's internalization of the strategies makes this fading possible. For example, if the client is saying each step aloud as it is completed, this will be faded to inner speech ("Say it in your head"). Similarly, the client may go from physically checking off each step on a checklist to using the list as a written reference when needed. It is critical to remember that some patients will *always* depend on external cues and prompts to use their strategies, particularly patients who have severe memory or executive function impairments and those who need to use the strategy in an unpredictable context. If an external cue or prompt is effective, efficient, and preferred by the client, there is no a priori reason to remove it.

Incorporating or Increasing Stimulus Variability

For most clients, unless their cognitive impairments are very mild, generalization or transfer of learning will need to be planned and trained explicitly. A main goal of this stage is to identify triggers that will facilitate the *initiation of strategy use* in the *target context*. These triggers are identified in the planning process and then incorporated during this phase of training. Examples of generalization training methods include:

- Varying training stimuli so that the strategy can be triggered by a variety of environmental cues.
- Involving people from the natural environment who will serve as "cues" in everyday life.

- Training strategy use in the target everyday context.
- Outlining a home program for practicing strategy use, in collaboration with client and home supports.
- Providing the client with everyday reminders to implement the strategy between therapy sessions, using cues such as voice mail, text messages, or e-mail.

Increasing Engagement

It may be difficult for the client to maintain motivation and interest in using the strategy beyond the clinic, particularly if it is difficult to use. Although this issue was addressed earlier in training by collaborating with the client in strategy selection, it also is important to consider strategies that will help the client maintain motivation and engagement after discharge. As discussed in Chapter 3, motivation and engagement are important predictors of long-term treatment adherence. Methods to increase self efficacy and commitment for implementing a strategy include:

- Creating a customized log to help client and/or support people record strategy use and impact, as a way to provide a concrete record of improved functioning with strategy use
- Conducting motivational interviewing (see Chapter 3; Miller & Rollnick, 2002) wherein the clinician asks questions that encourage the client to explore situations when the strategy would have been useful, even if the client was not able to implement it.
- Collaborating with the client to identify potential benefits and barriers to strategy use in daily living and developing alternative plans.
- Developing a record sheet showing the benefit of strategy use (e.g., time saved, number or type of goals completed, improvements in task accuracy, duration of time devoted to target task).

Maintenance Phase

As described in earlier chapters, the maintenance phase employs therapy methods that increase the likelihood that a rehabilitation target will be retained after therapy ends. To accommodate this phase, the clinician actively plans how to avoid abandonment of strategy use once therapeutic support is no longer available. For a strategy to be maintained, it must become automatic and internalized—two processes that require high-frequency practice. The primary methods that promote ongoing implementation of a strategy are the *incorporation of natural supports* and *cumulative review* (see Chapter 4). The techniques listed above for increasing metacognitive engagement facilitate the involvement of natural supports and provide a mechanism for checking in on strategy use. The use of diaries, logs, and "check-ins" can be very helpful for maintaining strategy use, particularly during the phase when therapy supports are withdrawn.

In terms of long-term strategy use, it is important to acknowledge that contexts and situations change; mechanisms need to be in place for reevaluating strategy effectiveness. Depending on the service delivery model and complexity of the strategy, the client may need follow-up visits or phone support to maintain strategy use over time.

PIE: EVALUATING OUTCOMES
OF METACOGNITIVE STRATEGY INSTRUCTION

This manual has emphasized the importance of multilevel outcome evaluation. As noted, the planning process results in a long-term outcome goal and short-term objectives. Examples of different types of data needed to evaluate outcomes are shown in Table 8.5, as previously noted, and provided in the following section on case applications.

As reviewed earlier under the planning section of this chapter, the clinician needs to measure progress toward the long-term goal and the short-term objectives by measuring the *accuracy, fluency, or efficiency in completing the components of the strategy* and by evaluating the *use of these skills in different contexts*. The clinician measures whether the client can implement the strategy with specific types of prompting and support; these comprise the session data. As strategy implementation becomes consistent, strategy use is measured under different conditions, including everyday environments; these are the generalization and maintenance data.

A clinician also measures *impact of strategy use* and determines whether the strategy achieved the desired functional impact in the client's everyday life. For example, if a client has learned a goal completion strategy and is implementing it in the target environments, the clinician should measure whether strategy use results in improved task completion. Similarly, if the client was taught a strategy to help remember specific information and was using it in the desired context, it is important to determine whether using this strategy resulted in improved recall of the target information. Data at this level of evaluation are often collected via home logs and interviews with the client and his or her natural support providers. A clinician may also use pre- and posttherapy impact by collecting baseline measures on task performance in the natural setting and then comparing those measures to performance after strategy training.

The *collection of efficacy data* is also an important evaluation component. In some cases, it may be expected that a client's cognitive processing will improve as a result of strategy training. If improved processing is an expectation, the clinician should collect pre- and postefficacy data using a relevant standardized test. For example, if executive function improvement is anticipated as a result of successful strategy instruction, the clinician may administer a standardized executive function test before and after training. To minimize the possibility that improvements are due to factors other than training (e.g., spontaneous recovery or improvements in mood), the clinician should collect data on some aspect of performance that was *not* targeted in treatment and therefore is not expected to change. For example, an expected result of training the use of a reading comprehension strategy would be improved retention of reading material, whereas improvement in reading fluency or speed would not be expected to change; hence both parameters might be measured to demonstrate therapeutic effectiveness. Effectiveness data are not only the cornerstone of ethical and efficient service delivery but are also essential for building a case for reimbursement. Data on untreated targets are relatively easy to collect, so the collection of these data should be a priority in treatment.

PUTTING IT ALL TOGETHER: CASE APPLICATIONS

In the remainder of the chapter we provide examples to show the application of the PIE framework to strategy training with actual clients. We begin by describing two examples from the research literature from the perspective of the PIE framework. We selected the imagery strategy training described by Kaschel and colleagues (2002), because it used a rigorous experimental design with detailed description of the training process and reported positive outcomes. We also summarize the strategy training curriculum evaluated in a pilot study by Huckans et al. (2010). This study offers a description of a curriculum with a logical scope and sequence for teaching a broad range of strategies to people with cognitive impairments. The research examples are followed by the description of two case applications that represent composite clients from our own practices.

Two Examples from the Literature

Kaschel et al. (2002)

Kaschel and colleagues (2002) conducted a randomized controlled clinical trial to evaluate a visual imagery training program. The goal of the imagery strategy was for patients to rapidly generate simple but distinct images of information that typically would be encoded verbally (e.g., conversations, text, lists of prospective actions to be completed) and use these images as retrieval cues for targets on prospective memory tasks. Treatment efficacy was measured by comparing recall in patients who received this training to that of patients receiving other types of memory treatment.

The program had two training phases. The first phase, analogous to the acquisition phase in the PIE framework, taught participants the basic skill of quickly generating images. There were three components: (1) eliciting motivation for imagery training by showing participants how generation of autobiographical images enhanced their recall; (2) providing practice with rapid generation of images for simple objects; and (3) providing practice with generation and retrieval of images for simple actions. Acquisition of the basic skill of generating images was hierarchically organized so that tasks systematically increased in difficulty. Initially objects and actions were presented visually, using video, then gradually the screen was withdrawn and object and action names were read to participants (no visual cues). In addition, the rate of stimulus presentation was gradually increased as participants became more adept at generating and recalling images. In the final step of the acquisition phase, participants recalled several objects and three complex actions. Once a participant could recall three complex actions using self-generated pictures, after a filled retention interval of 90 seconds, he or she was considered to have met the learning criteria for the acquisition phase. Acquisition criteria were established for each level of difficulty, and, if failures occurred, the training continued at the same level until criteria were reached. As such, this procedure followed the instructional principles described throughout this manual of aiming for high rates of correct practice and using distributed practice.

The second phase of training, the individualized transfer period, was analogous to the generalization and mastery phases of the PIE framework. The researchers selected individualized verbal targets and prospective memory tasks that were relevant to each participant (e.g., books related to the person's job, newspapers that an individual read, or an individual's appointments or target things to do). Participants were taught to identify the target information to be remembered, consider how imagery could be used to remember this information, and then practice using the imagery. Each participant's recall was recorded.

The researchers described multiple types of evaluation, another component of the

PIE framework. They recorded session data on the accuracy of recall using imagery during the acquisition and transfer phases of learning, and these data were used to determine when the participant could advance to the next level of difficulty. The efficacy of the intervention was evaluated using standardized neuropsychological tests, including a story recall test and an "appointments" test. Generalization was measured by relatives' ratings of frequency of memory problems. Researchers also collected control data on neuropsychological functions not expected to improve with treatment (e.g., selective attention). Maintenance data were collected at a 3-month follow-up visit. Results showed that patients with mild memory impairments learned to generate distinct images rapidly and use them successfully to remember either information they had read or actions they intended to carry out. There was specific improvement on neuropsychological tests related to verbal recall and prospective memory but not on tests of selective attention. Relatives reported decreased frequency of memory failures in everyday life, and all of these effects were maintained over 3 months.

In summary, a metacognitive strategy employing visual imagery was shown to be highly efficacious when training was systematic and incorporated motivation and skill acquisition, generalization, and maintenance. This program provides a training model for any type of metacognitive strategy.

Huckans et al. (2010)

Huckans and colleagues (2010) conducted a pilot study to examine the effects of a group-based cognitive strategy training (CST) on reported cognitive problems, psychiatric symptoms, daily functioning, and compensatory strategy use in veterans with persistent mild cognitive disorder due to combat-related traumatic brain injury. Participants were 21 veterans randomized to five separate groups, 16 of whom completed the group therapy. One purpose of the study was to evaluate whether the intervention was feasible in the Veteran's Administration service-delivery model and whether veterans would enroll in and attend the group. The first two groups were conducted in six weekly 2-hour sessions. Participants said they wanted a slower pace that allowed for more discussion and clarification of information, and based on their feedback, the last three groups were conducted in eight weekly 2-hour sessions.

The CST treatment provided training in both internal strategy use such as employing visual imagery to facilitate verbal recall, and also formal problem-solving strategies to compensate for executive dysfunction. Many of the strategies were similar to the attention, memory, and problem-solving strategies described earlier in this chapter. Treatment also included training in the use of external aids, as described in Chapter 7, including advanced organizers and assistive devices to promote completion of daily tasks, including planning activities and routines to encourage a healthy lifestyle (e.g., exercise, social activities, diet).

The instructional approach was a semimanualized curriculum with training organized into a series of six modules: (1) course overview and psychoeducation; (2) lifestyle strategies; (3) organizational strategies, routines, and prioritization; (4) attention strategies; (5) memory strategies; and (6) goal-planning and problem-solving strategies. The curriculum was sequenced from simple to complex with periodic cumulative review. The facilitator first presented the concept and rationale for the strategies being taught in that module, and then modeled them. The group then practiced one strategy in class, again at home, and discussed the results at the next session. Each session was structured in four parts: (1) review of home practice of strategies from the previous week and provision of feedback and encouragement; (2) interactive didactic presentation of new information and strategies; (3) class activities and discussion to model and practice that week's target strategy; and (4) assignment of home practice exercises for new strategies.

Treatment effects were measured via a battery of questionnaires, given pre- and posttreatment to assess the generalized use of strategies taught and their perceived utility, in addition to measures of psychiatric and cognitive symptom severity, adaptive functioning, and life satisfaction. Following the group CST treatment, veterans reported significantly increased use and perceived usefulness of cognitive strategies and compensatory aids, reduced depression and cognitive symptom severity, and increased life satisfaction. The authors commented that the reduction in depression and increase in life satisfaction were noteworthy given that treatment focused only on cognitive compensatory strategies and the emotional difficulties that often co-occur with brain injury. The study supports the implementation of systematic instruction that provides modeling, practice, and generalization training. The in-clinic session allowed for the acquisition phase of training, and home practice and follow-up discussions promoted generalization. The curriculum also provided instruction in strategy knowledge and purpose when first introducing each strategy. Thus, the overall treatment approach provides indirect empirical support for the techniques reviewed in this chapter.

Case 1: Esther

Description of Client

The client, Esther, was a 54-year-old woman referred for cognitive rehabilitation 2 years after surgical resection, chemotherapy, and radiation to treat brain cancer. Although the treatment was successful in treating the cancer, it had left her with cognitive impairments. She was receiving outpatient services from a speech–language pathologist because she complained of not being able to organize and complete tasks. She ran a small bookkeeping business from her home and reported difficulty meeting deadlines. She also described frustration about the messy state of her home. She lived with her husband, who was retired, and had two grown children who lived out of state. Esther's insurance provider authorized one outpatient visit for assessment and five visits for treatment.

Planning Phase

The speech–language pathologist initiated a needs assessment to address the four PIE planning considerations (*Who*, *What*, *Where* and *Why*). Results of the interview with the client and her husband, as well as supplementary cognitive testing to evaluate memory, attention, and executive functions, revealed the following client profile:

- *Key cognitive findings.* Esther's scores on standardized memory and attention tests were within normal limits. Scores on tests of executive function were in the moderately impaired range, particularly on tests requiring self-regulation and the ability to monitor completion of multiple tasks. She was observed to respond impulsively on some tests. In regard to daily cognition, Esther's premorbid knowledge of bookkeeping and domestic tasks (e.g., cleaning the bathroom, organizing the mail) was intact. She was proficient in using a computer and fluently used multiple applications on her cell phone.

• *Key affective variables.* Esther reported that she was frustrated by negative changes in her performance on home and work tasks, and she appeared highly motivated to improve her situation. Her husband stated that although Esther was self-aware and frustrated by her difficulties, this awareness tended to occur after a task or activity had not gone well. She tended to be overly optimistic and dive into tasks with limited self-regulation, and not use her prior negative experiences to guide future behavior. He said that Esther became resentful if he tried to assist.

• *Environmental variables.* Esther's husband kept the home environment organized and typically cleaned up the multiple projects Esther started but did not complete.

Esther's goal was to improve task completion for home and work activities and eliminate the problem of "multiple things started and nothing completed." Based on the results of the interview and testing, it was clear that Esther needed a strategy that would provide structure, help her control her impulsivity, and improve her task persistence. As shown in Figure 8.2, the clinician synthesized key information gathered in the assessment and followed a strategy selection process. Working together, Esther and the clinician identified a goal of developing a strategy to improve executive functions, specifically the ability to improve persistence on home and work tasks. The clinician then documented the key variables important to consider when selecting a strategy and using this information, and presented a number of different types of goal completion strategies to Esther and her husband. Two strategies were of most interest to them: (1) goal management training (GMT; Levine et al., 2000) and (2) a customized, self-monitoring, task-persistence strategy using Esther's cell phone alarm and the Notes application. The second strategy is based on principles of teaching self-monitoring that encourage goal setting, self-evaluation and error correction (e.g., Cicerone & Giacino, 1992). After discussion it was decided that the most useful approach would be a customized strategy that helped Esther set goals, monitor progress, and reflect on performance. It was felt that this approach would provide more structure and accountability than a goal management strategy that might not address her tendency to stray from a target task and begin something new. Esther and her husband collaborated with the therapist to design a strategy that would build on her strengths in technology use and compensate for her difficulties with self-monitoring and task persistence. To do this, it was necessary for Esther to identify the target goal, monitor progress at a specified time, record performance, and reflect on her temptation to start a new project. The strategy steps, long-term goals, short term acquisition objectives are documented on the instructional planning worksheet shown in Figure 8.4.

A multilevel evaluation was planned. It was determined that the ultimate outcome measure for impact of the strategy would be the number of home and work tasks completed. Esther and her husband kept a "task journal" for a 1-week period that documented tasks started and completed as intended; interfering tasks that Esther started and that interrupted the completion of the target task; and Esther's and her husband's frustration levels using a 1–4 rating scale and the couple's own rating descriptors (e.g., 1 = no problem; 4 = feel like yelling). It was also predicted that if Esther became proficient at using the self-monitoring strategy, generalization of task completion would occur; hence the executive function tests administered in the assessment were considered preefficacy tests.

Implementation Phase

The acquisition phase of training initially focused on motivational variables and increasing Esther's knowledge of how her self-monitoring strategy might help some of the problems identified in the "task journal." Esther was able to describe how her strategy might have allowed her to complete specific bookkeeping tasks. For example, she described how the strategy would have helped her continue entering account data and resisting checking e-mail—a scenario that had resulted in her not entering target account data. Esther was able to verbalize the steps of the strategy after several demonstrations and made herself a small cue card to post at her computer. Esther then practiced using the strategy in the clinic for three sessions, taking examples from her task journal. She was independent in implementing the strategy and demonstrated proficiency in setting the alarm on her cell phone, checking her task performance when the alarm came, entering "temptation to stray from task" ratings on her Notes application of her cell phone, and then continuing her task. (The temptation to stray rating was a 1–5 scale where 1 = no temptation and 5 = gave in to temptation and started an unplanned task). In the second session Esther demonstrated the six steps of the strategy without prompting, while completing her computer bookkeeping tasks in the clinic.

The generalization phase of training focused on increasing the range of tasks that Esther practiced in the clinic and reinforcing her use of the strategy at home. Initially, she practiced using the strategy on bookkeeping tasks as she could do those on the computer during the therapy session. During Sessions 3 and 4, the clinician began alternating these computer tasks with home tasks such as folding laundry and writing out grocery lists from the week's recipe plans. Esther brought materials from her home (e.g., basket of laundry, cookbooks/paper/pencil) to therapy and practiced the strategy in relation to this variety of tasks. Esther's husband came to therapy during the third session and was trained to complete performance logs to measure her generalization of strategy use at home. Because Esther felt sensitive about her husband overseeing her performance, she and the clinician decided that Esther would complete the performance logs in the task journal and her husband would just add comments from his perspective. According to performance logs Esther brought to the fourth session, she was using the strategy successfully at home.

Evaluation

The fifth and last treatment session was used both as a maintenance/follow-up session and to administer outcome measures. It was scheduled 4 weeks after the fourth session. Esther and her husband brought in the performance logs and reported that the strategy was working well. The performance logs showed that Esther was implementing the strategy successfully to complete four to six goal tasks per day. She rarely recorded a "temptation to stray" rating of greater than 1. The couple had made one adjustment to the strategy. Esther decided to set the alarm for 30-minute rather than 15-minute intervals, as she was now able to stick to the task for this amount of time, and a longer task interval allowed her to make more progress and to feel reinforced for her persistence. At this final session, the executive function battery was readministered, and Esther had improved one standard deviation on the two subtests requiring multitasking and self-monitoring.

Case 2: Anders

Description of Client

Anders, a 24-year-old male combat veteran, was referred for outpatient cognitive rehabilitation services for impairments due to a mild TBI that resulted from repeated blast injuries incurred during a 3-year combat tour. He was also diagnosed with posttraumatic stress disorder (PTSD). Anders had completed high school and had no previous learning difficulties, although he reported being unmotivated in school as an adolescent and had mostly C's and D's as grades. At the time of therapy, he was enrolled in several general studies courses at the local community college in preparation for transfer to a 4-year university to pursue a teaching credential. He was living independently with his girlfriend. Anders had received counseling to manage anxiety symptoms, and the counselor referred him to a psychologist for cognitive rehabilitation when Anders reported difficulties recalling what he read in his school textbooks. During the initial interview, Anders reported that he completely understood his textbook assignments while he was reading, but later could not recall the information sufficiently to answer questions on a quiz. He had tried using extensive repetition and note taking, but these methods had not improved his performance.

Planning Phase

The psychologist initiated a needs assessment following the four planning considerations (*Who*, *What*, *Where*, and *Why*). Results of the initial interview with Anders and subsequent neuropsychological testing revealed the following key findings:

• *Key cognitive findings.* Anders's IQ was within normal limits. The only cognitive deficits were a moderate impairment in working memory and a mild impairment in new declarative learning for verbal information. A reading assessment revealed immediate comprehension of paragraph-length material to be within normal limits, but moderate impairments in delayed recall.

• *Key affective variables.* Anders described significant anxiety symptoms that were characterized by profuse sweating, rapid heart rate, and a sense of needing to urgently relocate. These symptoms often occurred when he was studying. His descriptions of difficulties suggested intact self-awareness and insight. Anders was very motivated to perform well in his classes and was eager to pursue a teaching career.

• *Environmental variables.* Anders described difficulty concentrating if he was near a window, if someone approached his table, or if he heard ambient noise. When his anxiety began, it would escalate and he would need to cease the study session.

Results of the interview and testing revealed the need for a reading strategy that would elaborate content and allow him to more deeply process information and connect it to existing semantic networks in order to compensate for impairments in working memory. It was also clear that the strategy would need to help him organize his study environment in order to manage anxiety. As depicted in Figure 8.3, the psychologist described options for several different reading strategies. These included use of a graphic organizer to "map" main ideas and supporting facts, and using the SQ3R strategy to structure a process of previewing, active reading, and reviewing. The psychologist observed Anders's attempt at both strategies using a dynamic assessment. The latter strategy, SQ3R, was clearly superior at helping Anders retain the content of a reading passage from one of his textbooks.

The psychologist mapped out the instructional plan, as shown in Figure 8.5. The first step of the strategy was to identify a study location that felt safe and would minimize the chance for anxiety symptoms to occur. The psychologist and Anders worked together to integrate the anxiety-management breathing strategies that Anders had been taught in counseling with establishing criteria for a location conducive to studying. The criteria were used to generate a list of places that could become routine spots that were quiet, had low traffic, and did not have windows, including library study rooms and the loft in his apartment. Breathing techniques were then used if he started to feel anxious while studying.

The evaluation plan was to collect (1) session data to measure Anders's learning of the strategy steps; (2) strategy generalization and maintenance data, by having Anders bring in homework agendas that he used to record where he studied and what he accomplished; and (3) impact data, by having Anders report his performance on class quizzes.

Implementation Phase

The acquisition phase of training initially focused on teaching Anders to describe and demonstrate each of the six steps of his reading strategy. Anders brought in his textbooks, and the psychologist selected different chapters to use as training stimuli in conjunction with a homework agenda form they had created. The form included a written list of the six strategy steps and a description of each. Initially Anders demonstrated each step by reading the step aloud and completing it. The written list was faded so that there was just an initial word or two: *Homework Space*, *Survey* (reading material), *Question*, *Read*, *Recite*, and *Review*. Accuracy data were kept on whether Anders could describe and complete each step with just this written cue list. Within three sessions over 2 weeks Anders was independent in implementing his strategy for selected passages. There was no need to provide initial training on motivational factors or strategy knowledge, as Anders presented with high motivation and awareness of how study strategies could help him meet his goals.

The generalization phase of training was concurrent with the acquisition phase, as Anders was asked to bring in his actual homework agendas from the very beginning of strategy instruction. Strategy successes and difficulties were reviewed using the homework agendas. As Anders became more efficient and independent in using his reading strategy during the therapy session, the clinician selected reading passages that were longer and more complex. As Anders began to successfully use his reading strategy, therapy was lessened to once every 2 weeks. Maintenance probes evaluating strategy use were taken by counting the number of times the strategy was used, as reported on the homework agenda.

Evaluation

The impact of strategy training was evaluated by examining Anders's performance on his class reading quizzes. He had received a C or D on all of his quizzes prior to his midterm (the first 2 weeks of therapy). He began to demonstrate independent, accurate use of his strategy during Week 3 of therapy, and his quiz averages improved. He received three B's and one C during the subsequent weeks of the term. Interestingly, Anders reported that his anxiety symptoms during study periods had greatly diminished. He shared that he no longer needed to be as rigid about selecting study spaces and was able to focus without anxiety when sitting at different study desks throughout the library. He felt that the self-regulation imposed by the reading strategy process provided him with a sense of control, and his improved reading performance helped mitigate anxiety.

SUMMARY

This chapter applied the PIE framework to the selection and training of strategies to help people monitor their own thinking or behavior. There is substantial research evidence supporting the training of metacognitive strategies or routines to help people regulate their own thoughts and behavior to improve goal completion or performance on target activities. The planning process emphasizes selecting strategies based on an identified need and the client's cognitive profile while considering various strategy characteristics such as complexity. Delineating the components or steps in the strategy and identifying outcome measures are other key planning considerations. The implementation process includes training knowledge about when, where, and why to use the strategy in addition to providing systematic instruction for how to implement the strategy with models and prompts during the acquisition phase and facilitated opportunities to practice using the strategy in naturalistic settings during the generalization phase. Evaluation will include monitoring the client's learning of the strategy components during the initial training and ultimately measuring strategy use and impact in the intended environment.

The steps are summarized in Figure 8.8.

Summary of Clinical Sequence to Train Metacognitive Strategies

1. Complete needs assessment and planning to identify client needs and effective strategy, define treatment goals, and establish training parameters (see instructional planning worksheet, Form 8.1).
2. Train strategy knowledge and requisite concepts for using strategy (see data sheet for measuring strategy knowledge, Form 8.2).
3. Begin each session with a probe to determine retention and where to begin therapy (see progress monitoring form, Form 8.3).
4. Use instructional techniques that match the phase of learning, with more prompts and cues during the acquisition phase, and structured opportunities to practice and reflect on the effects of using strategy in natural contexts in the generalization phase of training.

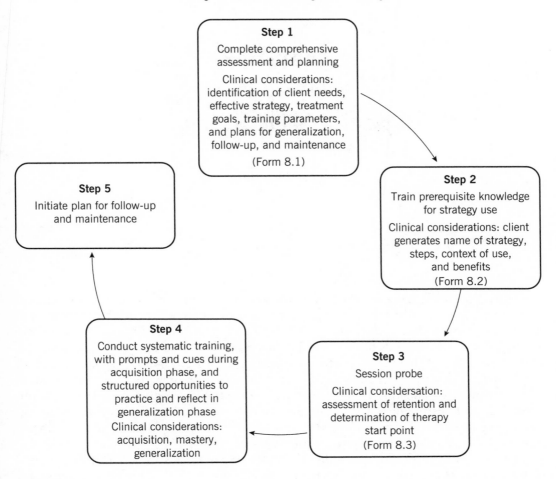

FIGURE 8.8. Summary of clinical training sequence for metacognitive strategy instruction.

APPLICATION EXERCISES

Carefully review the first case describing the clinical program for Esther. Rethink the case application selecting a different strategy that would also be a match to the information provided in the case study. For example, you might select one of the problem-solving or goal management strategies listed in Table 8.1. After selecting the strategy, answer the following questions.

1. Provide a rationale for the strategy you selected based on the information provided in the case application. Why might the strategy you selected also be a good match for Esther?

2. Complete the instructional planning worksheet (Form 8.1) with hypothetical information that would be reasonable in this case.

3. Develop a set of questions to assess strategy knowledge (see Form 8.2).

4. Generate hypothetical data to complete progress monitoring probes for two sessions (see Form 8.3). Write a paragraph interpreting the data you created.

CHAPTER 9

Social Skills Training

Changes in social functioning are among the most common and disabling consequences of acquired brain injury (ABI) and can have a major influence on work outcomes and independent living. As a result, social skills are a common target of rehabilitation. There are literally hundreds of books and electronic media dedicated to social skills training, and almost none of them is supported by evidence from studies of individuals with ABI (Ylvisaker, Turkstra, & Coelho, 2005). This limitation is important to keep in mind when planning social skills intervention: what works with children who have developmental disabilities might not work for individuals who had normal premorbid social development. It also is important to remember that improvements in social *skills* do not automatically translate into improvements in social *life* (Cavell, 1990), which is the ultimate goal of therapy. Therefore, rather than focusing only on social skills training, this chapter presents an overall framework for intervention aimed at fostering meaningful improvement in clients' social lives.

A FRAMEWORK FOR IMPROVING SOCIAL FUNCTIONING

Three themes in the cognitive rehabilitation literature have particular relevance for treating social functioning:

1. There is clear evidence across cognitive domains that *treatment must be individualized* to be effective.
2. For individuals with acquired cognitive disorders, there is *little evidence that discrete social skills training automatically generalizes to untreated skills and contexts*. Skills required for learning social behaviors (e.g., procedural learning) are not the same skills needed to generalize behaviors to novel contexts (e.g., executive functions and declarative memory; see Chapter 1 for a discussion of different memory types).
3. For highly proceduralized (i.e., automatic, routine) behaviors like social skills, *change requires many repetitions*.

In other words, training discrete skills such as turn taking or eye contact is unlikely to be effective unless those behaviors are directly relevant to the client's social life, and therapy is delivered with high frequency in the target context. Traditional training often relies on didactic instruction (e.g., "A good listener sits upright, turns toward the speaker, and makes good eye contact"), but knowledge about social skills is only a small piece of the puzzle. Success in social interactions relies on many skills, including social perception, declarative and procedural memory, working memory, and executive functions. The client needs to identify the appropriate time to use the skill, remember the correct skill to use, and be able to execute it in a timely and flexible manner, modifying goals and behavior based on ongoing feedback from others. Many clients with ABI have impairments in all of these functions, so it is no surprise that this traditional didactic approach has been generally ineffective in improving their social lives (Ylvisaker & Feeney, 1998).

An alternative to the traditional didactic training approach uses the International Classification of Functioning, Disability, and Health (ICF), which was presented in Chapter 4 and has been a theme throughout this book. Figure 9.1 applies the ICF model to Jay, a 25-year-old male who, 5 years after sustaining a TBI, sought therapy to help him "meet people." We return to Jay in the case example at the end of this chapter, but for now consider his strengths and limitations and the required elements for his intervention plan. Jay was highly motivated to seek therapy—to the point that he referred himself to the clinic—and had a clearly articulated goal and measurable deficits in social functions that could be remediated. The likelihood of reaching his goal was greatly reduced, however, by his lack of access to social activities. He also lacked a regular social partner with whom to practice his new skills and who could provide support and cues to help him behave appropriately. Compare this client to Ned, also age 25 years, whose ICF profile appears in Figure 9.2. Ned had more severe impairments in behavior regulation than Jay did and consistently made inappropriate comments in social interactions. He was equally motivated to improve his life in general, but was quite happy with his social network. He was charismatic and engaging in first encounters, and although he was underemployed (working part-time as a volunteer), employees in his chosen line

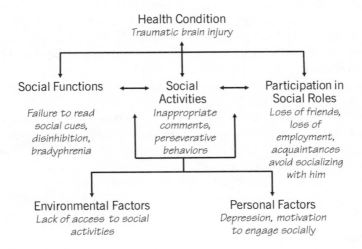

FIGURE 9.1. ICF framework applied to Jay.

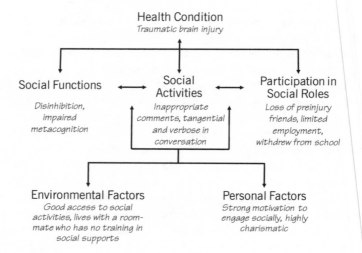

FIGURE 9.2. ICF framework applied to Ned.

of work had a high tolerance for disinhibited language, and the workplace was not open to the public. According to a traditional medical model, both of these individuals would be candidates for social skills training, as both have impairments in social behavior. For Jay, however, social skills training would be of limited benefit if he was not able to access social activities, and Ned did not need social skills intervention because he was generally happy with his social life and in a supportive context. These examples show how social skills training must occur in context, and they illustrate factors to be considered in intervention planning.

ASSESSMENT OF SOCIAL FUNCTIONING

Intervention planning always begins with assessment. Unlike cognitive functions, which typically are assessed by specialized practitioners such as neuropsychologists or speech–language pathologists, social functions are evaluated by everyone who comes into contact with the person with ABI. Social functioning is so integral to human interaction that we all feel qualified to render an opinion. This makes sense, however, as social "appropriateness" is a subjective, context-specific judgment. Because it is hard to imagine a standardized test that would capture the wide variety of social norms and complexities in everyday life, most assessment is informal. To help readers conduct this informal assessment, the following sections suggest guidelines for evaluating social functioning at each level of the ICF framework. Form 9.1 is a blank worksheet in the Appendix (an enlarged version is on the book's page on The Guilford Press website) for using the ICF. The results of this evaluation form the basis for the needs assessment, conducted below in Consideration 2 of the PIE approach.

Social Functions

Social functions can be divided into two domains: *social understanding* and *social behavior*. The term *social understanding* refers to knowledge of social norms (e.g., knowing culture-specific rules for politeness) and to the ability to "read" verbal and nonverbal social cues. Traditional didactic social skills training models assume that the person with ABI has intact social understanding but lacks the knowledge and skills to produce appropriate behaviors. Recent research has shown, however, that many individuals with acquired neurological disorders have marked impairments in aspects of social understanding. The two functions that have received the most attention are *emotion recognition* and *theory of mind* (ToM). In regard to emotion recognition, it is now clear that individuals with a variety of acquired neurological disorders have impairments in identifying emotions from facial expressions. Impairments in this domain have been observed in children and adults with TBI (Henry, Phillips, Crawford, Ietswaart, & Summers, 2006; Tonks, Williams, Frampton, Yates, & Slater, 2007; Turkstra, McDonald, & DePompei, 2001; Young, Newcombe, de Haan, Small, & Hay, 1993); in adults with multiple sclerosis (Krause et al., 2009); and in adults with focal lesions due to stroke, herpes encephalitis, or temporal lobectomy for epilepsy (Philippi, Mehta, Grabowski, Adolphs, & Rudrauf, 2009). Individuals in these groups may make errors of *valence*, confusing positive and negative emotions (e.g., mistaking angry for enthusiastic), and also errors of *magnitude* (e.g., mistaking angry for irritated). In general, recognition of basic emotions like "happy" is more likely to be intact, whereas recognition of subtler and more complex emotions, such as embarrassment or annoyance, are more likely to be impaired.

ToM is the ability to recognize that others have thoughts that differ from one's own, and that these thoughts influence others' actions (Premack & Woodruff, 1978). ToM impairments are a core deficit in autism (Baron-Cohen, Leslie, & Frith, 1985) and are common in disorders such as schizophrenia (Bora, Yucel, & Pantelis, 2009; Craig, Hatton, Craig, & Bentall, 2004) and frontotemporal dementia (Lough et al., 2006). It is only recently that ToM has been studied in individuals with ABI, including children, adolescents, and adults with TBI (Muller et al., 2009; Turkstra, 2008; Turkstra, Dixon, & Baker, 2004; Walz, Yeates, Taylor, Stancin, & Wade, 2010); and adults with right-hemisphere stroke (Surian & Siegal, 2001). Although the results in adults with right-hemisphere stroke continue to be debated (e.g., see Tompkins, Scharp, Fassbinder, Meigh, & Armstrong, 2008), there is consistent evidence that ToM is impaired in many individuals with ABI, and that this impairment cannot be explained by general cognitive deficits.

Emerging data on social understanding suggest that assessment of this aspect of social functioning should be the first step in intervention, as the client is unlikely to know which behavior to use if he or she doesn't recognize social cues. At the time of publication of this book, however, there was only one standardized test of emotion recognition, or ToM, for individuals with ABI: the Test of Awareness of Social Inference (TASIT; McDonald, Flanagan, & Rollins, 2002), a test of sarcasm comprehension and emotion recognition that uses videos of Australian speakers. Until more tests become available, informal assessment will remain the primary option for clinicians.

Additional cognitive functions should be considered when assessing social functioning. If a client with TBI asks the same question repeatedly, perhaps his declarative memory is impaired and he can't recall the answers. A client with poor executive function might make inappropriate comments because she's not able to inhibit the expression of her every thought. A client with poor working memory might miss the point of a story because he can't keep the relevant details in mind long enough to put it all together. Impairments in divided attention might make a person seem tangential or egocentric, because she is unable to focus on both a conversation and the work task she is performing. Another common reason for poor social functioning is cognitive fatigue: Good social behavior takes mental energy, and when we are mentally fatigued it is difficult to be on our best behavior (Kennedy & Coehlo, 2005). People with ABI are particularly vulnerable to cognitive fatigue, so if social problems tend to occur after a cognitively demanding task or near the end of the day, cognitive fatigue should be considered as a possible explanation.

It is impossible to list all of the social behaviors that could be assessed, as they include greetings, farewells, and everything in between. Basically, the clinician considers any behavior that serves a social function and is limiting the social participation of that person. These might be negative behaviors—such as disinhibited language, sexually inappropriate behavior in public, repetitive questioning, talking off topic, or monopolizing a conversation—and also lack of positive behaviors—such as failure to join social activities, participate in a conversation, or acknowledge the wants and needs of others. Clinicians are likely to have different social standards than their clients, and expectations for social behavior change with age, culture, and context, so in general the determination of what constitutes a social problem will depend on the report of the client and people in his or her social life rather than on a standardized test score.

Although all members of the team participate in an evaluation of social functioning, its relation to everyday communication typically is assessed by speech–language pathologists when they evaluate *pragmatic communication ability*. A discussion of methods for evaluating pragmatic communication is beyond the scope of this book, but in general this assessment uses a combination of questionnaires, such as the LaTrobe Communication Questionnaire (LCQ; Douglas, Bracy, & Snow, 2007) or the Profile of Functional Impairment in Communication (PFIC; Linscott, Knight, & Godfrey, 1996), and detailed examination of communication behaviors such as turn taking, topic maintenance, and other interpersonal behaviors that typically occur in social interactions (Snow & Ponsford, 1995; Turkstra, McDonald, & Kaufmann, 1996). For children and adolescents with ABI, some standardized tests can be useful for evaluating core skills underlying pragmatic communication, such as inference ability (e.g., the Comprehensive Assessment of Spoken Language; Carrow-Woolfolk, 1999). For adults with ABI, however, as with the other aspects of social functioning discussed above, no well-validated standardized tests of pragmatic communication have been published to date. As noted above, this absence is actually appropriate given the context dependence of pragmatic communication and the subjective nature of judgments of social appropriateness.

Social Activities

Assessment of social activities involves observation of the client as he or she is engaged in a social interaction. This is often accomplished either by role-playing situations that are typical for the client in everyday life (e.g., pretending to greet a new person), or observing the client in daily social interactions with caregivers and others. Some standardized caregiver checklists include questions about social performance in activities, such as the Pediatric Assessment of Disability Inventory (Haley, Coster, Ludlow, Haltiwanger, & Adrellos, 1992); the Functional Assessment of Communication Skills for adults (Frattali, Thompson, Holland, Wohl, & Ferketic, 1995); and the Behavior Rating Inventory of Executive Function (Roth, Isquith, & Gioia, 2005), which has child, adolescent, and adult versions. In general, however, social activities are assessed using informal measures. When assessing performance by role playing, it is important to keep in mind that clinical interactions differ from everyday social life in important ways. Clinicians tend to provide structure and support that is absent in everyday life. Our interactions with clients often occur around a predetermined topic and have a question-and-answer format (Turkstra, 2001), which gives artificial structure to the conversation. We also typically evaluate clients in quiet settings with few distractions. As a result, assessment in the clinic setting might overestimate the client's social ability. On the other hand, clinicians lack shared history that can support conversations with friends and family. We also have a status relationship with the client, a factor that is known to have a negative effect on aspects of social interaction (Togher, Hand, & Code, 1996). Thus, the best way to evaluate performance in social activities is to observe the client in everyday social interactions, and to ask caregivers and other communication partners to rate behaviors in these settings.

Social Participation

In recent years, individuals with disabilities have advocated for treatments that improve their life participation and not just performance on standardized tests in the clinic (Hartley, 1995). This advocacy has led to the development of standardized tools with items that specifically address participation in social life. Social participation can be assessed using either *objective* measures, which ask about outcomes that society in general would consider to be desirable (e.g., having friends, being involved in the community), or *subjective* measures, which ask about outcomes specific to the client (e.g., "Is your social life satisfactory to you?"). Most current scales are objective. These include the Pediatric Quality of Life Inventory (PedsQL; Varni, Seid, & Rode, 1999) for children, and the Craig Handicap Assessment and Reporting Technique (CHART; Whiteneck, Charlifue, Gerhart, Overholser, & Richardson), the Community Integration Questionnaire (CIQ; Willer, Rosenthal, Kreutzer, & Gordon, 1993), and the Quality of Communication Life Scale (Paul et al., 2005) for adults. The objective nature of these instruments should be kept in mind: Each client has his or her own unique goals for social participation, so when the client answers "Never" or "Not often" to a question such as "Do you go to the movies with friends?", the clinician should ask if this particular outcome is important to that client. People vary in the extent to which they seek social engagement, and there are marked differences across cultures as well (Larkins, Worrall, & Hickson, 2004), so not all items will apply to all clients.

Environmental Factors

The most important environmental factors in regard to social functioning are the people with whom the client interacts. Because we, as clinicians, rely on these individuals to provide cues and supports in everyday life, we need to know their willingness and ability to do so. There are, however, no standardized methods for evaluating these social partners (the lack of validated, standardized measures is definitely a theme of this chapter!). Thus, we rely on discussions with, and observations of, social partners and their stated willingness to be part of the intervention process.

Environmental assessment also includes identification of social opportunities available to the client, including both the activities themselves and also practical factors such as transportation and funds. Additional environment-related questions include whether the target social context is private or public, the number of people and distractions involved, and the standards for social behavior (or costs of misbehavior) in that context. Answers to these questions will shape treatment goals.

Personal Factors

When a person has new cognitive impairments, it may take time before he or she is ready to be out in public or seeing premorbid friends. Readiness to be out in the social world and to use strategies and supports might be the greatest predictors of response to therapy. Thus, attention to factors discussed in Chapter 3 is critical for intervention planning. It is common for adolescents and adults with ABI to experience depression because of changes in their social abilities and social lives, particularly when some time has passed and premorbid friends have, as one man with TBI eloquently put it, "fallen away" (McWreath, 2005). As noted above, premorbid social style, skills, attitudes, and interests also must be considered when designing treatment, so that goals are feasible and meaningful to that person.

PIE: PLANNING FOR INTERVENTION TO IMPROVE SOCIAL FUNCTIONING

Intervention for social functioning typically includes a combination of training social routines and compensatory strategies, making environmental modifications, and identifying or training caregiver supports. The assessment results will dictate the combination of these that is appropriate for any given client. For example, Ted, a man with a severe TBI, had problems in his group home because he would yell at other residents when they changed the channel during his favorite television program. Ted had poor declarative memory but good procedural learning, so he needed an intervention that gave him a new routine and external memory supports as cues. Thus, intervention included training Ted in a script to tell, rather than yell at, someone who had changed the channel; posting a television-watching schedule in a highly visible location so that other residents could easily remember Ted's and their viewing times, training care staff to stick to the viewing schedule and cue Ted's script, and planning to purchase video-recording capability for the television so that Ted could watch his program whenever he wished.

In this section, we use the PIE framework to review the key planning considerations specific to social functioning. The "Plan" and "Prognosis" sections of Form 9.1 can be used to summarize the results. We then return to the example of Jay as an illustration of the PIE process.

Consideration 1: Who Is the Learner?

The clinician first considers the client's social skills (including social understanding) and also cognitive, physical, and sensory abilities. As discussed above, assessment of learner characteristics may occur through standardized testing, observation in social activities, or interviews with the client and relevant support people. Some of this assessment can be done out of the social context, such as testing of cognitive functions. Assessment of social functions, however, is best done in context, as described above.

In terms of candidacy for intervention, in general the client must have motivation and readiness to improve social functioning. The extent to which the client needs awareness and insight depends on the nature of the intervention. If intervention is mostly focused on training social scripts (Chapter 5), structured multistep routines (Chapter 6), or the use of external cognitive aids (Chapter 7), these can be learned as automatic behaviors without significant client insight. On the other hand, if the client will be using a metacognitive strategy (Chapter 8), such as "When I meet a new person, I will shake hands, not hug," good awareness is a prerequisite.

Consideration 2: Selecting the Target and Training Method (What? Where? When? How?)

Once the client's strengths and limitations are identified, the next step is to match that profile to specific intervention strategies. As discussed in earlier chapters, this process is referred to as a *needs assessment* and begins with identifying the client's goal and relevant context factors, then using task analysis to identify components that will be addressed in intervention. To the extent possible, this is done in collaboration with the client and his or her social interaction partners. The following planning questions help to guide this process:

What Is the Specific Need?

The question *"What is the specific need?"* concerns the client's goal. Is the client a nursing-home resident who wants to increase engagement in social activities, or is he living at home with a family who is embarrassed by his behaviors out in the community? Is she a child who laughs when another child gets hurt in school, or an adolescent who wants to "fit in" socially with her preinjury peer group? Intervention for social functioning is always client-centered, as the client is unlikely to work on goals that are not personally meaningful and relevant, so collaboration with the client and his or her everyday support people is essential in identifying intervention goals.

Where Is the Target Environment?

The answer to the question *"Where is the target environment?"* will help determine where training takes place, particularly if the client has poor executive function and declarative memory and thus is unlikely to generalize the behavior. This question also aims to identify available social supports, including people, as well as environmental modifications needed and standards for social behavior. It is cost-efficient for the clinician to see the target environment firsthand, as context factors will have a critical influence on the success of intervention. Money spent training social skills that require cues from nursing home staff will be wasted if staff members are not available during social activities. The target environment may be something related to that person. We once identified a goal of training a client to read a social script that he kept in his wallet, to reduce his long monologues about his accident (a complaint of his family when they were out in public), then discovered that he typically wore sweatpants with no pockets!

When Will the Client Implement the Strategy?

The question *"When will the client implement the strategy?"* also addresses the context, in this case the timing of the goal behavior. It is important to know if the client is expected to independently identify when he or she should use a target social behavior, because impairments in social understanding and metacognitive skills will influence the likelihood of success. Unlike other types of behavior, such as work routines, social behaviors tend to be unpredictable and variable, so it is very helpful to know if there are any environmental cues that will help the client identify when he or she needs to execute a behavior. In general, low-frequency targets are more difficult to learn, as discussed in Chapter 5. If the client wishes to learn a joke to tell at parties, but only attends one party per year, there is not much opportunity to practice. This is not to say that low-frequency events are always poor treatment targets. A client may have an important upcoming event, such as the wedding of a child or an outing with a group, and learning a strategy or script for this type of event may be the most meaningful social intervention for that client.

How Will the Intervention Be Implemented?

The first answer to *"How will the intervention be implemented?"* is *"In collaboration with the client."* Social goals are guaranteed to be idiosyncratic, so no plan will succeed if the client is not invested in the outcome. The rest of the answer to this question depends on the results of the assessment, the answers to the three preceding questions, and the intervention goals. Use of the decision tree in Figure 5.1 (p. 92) may be helpful here. If the focus of intervention is on changing the client's behavior (vs. the environment), then training will use declarative and procedural learning techniques, as described in Chapters 5 and 6. The extent to which each is used will depend on the client's declarative memory and executive function ability. If the client has good insight and relatively good executive function, then metacognitive strategies can be used (Chapter 8). By contrast, if procedural memory is the client's main route to new learning, then errorless learning and spaced retrieval are more appropriate, and the client will need high-frequency practice of correct responses (Chapters 5 and 6). In the latter case, if the target is to be used in multiple contexts, stimulus variability will need to be built in to the intervention plan.

If the focus of intervention is on environmental adaptations and modifications, the method for achieving these will depend on the goals. One general recommendation is to formally involve stakeholders in the process, and to consider the burden on families and care providers when asking them to provide supports. The literature suggests that lack of meaningful social interaction with the person with ABI is a significant source of long-term stress for families (Verhaeghe, Defloor, & Grypdonck, 2005), so families are likely to be motivated to participate in intervention that aims to improve social functioning. There is no strong evidence to support any particular methods for training caregivers (Boschen et al., 2007), however, and it may add to stress levels to expect families to change their own social behaviors to accommodate the person with social impairments.

When stakeholders are employers, they may need education about the potential benefits of providing social supports at work. Moving a person with ABI to a private workspace, so he or she is not engaged in distracting social conversations, may be an inconvenient and expensive undertaking for a business, and the clinician may need to provide concrete evidence of the potential for this arrangement to increase worker productivity. This is similar in school settings: Some students with ABI need structure and advanced preparation to act appropriately when working in groups in class. This need places an added burden on the teacher, but it might benefit all students in the class.

Consideration 3: Specifying the Desired Outcomes (Why?)

As in all aspects of intervention, the clinician must be clear on the rationale for the intervention goal and how outcome will be measured. As described in Chapter 4, treatment effectiveness is determined using a multilevel evaluation that considers not only within-session progress (if the plan includes teaching specific skills to the client or social interaction partners) but also the extent to which change is observed in the target context and maintained over time. The answer to the "Plan" in Form 9.1 must include a rationale that clearly states why this goal is relevant to social participation. A benefit of using the ICF as a treatment-planning framework is that the *Why* of intervention is transparent from the outset, and the level at which outcome can be measured is easily observable. The specification of environmental and personal factors in this framework also helps to identify factors that are beyond the clinician's control. For example, if a person needs workplace social skills but is no longer employed, is unable to attend social events because of transportation, or is socially withdrawn because of depression, then the intervention plan may focus on referral to other specialists, rather than on direct intervention, and successful referral will be the criterion for successful outcome.

Consideration 4: Designing the Individualized Plan

By now the clinician has gathered the information necessary to design an individualized instructional plan. Form 9.1 provides a worksheet to help design an instructional plan that incorporates the information collected during the evaluation.

PIE: IMPLEMENTING SYSTEMATIC INSTRUCTION FOR SOCIAL FUNCTIONING

The planning process reviewed in the above section lays the groundwork for training that is carried out in the implementation phase. The planning process has generated (1) the client's or stakeholder's skills and knowledge, environmental modifications, or referrals that will meet the client's social participation goals; (2) measurable objectives to monitor performance; and (3) training stimuli to facilitate learning social skill components. The next phase is to implement the plan, make sure that target behaviors are mastered and generalized, complete a multilevel assessment, and plan for maintenance over time. The specific procedures to be used for each element of the plan will depend on the nature of the target. If proceduralized social skills are to be trained, then the clinician uses Figure 5.2 to guide the selection of a training method. If external aids will be used, the clinician follows procedures in Chapter 7. If facts and concepts are part of the training—such as information that will be included in a conversation script to use in social situations—then Chapter 5 procedures can guide intervention. The most important element of training to keep in mind is that it is multifactorial and must directly address improvements in social life.

PUTTING IT ALL TOGETHER: CASE APPLICATIONS

In the remainder of the chapter we provide examples to demonstrate the application of the PIE model to social functioning intervention with actual clients. The first two examples are group studies by McDonald and colleagues (2008) and Dahlberg and colleagues (2007), which to date are the only randomized controlled clinical trials of social skills intervention for individuals with TBI. In the third example, we revisit Jay, who was described in the introduction to this chapter.

Examples from the Literature

McDonald and colleagues (2008) conducted a study aimed at (1) improving social behaviors and social understanding in adults with TBI and (2) also reducing anxiety and depression—thus addressing both social functions and personal factors from the ICF framework. Participants, 51 adults in the chronic stage postinjury, were assigned to one of three conditions: (1) a 12-week social skills training program; (2) a 12-week nontherapy program that included social activities such as cooking and outings; or (3) a wait-list control group. The primary outcome measures were *social understanding*, *social behaviors*, and *emotional adjustment*, measured by researchers. To assess social understanding, participants completed the TASIT (McDonald, Garg, & Haynes, 2002). For assessment of behaviors, participants were videotaped before and after treatment in a conversation with a male and female confederate (professional actors), and raters blinded to the treatment conditions scored each video for behaviors such as self-centered behavior, social manners, and humor. Emotional adjustment was measured by self-report. Secondary outcome measures included self- and caregiver reports of participants' social behavior and social participation in everyday life, measured with the LCQ, the Katz Adjustment Scale (Katz & Lyerly, 1963), the Social Performance Survey Schedule (Lowe & Cautela, 1978), and the Sydney Psychosocial Reintegration Scale (Tate, Hodgkinson, Veerabangsa, & Maggiotto, 1999).

The social skills treatment group completed 12 weekly 3-hour group sessions with three to five other participants with TBI and two therapists, as well as 1 hour per week of individual counseling with a clinical psychologist. Two hours of each group session focused on didactic training of social skills, such as starting a conversation or choosing topics. Participants chose individual goals for training. Each session included warm-up games, a review of homework assigned to each participant the previous session, introduction of a target skill, discussion of potential issues and solutions, therapist modeling of appropriate and inappropriate behavior, and role playing. Participants were taught the acronym WSTC (What am I doing? Select a strategy? Try it. Check it out!) and encouraged to use it consistently. The clinicians provided high levels of social reinforcement to aid participants' confidence and motivation, gave immediate and primarily positive feedback, and provided many opportunities for repetition of target behaviors. The authors did not provide information about specific training strategies used, such as elaborative encoding, visualization, or errorless learning. The 1-hour counseling sessions were individualized and used standard cognitive-behavioral therapy techniques such as relaxation and assertiveness training, modified to fit the cognitive profile of each participant.

Analysis of the primary outcome measures showed improvement in social behaviors in the treatment group but not the other two groups, and no change in social understanding or social adjustment in any group. There also were no significant changes in any group in caregiver reports of behavior or community outcomes.

Dahlberg et al. (2007) completed a similar study and obtained similar results. This study addressed a limitation of the study by McDonald and colleagues, who noted that small sample sizes might have been the reason for the lack of significant group differences on some measures. There were 52 participants in the Dahlberg et al. study, 26 in the treatment group and 26 in a delayed treatment group, who crossed over to receive treatment in the second phase of the study. As in the study by McDonald et al., group social skills training was delivered weekly for 12 weeks, in this case for 1.5 hours per week. Outcome measures included scores on the PFIC (Linscott et al., 1996), analyzed by a rater blinded to treatment condition; the Social Communication Skills Questionnaire (McGann, Werven, & Douglas, 1997), completed by the participant and a family member or significant other; the CHART (Whiteneck et al., 1992); the CIQ (Willer et al., 1993); and the Satisfaction with Life Questionnaire (Diener, Emmons, Larsen, & Griffin, 1985). Progress also was measured using goal attainment scaling (GAS), a process used often in rehabilitation for TBI (Malec, Smigielski, & DePompolo, 1991), whereby each participant's goal is broken down into incremental steps that can be measured. For example, one participant had the goal of asking more questions in conversations. This target behavior was divided into five steps, beginning with "I will ask questions in 10% or less of conversations" and working up to "I will ask questions in 90% or more of conversations."

Group therapy sessions followed a manualized social skills curriculum, which included instruction about the skills of a good communicator, and topics such as starting conversations, being assertive, respecting social boundaries, and conflict resolution. Groups were facilitated by a speech–language pathologist and a clinical social worker, to provide two perspectives on social functioning and two models of social behavior. Participants were supported in developing personal goals through self-reflection, with input from caregivers and clinicians, and the group format provided a vehicle for natural feedback and practice. Although the intervention included both social skills training and procedures for generalization, specific training methods were not described.

Results showed improvements primarily in PFIC and GAS scores, with improvements in self-report on the Satisfaction with Life Questionnaire as well. Of the ratings by caregivers, only GAS scores showed significant improvements with treatment. All of these changes remained significant at 6 months posttreatment.

In both of the studies just discussed, social skills training led to improvements in discrete social behaviors, and these improvements were maintained over time. In both studies, however, there were no significant changes in social activities, as rated by others, or in social participation. The one exception was a positive change in perceived satisfaction with social life in the study by Dahlberg et al., which was an important outcome. The overall lack of change in social activities and participation underscores the importance of considering all elements of the ICF framework when planning intervention and measuring outcomes. As McDonald et al. noted, unrelated life events can have a significant influence on social participation, and participants might not have a range of opportunities to practice skills learned in therapy. This point underscores our contention that identification of environmental and personal factors, as well as of limitations in activities and participation, is a critical element of intervention planning. In addition, perhaps the skills trained in these studies were not the most important reasons for participants' social problems in everyday life. It was commendable that caregivers collaborated in choosing goals, but that does not guarantee that changing one or two individual behaviors will have a positive effect on overall social interactions.

Case Application: Jay

Description of Client

Jay was a 25-year-old man who referred himself for therapy 5 years after he sustained a TBI. Jay had received in- and outpatient rehabilitation for a few weeks after his injury, but had not received any services for more than 4 years. As stated at the beginning of this chapter, Jay's goal was to meet people, and his opinion was that social skills training would help this happen. Jay was unemployed, although he very much wanted to work. He lived alone on the other side of town from his parents, a situation that appeared to suit them both.

Planning Phase

The speech–language pathologist initiated a needs assessment following the four planning considerations (Who, What, Where, and Why). Results of the interview with the client, as well as supplementary cognitive testing to evaluate memory, attention, and executive functions, revealed the following client profile:

• *Cognitive and social functioning.* Jay's scores on the Repeatable Battery for Assessment of Neuropsychological Status (Randolph, 2001), a screening test of cognitive functions, were at the bottom of the normal range. In everyday life, he appeared to have relatively good declarative memory: He remembered upcoming therapy appointments and had learned the bus arrival and departure schedule. By contrast, he showed poor executive function, at least in some contexts: He perseverated on topics and comments, called the clinician repeatedly between therapy sessions, and was often tangential and distractible. He also had mild word-finding difficulties in spontaneous social interaction. Jay lived independently, with no family or paid assistance, and managed to get to clinic and social activities on time, so planning and organization appeared to be strengths. In terms of social understanding, Jay showed consistent evidence of impairment in reading social cues. He was considered "overly friendly" with strangers, frequently made flirtatious comments to students in the clinic, and did not appear aware of the effects of his behavior on others. He made errors in both verbal inference (e.g., if the clinician said, "I'll talk to you next week," he did not infer that this meant they would *not* be talking in the interim) and social inference (e.g., inferring that different behaviors were expected with a clinician vs. a stranger).

• *Social activities and participation.* Jay's neighbor reported that she occasionally took him to community social events, but he otherwise stayed at home, attended the monthly TBI support group, or came for therapy. He did not appear to seek social interaction with his parents, and vice versa. Increasing his range of social activities was a major goal for him (particularly, meeting women). Overall Jay was not an active member of his desired social community.

• *Environmental factors.* Positive environmental factors included access to the bus (Jay did not drive because of TBI-related sensory, cognitive, and motor limitations, but he walked without assistance), a neighbor who would take him places and was genuinely interested in helping him, and contact with the local brain injury association chapter, which provided opportunities for social outings. Negative environmental factors included Jay's lack of employment and the limitations inherent in relying on public transportation in a city where many social events are not at times and locations easily served by the bus.

• *Personal factors.* Jay was highly motivated to improve his social life. He had a great sense of humor and a generally outgoing and positive personality. Jay stated that he attended therapy at our university clinic "to help teach the students." This was something we should have heard more clearly at the beginning, because it later became apparent that Jay believed he was attending therapy as an instructor, with the added benefit that it gave him opportunity to socialize with lots of people in the waiting room (and female students).

Acquisition and Mastery Phase

Jay's long-term goal was to improve social functioning. Jay and his clinician collaborated to develop an acronym that described his target behavior in social situations, PRWD (pronounced *proud*), which stood for Plain language and tone, Respect other's space, Wait until you know the person better, and Don't mock. Jay used overt self-talk to cue himself to use these behaviors. Because the initial assessment revealed that Jay could implement these behaviors accurately with explicit social cues, he moved immediately to the generalization stage with no need for acquisition or mastery training for the behavior. The acronym itself was trained using SR training with high-prompt variability, and in two sessions Jay learned to cite the acronym in response to a variety of social queries (e.g., "What would be appropriate in that situation? How could you have acted in that situation?").

Generalization Phase

The next step was for Jay to use PRWD in everyday life. The first objective was for Jay to identify opportunities outside of therapy where he potentially could use his PRWD strategy. This was done by planning social encounters that could be observed by the clinician, discussing that situation with Jay immediately after it occurred, and then recording the number of times Jay accurately identified the need for the PRWD behaviors. Next, Jay recorded PRWD opportunities in everyday life (Jay was independent in using a planner, as this had been trained in previous sessions). He brought these notes to therapy for discussion with the clinician. The next step was learning to anticipate times when PRWD should be used, which was addressed by video modeling, with Jay making predictions about appropriate behavior based on the scenario described, then judging the actors' subsequent behavior. The last step was for Jay to consult his planner in advance to identify upcoming social events where PRWD could be used, use the strategy at those events, and then record the outcomes. A sample plan is shown in Figure 9.3 adapted from Form 5.2.

Multilevel Outcome Evaluation

Session data indicated that Jay was able to use his PRWD strategy consistently with minimal cues (e.g., a glance from the therapist). He also described events in which he had used it in social life. This was partially confirmed by his neighbor, who often attended social events with him: She said that Jay often verbalized the strategy at appropriate times, but still crossed personal boundaries when out in public. The clinician also noted that Jay's word-finding problems sometimes limited his ability to initiate an appropriate topic of conversation when his automatic topics were inappropriate. This suggested that conversation script training (Manheim, Halper, & Cherney, 2009) might have been an effective intervention approach, as this would have given Jay behavioral alternatives.

The most important data were at the level of life participation: Jay decided that he had enough social skills and did not see the need to have new scripts or further therapy. He had made a contribution to student education, and mostly liked being in the waiting room and meeting new people. Therefore, he was discharged from therapy and continued to pursue social opportunities via Brain Injury Association functions and outings with his neighbor. Form 9.2 in the Appendix is a blank instructional planning worksheet for social skills (an enlarged version is on the book's page on The Guilford Press website).

SUMMARY

This chapter applied the PIE framework to intervention for problems in social interaction. Three general principles guide intervention in this domain: the importance of individualizing treatment, the lack of evidence that training discrete social skills will generalize to novel situations, and the importance of high-frequency repetition to mastery and maintenance of social goals. We propose a framework that considers not only basic social skills, such as theory of mind, but also performance in everyday social activities and, most important, full participation in social life. In the social domain, perhaps more than any other, individuals with acquired cognitive impairments report chronic, life-limiting disability that is not addressed adequately in therapy. Consideration of life goals as the first step in treatment planning will help remedy this gap in our service delivery. This approach is exemplified by the modified versions of World Health Organization Classification of Functioning, Disability, and Handicap, shown in Figures 4.2 and 9.1. Intervention planning must consider not only the patient's cognitive strengths and limitations, but also his or her personality and priorities, as well as available social supports and opportunities for socialization. As Ylvisaker and Feeney (1998, 2000) often stated, this planning process must be a *collaborative* process. Patients with acquired brain injury often have social goals that differ substantially from those of their

WHAT will I teach the client?

Long-Term Goal: | Improve social life

Initial Acquisition
Objectives: | Every morning after breakfast, independently check planner and note opportunities to use
PRWD strategy

(Specify target, approach, objective performance, independence, criterion, and context/conditions.)

HOW will I train the skill?

(Specify method; e.g., MVC, SR, elaboration, visualization,
mnemonics, strategy training.)

SR training

☑ It is a functional target

☑ It is customized to client

☑ The context is specified

☑ Progress measurement specified in long-term goal
and/or acquisition goal

Plan to enhance client motivation/engagement: | Goal and strategy chosen by client, SR has high
success rates

WHEN will I teach the target?

Therapy Frequency: ____4____ / week (2 FTF, 2 via phone)
Session Duration: ____30____ min
Therapy Duration: ____1____ Sessions, (Weeks,) Months

☑ There is opportunity for sufficient practice within sessions
☑ There is opportunity for sufficient practice across sessions

To be used in same context or novel context?

Same context: Fixed stimuli = use same planner each time

Novel contexts: Varied stimuli = different prompts to check planner

Nature of information to be learned

Simple: Plan for spaced presentation is prompt = version of "What's on your schedule today?"

Response = Client checks planner and identifies PRWD opportunities

Complex: Plan for massed presentation is _____

WHO will implement training outside of session?

☑ Support person identified to provide additional practice between sessions   attendant

☑ Sufficient variety of people identified to provide stimuli to allow generalization   per attendant, client has
interactions with 1 acquaintance/new person each day in job placement, residence, or outings.

Describe plan to *train* support person/people: 30 min in-service training residence

FIGURE 9.3. Instructional planning worksheet for Jay.

clinicians, and collaborative planning will help our clients achieve meaningful gains in their everyday social lives.

APPLICATION EXERCISES

1. Identify a successful social interaction in your own daily life. Using the ICF worksheet in Form 9.1, deconstruct this activity into the social skills, general cognitive skills, personal factors, and environmental factors that contributed to your positive performance. Identify any positive participation-level outcomes associated with this event. Repeat the process for a social interaction in which you feel you performed poorly. Using these data, consider what a clinician would need to evaluate to capture your performance and outcomes in these different settings. The goal of this exercise is to practice using task analysis and the ICF framework to identify relevant intervention targets.

2. Identify a target activity in which you would like to change your social behavior. Be sure to choose an activity that is relevant and has the potential to improve your overall social participation. Using the PIE framework, develop a plan to reach your target. Specify any supports you might need, such as notes or cues from peers, and set criteria for measuring outcome (e.g., a peer's rating of your success). Implement your plan and evaluate the outcome, then answer the following questions:

   a. Could this goal be achieved by work done in a therapy setting?

   b. How would a therapist obtain the information necessary to plan and implement intervention?

   c. What were the unexpected barriers and supports you encountered when developing and implementing your plan?

   d. What elements of this experience will inform your clinical practice?

   The goals of this exercise are to reflect on supports and challenges in changing everyday social behavior and to identify goal-setting and implementation strategies you can use in your clinical practice.

CHAPTER 10

Conclusion
Now What?

You did it. You read a book detailing instructional practices to optimize your rehabilitation outcomes. We commend you. Theoretically you now know what to do, or you at least have a reference to use as a guide when planning and implementing your therapy. Perhaps the hardest part is yet to come—it is where the rubber hits the road, that is, the implementation of treatment practices that may not currently be part of your repertoire. Those of you who are seasoned practitioners, have the advantage of experience and can adapt procedures and apply the research for your clinical context. However, you have the disadvantage of having internalized and established clinical routines, some of which you may want to abandon. Change can be hard when habits have been formed. Those of you who are students or early practitioners, have a fresh slate to facilitate adoption of these techniques, but are disadvantaged by having less knowledge to integrate with your new learning. Regardless of years of experience, we are no different from our patients. We need practice at learning new techniques and becoming fluent in their use.

In these concluding pages we attempt to help you set some personal clinical goals and make a plan to practice the desired skills. You have made an investment by reading about instructional practices. The best way to actualize your return and improve your clinical delivery is to develop and follow a practice plan: Plan, Implement, and Evaluate. We end by offering you your own personal clinical PIE process in Table 10.1. If you have a colleague who is interested in increasing his or her instructional skills, we suggest forming a partnership to share your plan and provide each other with feedback.

The likelihood that you will use the skills and techniques in this book depends in part on four factors that are unique to you:

1. Your self-efficacy, or your belief that you have or can develop the necessary skills.
2. Your locus of control, or the extent to which you believe changes are within your control.

TABLE 10.1. 25 Clinician Skills and Behaviors That Enhance the Client's Engagement in Therapy

To enhance personal factors:

1. My goal is to support clients in managing their own daily lives. To foster each client's self-efficacy (belief in being able to achieve goals), I will make sure my treatment decisions fit the client's belief system, and I will show the client early success in therapy.
2. I will provide clients with tools to evaluate their current performance relative to their future goals, rather than focusing on their pre-injury status.
3. I will help motivate clients by exposing them to successful examples, such as clients who are similar in cognitive strengths and limitations and have achieved their goals.
4. I will use incentives, rewards, and reinforcements, verbal or tangible, as encouragement for clients.
5. I will remind clients early and often of the goals and benefits of the therapy program, from their perspective, not mine (or a third-party payer's).
6. I will prepare clients to cope with temporary lapses and challenges by anticipating them and making alternate plans in advance.
7. I will minimize potential anxiety by instructing clients about upcoming activities and possible physiological or psychological responses (e.g., frustration, pain, or fatigue).
8. I will conduct a thorough cognitive assessment to ensure clients possess requisite cognitive abilities to actively participate in their treatment.
9. I will make sure treatment has enough variety to engage the client, without overwhelming him or her with choices or changes.

To enhance the environment:

10. I will review how services are being delivered and consider alterations to the environment, schedule, or transportation that will maximize the patient's ability to participate.
11. I will review the environment and ask myself whether environmental or internal distractors are influencing the client's performance.
12. To prompt target behavior, I will use environmental cues such as stickers, reminder notes, and calendars, when appropriate.
13. I will collaborate with important people in the client's life as true rehabilitation partners. This might include asking them to assist with observations, collaborate in the development of management strategies, and give the client feedback (including praise and support). I will provide sufficient training for these stakeholders.
14. As Ylvisaker and Feeney (1998) recommended, I will aim for therapy to be "social" not "solo."

To maximize the success of the therapy program:

15. I will individualize therapy programs and try multiple strategies to find the best "fit" for the client.
16. I will collaborate with the client to create programs that accommodate to that client's lifestyle, using motivational counseling strategies when possible.
17. I will ensure activities and materials are age appropriate.
18. I will help the client establish a routine to fit a therapy program into his or her schedule.
19. I will provide clear, ongoing instructions and feedback about therapy performance and progress.
20. I will make sure that activities are within the patient's ability to achieve independently, if independent practice is a goal.
21. I will consider error-control techniques, teaching prerequisite knowledge or skills and breaking down multistep tasks into component steps using task analysis.
22. I will use written goal logs and provide regular feedback on completion of goals to increase accountability.
23. I will monitor participation regularly and attempt to resolve challenges to program participation.
24. I will provide personalized attention, education, and support as needed for the client and other stakeholders.
25. I will record and review examples of successful in-session mastery of tasks with the client as a "self-as-model" intervention. If possible and appropriate, I will provide a copy of this video for home review and self-encouragement.

3. Your belief system, whether you believe the principles we have presented in this book.
4. Your willingness to practice the techniques.

As "senior" clinicians, we appreciate the challenges in these four domains. We have experienced firsthand the challenges of delivering the highest standard of care when resources are limited. It is up to us, however, to advance rehabilitation standards for our patients, and we believe in you.

My Plan

1. I have read the list of clinicians skills and behaviors in Table 10.1 and identified the following skill(s) that I want to incorporate into my therapy and therefore need to practice.

_____

_____

_____

2. I have identified descriptions and forms in this manual that will be helpful references for me in my clinical work. Here are my top five:

Page	Item

3. I have identified a client whom I treated in the past and whose program would have been enhanced if I had used the instructional skills in Table 10.1. My first practice of my new skills will be a retrospective application of these skills to this client. Below, I describe how I would have used these skills had I known about them at that time. I will locate the corresponding worksheets in the book or on The Guilford Press website and fill them out with the clinical data that I would have expected.

_____

_____

_____

_____

4. I plan to use the following skills in my next sessions:

Session date	Skill I need to master before that session

5. I implemented the skills above, and here is my evaluation of my performance:

_____

_____

_____

_____

6. Having reflected on my own performance, I believe I can improve my performance in the next session in the following ways:

_____

_____

_____

_____

_____

_____

_____

_____

7. I will go through steps 5–7 once again.

APPENDIX

REPRODUCIBLE FORMS

Individualized Training Plan: Generic Planning Sheet

SPECIFY THE TARGET
WHAT will I teach the client to do?

☐ Is it a functional target that is meaningful to the client and to relevant stakeholders and was developed in collaboration with the client? How will it enhance the client's life participation?

☐ Is the client motivated to address this goal? How can I optimally engage my client?

☐ Do I need to teach any prerequisite skills?

☐ Have I specified the component steps or skills (i.e., task analysis)? Did I work with the client to identify these steps, so that the client understands the process?

☐ Have I considered the learner's strengths and weaknesses that impact this target?

☐ Have I considered natural facilitators and barriers in the environment?

☐ How will I measure progress toward learning this target? What is the desired criterion?

SPECIFY THE CONTEXTS
WHEN and HOW will I teach the instructional target?

Therapy Frequency: _____ / week	
Session Duration: _____ min	
Therapy Duration: _____ Sessions, Weeks, Months	

☐ What materials do I need for stimuli to prompt the learner to practice the target?

☐ Is there opportunity for sufficient practice within sessions?

☐ Is there opportunity for sufficient practice across sessions?

☐ What is the plan for progressing from modeling to distributed practice?

☐ What is the plan for varying stimulus–response set—do I have enough examples?

☐ Have I planned for follow-up?

WHERE will I address this goal?

☐ Have I planned for generalization to different settings?

☐ How will I measure generalization, maintenance, and impact of training?

☐ Is someone available to support additional practice between sessions?

☐ How will I train this person to carry out a home program using proper techniques?

Client Goal and Spaced Retrieval Data Sheet (I)

Client Name: _____ Type of Therapy: _____

Date: _____

Training Phrase: _____

Information Client is Learning: _____

Longest Time Between Successful Recalls Achieved Last Session: _____

Successful Recall at the Beginning of This Session? Yes No

The numbers below represent the minutes between recall of information. Circle the time interval completed and indicate if the recall was correct or incorrect by placing a plus (+) or minus (-) sign in the last box.

1	2	3	4	5	6	8	10	12	14	15	16	18	20	22	24	25	26	28	32	
1	2	3	4	5	6	8	10	12	14	15	16	18	20	22	24	25	26	28	32	
1	2	3	4	5	6	8	10	12	14	15	16	18	20	22	24	25	26	28	32	
1	2	3	4	5	6	8	10	12	14	15	16	18	20	22	24	25	26	28	32	
1	2	3	4	5	6	8	10	12	14	15	16	18	20	22	24	25	26	28	32	
1	2	3	4	5	6	8	10	12	14	15	16	18	20	22	24	25	26	28	32	
1	2	3	4	5	6	8	10	12	14	15	16	18	20	22	24	25	26	28	32	
1	2	3	4	5	6	8	10	12	14	15	16	18	20	22	24	25	26	28	32	
1	2	3	4	5	6	8	10	12	14	15	16	18	20	22	24	25	26	28	32	
1	2	3	4	5	6	8	10	12	14	15	16	18	20	22	24	25	26	28	32	
1	2	3	4	5	6	8	10	12	14	15	16	18	20	22	24	25	26	28	32	
1	2	3	4	5	6	8	10	12	14	15	16	18	20	22	24	25	26	28	32	

Therapy Goals	**Current Status**

Functional Progress/Status:

_____

_____

_____

_____

_____

Signature: _____

Client Goal and Spaced Retrieval Data Sheet (II)

Client Name: _____ Type of Therapy: _____

Date: _____

Training Phrase: _____

Information Client is Learning: _____

Longest Time Between Successful Recalls Achieved Last Session: _____

Successful Recall at the Beginning of This Session? Yes No

> The numbers below represent the minutes between recall of information. Circle the time interval completed and indicate if the recall was correct or incorrect by placing a plus (+) or minus (-) sign in the last box.

1	2	3	4	5	6	8	10	12	14	15	16	18	20	22	24	25	26	28	32	
1	2	3	4	5	6	8	10	12	14	15	16	18	20	22	24	25	26	28	32	
1	2	3	4	5	6	8	10	12	14	15	16	18	20	22	24	25	26	28	32	
1	2	3	4	5	6	8	10	12	14	15	16	18	20	22	24	25	26	28	32	
1	2	3	4	5	6	8	10	12	14	15	16	18	20	22	24	25	26	28	32	
1	2	3	4	5	6	8	10	12	14	15	16	18	20	22	24	25	26	28	32	
1	2	3	4	5	6	8	10	12	14	15	16	18	20	22	24	25	26	28	32	
1	2	3	4	5	6	8	10	12	14	15	16	18	20	22	24	25	26	28	32	
1	2	3	4	5	6	8	10	12	14	15	16	18	20	22	24	25	26	28	32	
1	2	3	4	5	6	8	10	12	14	15	16	18	20	22	24	25	26	28	32	
1	2	3	4	5	6	8	10	12	14	15	16	18	20	22	24	25	26	28	32	
1	2	3	4	5	6	8	10	12	14	15	16	18	20	22	24	25	26	28	32	

Therapy Goals	Correct Trials	Incorrect Trials	%

Functional Progress/Status:

_____

_____

_____

_____

_____

Signature: _____

WHAT will I teach the client?

Long-Term Goal:

Initial Acquisition Objectives:

(Specify target, approach, objective performance, independence, criterion, and context/conditions.)

HOW will I train the fact/concept?

(Specify method; e.g., MVC, SR, elaboration, visualization, mnemonics, strategy training.)

☐ It is a functional target

☐ It is customized to client

☐ The context is specified

☐ Progress measurement specified in long-term goal and/or short-term acquisition objectives

Plan to enhance client motivation/engagement:

WHEN will I teach the target?

Therapy Frequency: _____ / week

Session Duration: _____ min

Therapy Duration: _____ Sessions, Weeks, Months

☐ There is opportunity for sufficient practice within sessions

☐ There is opportunity for sufficient practice across sessions

To be used in same context or novel context?

Same context: Fixed stimuli = _____

Novel contexts: Varied stimuli = _____

Nature of information to be learned

Simple: Plan for spaced presentation is _____

Complex: Plan for massed presentation is _____

WHO will implement training outside of session?

☐ Support person identified to provide additional practice between sessions

☐ Sufficient variety of people identified to provide stimuli to allow generalization

Describe plan to *train* support person/people: _____

Instructional Planning Worksheet for Multistep Routines

Long-Term Goal:

Initial Acquisition Objectives:

(Specify target, approach, objective performance, independence, criterion, and context/conditions.)

Prerequisite Skills:

WHAT will I teach the client to do?

Task Analysis (List Steps)

☐ It is a functional target

☐ It is customized to client

☐ Context/antecedent specified

☐ Progress measurement specified in long-term goal and/or acquisition objectives

_____

_____

_____

_____

_____

_____

_____

_____

_____

_____

Plan to enhance client motivation/engagement:

WHEN and HOW will I teach the instructional target?

Therapy Frequency: _____ / week

Session Duration: _____ min

Therapy Duration: _____ Sessions, Weeks, Months

☐ There is opportunity for sufficient practice within sessions

☐ There is opportunity for sufficient practice across sessions

(cont.)

List materials needed to elicit routine and plan for varying stimuli with sufficient examples:

What is the plan for progressing from modeling to distributed practice?

WHO will help training outside of session?

☐ Support person identified to provide additional practice between sessions

☐ Sufficient variety of people identified to provide stimuli to allow generalization

Describe plan to train support person/people:

WHERE will I address this goal?

☐ There is a plan for generalization to different settings

☐ Measures of generalization across settings are incorporated into long-term goal

Initial Assessment Worksheet for Multistep Routines

Initial Assessment		
Client: _____		Date: _____
Target Routine: _____		
Antecedent to Start Routine: _____		
LIST STEPS	**ACCURACY (+/–/ cued)**	**COMMENTS**
Baseline: ____/____		

(cont.)

Dynamic Assessment to Establish Cue Hierarchy		
STEPS/ANTECEDENT	TYPE OF PROMPT/CUE	PERFORMANCE EFFECT

Recommended Cue Hierarchy:

Level I _____

Level II _____

Level III _____

Level IV _____

Level V _____

Progress Monitoring Form for Multistep Routines

Routine:

Long-Term Goal:

Initial Acquisition Short-Term Objective(s):

Steps	Session Probe Data					
Completion Time:						
Engagement Strategies:						
Generalization Programming during Training:						
Comments:						

Note: Graph the number of steps performed successfully each time the routine is probed.

Session Data Form for Multistep Routines

Client:			Date:
Step	Number of Massed Practice Trials and Level of Cueing	Duration and Number of Distributed Practice Trials	Comments
1.			
2.			
3.			
4.			
5.			
6.			
Summary			
Recommendations for next session			

Note: + correct; – incorrect; M = model; C = cued

Instructional Planning Worksheet for External Cognitive Aids

External Aid: _____

Primary Function	Requisite Skills	Impact/Goal	
		Short-term	Long-term

Long-Term Goal:

Initial Acquisition
Objectives:

(Specify target, approach, objective performance, independence, criterion, and context/conditions.)

WHAT will I teach the client to do? (Use of Tool)

Task Analysis (List Steps)

_____   _____

_____   _____

_____   _____

_____   _____

☐ Plan is customized to client
☐ Context/antecedent specified
☐ Progress measurement specified in long-term goal and/or acquisition objectives

Plan to enhance client motivation/engagement:

(cont.)

Plan to involve environmental supports:

WHEN and HOW will I teach the instructional target?

Therapy Frequency: _____ / week	
Session Duration: _____ min	
Therapy Duration: _____ Sessions, Weeks, Months	

☐ There is opportunity for sufficient practice within sessions
☐ There is opportunity for sufficient practice across sessions

List materials needed to practice using tool and plan for varying stimuli with sufficient examples:

What is the plan for progressing from modeling to distributed practice?

WHERE will the tool ultimately be used?

WHO will support training and tool use?

Describe context:

Describe plan to train support people:

Initial Assessment		
Client:		Date:
External Aid:		
Antecedent to Use Aid:		
LIST STEPS	**ACCURACY (+/–/cued)**	**COMMENTS**
Baseline: ____/____		

(cont.)

Dynamic Assessment to Establish Cue Hierarchy		
STEPS/ANTECEDENT	**TYPE OF PROMPT/CUE**	**PERFORMANCE EFFECT**
Recommended Cue Hierarchy:		
Level I _____		
Level II _____		
Level III _____		
Level IV _____		

Progress Monitoring Form for External Cognitive Aids

External Aid:

Long-Term Goal:

Initial Acquisition Short-Term Objective(s):

Strategy Steps/Component	Session Probe Data				
Completion Time:					

Supports:

Motivational/Engagement Strategies:

Generalization Programming:

Comments:

Note: **Graph the number of steps performed successfully each time the routine is probed.**

Session Data Form for External Cognitive Aids

Client:		Date:	
Step	Number of Massed Practice Trials and Level of Cueing	Duration and Number of Distributed Practice Trials	Comments
1.			
2.			
3.			
4.			
5.			
6.			
Summary			
Recommendations for next session			

Note: + correct; − incorrect; M = model; C = cued

Follow-Up Form to Collect Maintenance Data

Date: _____

_____ week follow-up

Dear _____,

This purpose of this letter is to check in and see how _____
is working. Please use the rating scales to indicate how much help is currently required to use the tool(s) learned in rehabilitation in comparison to how much you anticipated needing to assist, in addition to rating the frequency of use. Thank you for completing the information and returning this follow-up letter so that we can track recovery and outcomes.

Level of Independence	Expected Level of Independence	Frequency of Use	Comments

Independence Rating:

1 = Unable

2 = Lots of help

3 = Occasional help

4 = Reminders only

5 = Independent

Frequency of Use:

0 = Never

1 = One time a week

2 = A few times a week

3 = Most days

Please call _____ if you have any questions or would like reminders about training or would like to schedule a follow-up visit.

Instructional Planning Worksheet for Strategy Instruction

Long-Term Goal:	

Initial Acquisition Objectives:	

(Specify target, approach, objective performance, independence, criterion, and context/conditions.)

WHAT will I teach the client to do?
Strategy (List Steps)

_____

_____

_____

_____

_____

_____

_____

_____

_____

Strategy (Checklist)

☐ Strategy addresses identified need(s)

☐ Client has sufficient insight/awareness

☐ Strategy is customized to client

☐ Context/antecedent specified

☐ Progress measurement specified in long-term goal and/or acquisition objectives

Plan to enhance client motivation/engagement:	

(cont.

WHEN and HOW will I teach
the strategy?

Therapy Frequency: _____ / week

Session Duration: _____ min .

Therapy Duration: _____ Sessions, Weeks, Months

☐ There is opportunity for sufficient practice within sessions

☐ There is opportunity for sufficient practice across sessions

List materials needed to elicit strategy
use and plan for varying stimuli with
sufficient examples:

What is the plan for progressing:

Data Sheet for Measuring Strategy Knowledge

	DATE					
Knowledge Questions						
What is the name of your strategy?						
Describe the steps in your strategy						
What are examples of when you would use your strategy?						
How can your strategy be useful to you?						

M = Modeled—presented entire answer

A = Assisted—gave partial response

I = Independent, no cues

FORM 8.3

Progress Monitoring Form for Strategy Instruction

Strategy:

Long-Term Goal:

**Initial Acquisition
Short-Term
Objective(s):**

Strategy Steps/Component	Session Probe Data				
Supports (e.g., written cues, checklist, say aloud, auditory prompts):					
Motivational/Engagement Strategies:					
Generalization Programming during Training:					
Comments:					

Note: Graph the number of steps performed successfully each time the routine is probed.

FORM 9.1

ICF Worksheet

Diagnosis:

Social Participation

Social Activities

Social Functions

Personal Factors

Environmental Factors

PLAN:

PROGNOSIS:

Instructional Planning Worksheet for Social Skills

WHAT will I teach the client?

Long-Term Goal:

Initial Acquisition
Objectives:

(Specify target, approach, objective performance, independence, criterion, and context/conditions.)

HOW will I train the skill?
(Specify method; e.g., MVC, SR, elaboration, visualization,
mnemonics, strategy training.)

_____

☐ It is a functional target

☐ It is customized to client

☐ The context is specified

☐ Progress measurement specified in long-term goal
  and/or short-term acquisition objectives

Plan to enhance client motivation/engagement:

WHEN will I teach the target?

| Therapy Frequency: _____ / week |
| Session Duration: _____ min |
| Therapy Duration: _____ Sessions, Weeks, Months |

☐ There is opportunity for sufficient practice within sessions
☐ There is opportunity for sufficient practice across sessions

To be used in same context or novel context?

Same context: Fixed stimuli = _____

Novel contexts: Varied stimuli = _____

Nature of information to be learned

Simple: Plan for spaced presentation is _____

Complex: Plan for massed presentation is _____

WHO will implement training outside of session?

☐ Support person identified to provide additional practice between sessions
☐ Sufficient variety of people identified to provide stimuli to allow generalization

Describe plan to _train_ support person/people: _____

_____

References

Ada, L., Dorsch, S., & Canning, C. G. (2006). Strengthening interventions increase strength and improve activity after stroke: A systematic review. *The Australian Journal of Physiotherapy, 52,* 241–248.

Alexander, S. C., Sleath, B., Golin, C. E., & Kalinowski, C. T. (2006). Provider–patient communication and treatment adherence. In H. B. Bosworth, E. Z. Oddone, & M. Weinberger (Eds.), *Patient treatment adherence: Concepts, interventions, and management* (1st ed., pp. 329–372). Mahwah, NJ: Erlbaum.

Anderson, N. D., & Craik, F. I. (2006). The mnemonic mechanisms of errorless learning. *Neuropsychologia, 44*(14), 2806–2813.

Andrewes, D., & Gielewski, E. (1999). The work rehabilitation of a herpes simplex encephalitis patient with anterograde amnesia. *Neuropsychological Rehabilitation, 9*(1), 77–99.

Baddelely, A., Eysenck, M., & Anderson, M. (2009). *Memory.* New York: Psychological Press.

Baddeley, A., & Wilson, B. A. (1994). When implicit learning fails: Amnesia and the problem of error elimination. *Neuropsychologia, 32*(1), 53–68.

Baker, S., Gersten, R., & Scanlon, D. (2002). Procedural facilitators and cognitive strategies: Tools for unraveling the mysteries of comprehension and the writing process, and for providing meaningful access to the general curriculum. *Learning Disabilities Practice, 17,* 65–77.

Baron-Cohen, S., Leslie, A. M., & Frith, U. (1985). Does the autistic child have a "theory of mind"? *Cognition, 21,* 37–46.

Bastian, L. A., Molner, S. L., Fish, L. J., & McBride, C. M. (2006). Smoking cessation and adherence. In H. B. Bosworth, E. Z. Oddone, & M. Weinberger (Eds.), *Patient treatment adherence: Concepts, interventions, and management* (1st ed., pp. 125–146). Mahwah, NJ: Erlbaum.

Baughman, F. D., & Thomas, M. S. C. (2008). Specific impairments in cognitive development: A dynamical systems approach. In B. C. Love, K. McRae, & V. M. Sloutsky (Eds.), *Proceedings of the 30th annual conference of the Cognitive Science Society* (pp. 1819–1824). Austin, TX: Cognitive Science Society.

Bellini, S., & Akullian, J. (2007). A meta-analysis of video modeling and video self-modeling interventions for children and adolescents with autism spectrum disorders. *Exceptional Children*, 73(3), 264–287.

Berg, J. S., Dischler, J., Wagner, D. J., Raia, J. J., & Palmer-Shevlin, N. (1993). Medication compliance: A healthcare problem. *Annals of Pharmacotherapy*, 27(9), S4–S19.

Bergquist, T., Gehl, C., Mandrekar, J., Lepore, S., Hanna, S., Osten, A., et al. (2009). The effect of internet-based cognitive rehabilitation in persons with memory impairments after severe traumatic brain injury. *Brain Injury*, 23(10), 790–799.

Bier, N., Van der Linden, M., Gagnon, L., Desrosiers, J., Adam, S., Louveaux, S., et al. (2008). Face–name association learning in early Alzheimer's disease: A comparison of learning methods and their underlying mechanisms. *Neuropsychological Rehabilitation*, 18(3), 343–371.

Bonaiuti, D., Rebasti, L., & Sioli, P. (2007). The constraint induced movement therapy: A systematic review of randomized controlled trials on the adult stroke patients. *Europa Medicophysica*, 43, 139–146.

Bora, E., Yucel, M., & Pantelis, C. (2009). Theory of mind impairment in schizophrenia: Meta-analysis. *Schizophrenia Research*, 109(1–3), 1–9.

Borkwoski, J., Carr, M., Rollinger, E., & Pressley, M. (1990). Self-regulated cognition: Interdependence of metacognition, attributions, and self esteem. In B. Fly & L. Idol (Eds.), *Dimensions of thinking and cognitive instruction* (pp. 53–93). Hillsdale, NJ: Erlbaum.

Boschen, K., Gargaro, J., Gan, C., Gerber, G., & Brandys, C. (2007). Family interventions after acquired brain injury and other chronic conditions: A critical appraisal of the quality of the evidence. *Neurorehabilitation*, 22(1), 19–41.

Bourgeois, M., Lenius, K., Turkstra, L., & Camp, C. (2007). The effects of cognitive teletherapy on reported everyday memory behaviours of persons with chronic traumatic brain injury. *Brain Injury*, 21(12), 1245–1257.

Bowman, I. L., Linberg, S. C., Hemmingsson, H., & Barfai, A., (2010). A training apartment with a set of memory aids for patients with cognitive problems. *Scandinavian Occupational Therapy*, 17(2), 140–148.

Bradley, V. A., Kapur, N., & Evans, J. (2003). The assessment of memory for memory rehabilitation. In P. Halligan & D. Wade (Eds.), *Effectiveness of rehabilitation for cognitive deficits* (pp. 115–134). New York: Oxford University Press.

Brown, M., Dihkers, M. P., Gordon, W. A., Ashman, T., Charatz, H., & Cheng, Z. M. A. (2004). Participation objective, participation subjective: A measure of participation combining outsider and insider perspectives. *The Journal of Head Injury Rehabilitation*, 19(6), 459–481.

Brush, J. A., & Camp, C. J. (1998). *A therapy technique for improving memory: Spaced retrieval.* Beachwood, OH: Menorah Park Center for the Aging.

Burbank, P. M., Padula, C. A., & Nigg, C. R. (2000). Changing health behaviors of older adults. *Journal of Gerontological Nursing*, 26(3), 26–33; quiz 52–53.

Burke, J. M., Danick, J. A., Bemis, B., & Durgin, C. J. (1994). A process approach to memory book training for neurological patients. *Brain Injury*, 8, 71–81.

Burke, L. E., Styn, M. A., Glanz, K., Ewing, L. J., Elci, O. U., Conroy, M. B., et al. (2009). SMART trial: A randomized clinical trial of self-monitoring in behavioral weight-management design and baseline findings. *Contemporary Clinical Trials*, 30(6), 540–551.

Burkhead, L. M., Sapienza, C. M., & Rosenbek, J. C. (2007). Strength-training exercise in dysphagia rehabilitation: Principles, procedures, and directions for future research. *Dysphagia*, 22, 251–265.

Bussman-Mork, B. A., Hildberandt, H., Giesselmann, H., & Sachsenheimer, W. (2000). Treatment of verbal memory disorders: A comparison of several methods. *Neurologie und Rehabilitation, 4,* 195–204.

Butler, R., Copeland, D., Fairclough, D., Mulhern, R., Katz, E., Kazak, A., et al. (2008). A multicenter, randomized clinical trial of a cognitive remediation program for childhood survivors of a pediatric malignancy. *Journal of Consulting and Clinical Psychology, 76*(3), 367–378.

Butters, M. A., Glisky, E., & Schacter, D. (1993). Transfer of new learning in memory-impaired patients. *Journal of Clinical and Experimental Neuropsychology, 15*(2), 219–230.

Campbell, L., Wilson, C. F., McCann, J., Kernahan, G., & Rogers, R. (2007). Single case experimental design study of carer facilitated errorless learning in a patient with severe memory impairment following TBI. *NeuroRehabilitation, 22,* 325–333.

Campbell, R., Evans, M., Tucker, M., Quilty, B., Dieppe, P., & Donovan, J. L. (2001). Why don't patients do their exercises?: Understanding non-compliance with physiotherapy in patients with osteoarthritis of the knee. *Journal of Epidemiology and Community Health, 55,* 132–138.

Cardol, M., Beelen, A., van den Box, G. A., de Jong, B. A., de Groot, I. J., & de Haan, R. J. (2002). Responsiveness of the Impact on Participation and Autonomy Questionnaire. *Archives of Physical Medicine and Rehabilitation, 83*(11), 1524–1529.

Carrow-Woolfolk, E. (1999). *Comprehensive assessment of spoken language.* Circle Pines, MN: American Guidance Service.

Cavell, T. A. (1990). Social adjustment, social performance, and social skills: A tri-component model of social competence. *Journal of Clinical Child Psychology, 19*(2), 111–122.

Chen, C., Neufeld, P. S., Feely, C. A., & Skinner, C. S. (1999). Factors influencing compliance with home programs among patients with upper-extremity impairment. *American Journal of Occupational Therapy, 53,* 171–180.

Cherney, L. R., Patterson, J. P., Raymer, A., Frymark, T., & Schooling, T. (2008). Evidence-based systematic review: Effects of intensity of treatment and constraint-induced language therapy for individuals with stroke-induced aphasia. *Journal of Speech, Language, and Hearing Research, 51*(5), 1282–1299.

Cherry, K. E., Hawley, K. S., Jackson, E. M., & Boudreaux, E. O. (2009). Booster sessions enhance the long-term effectiveness of spaced retrieval in older adults with probable Alzheimer's disease. *Behavior Modification, 33*(3), 295–313.

Cicerone, K. D., & Giacino, J. T. (1992). Remediation of executive function deficits after traumatic brain injury. *NeuroRehabilitation, 2,* 12–22.

Cicerone, K. D., & Tupper, D. (1991). *The Neuropsychology of Everyday Life: Issues in Development and Rehabilitation.* Norwell, MA: Kluwer Academic.

Cicerone, K. D., & Wood, J. C. (1987). Planning disorder after closed head injury: A case study. *Archives of Physical Medicine and Rehabilitation, 68,* 111–115.

Clare, L., Roth, I., Wilson, B., Carter, G., & Hodges, J. (2002). Relearning face–name associations in early Alzheimer's disease. *Neuropsychology, 16*(4), 538–547.

Clare, L., Wilson, B. A., Carter, G., Breen, K., Gosses, A., & Hodges, J. R. (2000). Intervening with everyday memory problems in dementia of the Alzheimer type: An errorless learning approach. *Journal of Clinical and Experimental Neuropsychology, 22*(1), 132–146.

Clark, H. M. (2003). Neuromuscular treatments for speech and swallowing: A tutorial. *American Journal of Speech–Language Pathology, 12,* 400–415.

Clinical Practice Guideline for Treating Tobacco Use and Dependence 2008 Update Panel, Liaisons, and Staff. (2008). A clinical practice guideline for treating tobacco use and dependence: 2008 update: A U.S. Public Health Service report. *American Journal of Preventive Medicine, 35*(2), 158–176.

Cole, E. (1999). Cognitive prosthetics: An overview to a method of treatment. *NeuroRehabilitation, 12,* 39–51.

Corrigan, J. D., & Bogner, J. (2004). Latent factors in measures of rehabilitation outcomes after traumatic brain injury. *Journal of Head Trauma Rehabilitation, 19*(6), 445–458.

Cream, A., O'Brian, S., Jones, M., Block, S., Harrison, E., Lincoln, M., et al. (2010). Randomized controlled trial of video self-modeling following speech restructuring treatment for stuttering. *Journal of Speech, Language, and Hearing Research, 53*(4), 887–897.

Cream, A., O'Brian, S., Onslow, M., Packman, A., & Menzies, R. (2009). Self-modelling as a relapse intervention following speech-restructuring treatment for stuttering. *International Journal of Language and Communication Disorders/Royal College of Speech and Language Therapists, 44*(5), 587–599.

Dahlberg, C. A., Cusick, C. P., Hawley, L. A., Newman, J. K., Morey, C. E., Harrison-Felix, C. L., et al. (2007). Treatment efficacy of social communication skills training after traumatic brain injury: A randomized treatment and deferred treatment controlled trial. *Archives of Physical Medicine and Rehabilitation, 88*(12), 1561–1573.

Dewar, B. K., Patterson, K., Wilson, B. A., & Graham, K. S. (2009). Re-acquisition of person knowledge in semantic memory disorders. *Neuropsychological Rehabilitation, 19*(3), 383–421.

Diener, E., Emmons, R. A., Larsen, R. J., & Griffin, S. (1985). The Satisfaction with Life Scale. *Journal of Personality Assessment, 49(1), 71–75.*

Dishman, R. K. (1994a). *Advances in exercise adherence.* Champaign, IL: Human Kinetics.

Dishman, R. K. (1994b). Motivating older adults to exercise. *Southern Medical Journal, 87*(5), S79–S82.

Dominick, K. L., & Morey, M. (2006). Adherence to physical activity. In H. B. Bosworth, E. Z. Oddone, & M. Weinberger (Eds.), *Patient treatment adherence: Concepts, interventions, and management* (1st ed., pp. 49–94). Mahwah, NJ: Erlbaum.

Donaghy, S., & Williams, W. (1998). A new protocol for training severely impaired patients in the usage of memory journals. *Brain Injury, 12,* 1061–1070.

Donovan, J. J., & Radosevich, D. J. (1999). A meta-analytic review of the distribution of practiceeffect: Now you see it, now you don't. *Journal of Applied Psychology, 84*(5), 795–805.

Dou, Z. L., Man, W. K., Ou, H. N., Sheng, J. L., & Tam, S. F. (2006). Computerized errorless learning-based memory rehabilitation for Chinese patients with brain injury: A preliminary quasi-experimental clinical design study. *Brain Injury, 20,* 219–225.

Douglas, J. M., Bracy, C. A., & Snow, P. C. (2007). Measuring perceived communicative ability after traumatic brain injury: Reliability and validity of the La Trobe Communication Questionnaire. *Journal of Head Trauma Rehabilitation, 22*(1), 31–38.

Douglas, J. M., & Spellacy, F. J. (2000). Correlates of depression in adults with severe traumatic brain injury and their carers. *Brain Injury, 14*(1), 71–88.

Driver, S. (2006). Applying physical activity motivation theories to people with brain injuries. *Adapted Physical Activity Quarterly, 23,* 148–162.

Dromerick, A. W., Lang, C. E., Birkenmeier, R. L., Wagner, J. M., Miller, J. P., Videen, T. O., et al. (2009). Very early constraint-induced movement during stroke rehabilitation (VECTORS): A single-center RCT. *Neurology, 73*(3), 195–201.

Dunlosky, J., Hertzog, C., Kennedy, M., & Thiede, K. (2005). The self-monitoring approach for effective learning. *Cognitive Technology, 10,* 4–11.

Dunlosky, J., & Metcalfe, J. (2008). *Metacognition.* Thousand Oaks, CA: Sage.

Dunn, J., & Clare, L. (2007). Learning face–name associations in early-stage dementia: Comparing the effects of errorless learning and effortful processing. *Neuropsychological Rehabilitation, 17*(6), 735–754.

Dzewaltowski, D. A. (1994). Physical activity determinants: A social cognitive approach. *Medicine and Science in Sports and Exercise, 26*, 1395–1399.

Easterling, C., Grande, B., Kern, M., Sears, K., & Shaker, R. (2005). Attaining and maintaining isometric and isokinetic goals of the Shaker exercise. *Dysphagia, 20*, 133–138.

Ehlhardt, L., Sohlberg, M. M., Glang, A., & Albin, R. (2005). TEACH-M: A pilot study evaluating an instructional sequence for persons with impaired memory and executive functions. *Brain Injury, 19*(8), 569–583.

Ehlhardt, L., Sohlberg, M. M., Kennedy, M., Coelho, C., Ylvisaker, M., Turkstra, L., et al. (2008). Evidence-based practice guidelines for instructing individuals with neurogenic memory impairments: What have we learned in the past 20 years? *Neuropsychological Rehabilitation, 18*(3), 300–342.

Elley, C. R., Dean, S., & Kerse, N. (2007). Physical activity promotion in general practice: Patient attitudes. *Australian Family Physician, 36*(12), 1061–1064.

Engberg, M. E. (2004). Improving intergroup relations in higher education: A critical examination of the influence of educational interventions on racial bias. *Review of Educational Research, 74*(4), 473–524.

Engelmann, S. E., & Carnine, D. W. (1991). *Theory of instruction: Principles and applications.* Eugene, OR: ADI Press.

Englert, C. S., Raphael, T. E., Anderson, L. M., Anthony, H. M., & Stevens, D. D. (1991). Making writing strategies and self-talk visible: Cognitive strategy instruction in regular and special education classrooms. *American Education Research Journal, 28*, 337–372.

Evans, J. J., Wilson, B. A., Schuri, U., Andrade, J., Baddeley, A., Bruna, O., et al. (2000). A comparison of "errorless" and "trial and error" learning methods for teaching individuals with acquired memory deficits. *Neuropsychological Rehabilitation, 10*(1), 67–101.

Fasotti, L., Kovacs, F., Eling, P. A. T. M., & Brouwer, W. H. (2000). Time pressure management as a compensatory strategy training after closed head injury. *Neuropsychological Rehabilitation, 10*(1), 47–65.

Fatouros, I. G., Kambas, A., Katrabasas, I., Nikolaidis, K., Chatzinikolaou, A., Leontsini, D., et al. (2005). Strength training and detraining effects on muscular strength, anaerobic power, and mobility of inactive older men are intensity dependent. *British Journal of Sports Medicine, 39*, 776–780.

Feeney, T. J., & Ylvisaker, M. (1997). A positive, communication-based approach to challenging behavior after ABI. In A. Glang, G. H. S. Singer, & B. Todis (Eds.), *Students with acquired brain injury: The school's response* (pp. 229–254). Baltimore: Brookes.

Fluharty, G., & Priddy, D. (1993). Methods of increasing client acceptance of a memory book. *Brain Injury, 7*, 85–88.

Frattali, C., Thompson, C., Holland, A., Wohl, C., & Ferketic, M. (1995). *American Speech Language Hearing Association functional assessment of communication skills for adults* (1st ed.). Rockville, MD: American Speech Language Hearing Association.

Friedrich, M., Gittler, G., Halberstadt, Y., Cermak, T., & Heiller, I. (1998). Combined exercise and motivation program: Effect on the compliance and level of disability of patients with chronic low back pain: A randomized controlled trial. *Archives of Physical Medicine and Rehabilitation, 79*, 475–487.

Gauthier, S., Reisberg, B., Zaudig, M., Petersen, R. C., Ritchie, K., Broich, K., et al. (2006). Mild cognitive impairment. *Lancet, 367*(9518), 1262–1270.

Gazzaniga, M. S., Ivry, R. B., & Mangun, G. R. (2002). *Cognitive neuroscience: The biology of the mind* (2nd ed.). New York: Norton.

Gentry, T., Wallace, J., Kvarfordt, C., & Lynch, K. (2008). Personal digital assistants as cognitive aids for individuals with severe traumatic brain injury: A community based trial. *Brain Injury, 22*(1), 19–24.

Giles, G. M., Ridley, J. E., Dill, A., & Frye, S. (1997). A consecutive series of adults with brain injury treated with a washing and dressing retraining program. *American Journal of Occupational Therapy, 51*, 256–266.

Glang, A., Singer, G., Cooley, E., & Tish, N. (1992). Tailoring direct instruction techniques for use with elementary students with brain injury. *Journal of Head Trauma Rehabilitation, 7*(4), 93–108.

Glisky, E. (1992). Acquisition and transfer of declarative and procedural knowledge by memory-impaired patients: A computer data-entry task. *Neuropsychologia, 30*(10), 899–910.

Glisky, E. (1995). Acquisition and transfer of word processing skills by an amnesic patient. *Neuropsychological Rehabilitation, 5*(4), 299–318.

Glisky, E. L., & Delaney, E. L. (1996). Implicit memory and new semantic learning in posttraumatic amnesia. *Journal of Head Trauma Rehabilitation, 11*(2), 31–42.

Glisky, E. L., & Schacter, D. L. (1987). Acquisition of domain-specific knowledge in organic amnesia: Training for computer-related work. *Neuropsychologia, 25*(6), 893–906.

Glisky, E. L., & Schacter, D. L. (1988). Long-term retention of computer learning by patients with memory disorders. *Neuropsychologia, 26*(1), 173–178.

Glisky, E. L., & Schacter, D. L. (1989). Extending the limits of complex learning in organic amnesia: Computer training in a vocational domain. *Neuropsychologia, 27*(1), 107–120.

Glisky, E. L., Schacter, D. L., & Tulving, E. (1986a). Computer learning by memory-impaired patients: Acquisition and retention of complex knowledge. *Neuropsychologia, 24*(3), 313–328.

Glisky, E. L., Schacter, D. L., & Tulving, E. (1986b). Learning and retention of computer-related vocabulary in memory-impaired patients: Method of vanishing cues. *Journal of Clinical and Experimental Neuropsychology, 8*(3), 20.

Graham, S., & Harris, K. R. (2003). Students with learning disabilities and the process of writing: A meta-analysis of SRSD studies. In H. L. Swanson, K. R. Harris, & S. Graham (Eds.), *Handbook of learning disabilities* (pp. 323–344). New York: Guilford Press.

Graham, S., MacArthur, C., & Schwartz, S. (1995). Effects of goal setting and procedural facilitation on the revising behavior and writing performance of students with writing and learning problems. *Journal of Educational Psychology, 87*, 230–240.

Greenberg, D. L., & Verfaellie, K. R. (2010). Interdependence of episodic and semantic memory: Evidence from neuropsychology. *Journal of International Neuropsychology Society, 1*–6.

Gumpel, T. P., & Nativ-Ari-Am, H. (2001). Evaluation of a technology for teaching complex social skills to young adults with visual and cognitive impairments. *Journal of Visual Impairments and Blindness, 95*, 95–107.

Gustafson, D. H., Hawkins, R. P., Boberg, E. W., McTavish, F., Owens, B., Wise, M., et al. (2002). CHESS: 10 years of research and development in consumer health informatics for broad populations, including the underserved. *International Journal of Medical Informatics, 65*(3), 169–177.

Haley, S. M., Coster, W. J., Ludlow, L. H., Haltiwanger, J. H., & Adrellos, P. J. (1992). *Pediatric Evaluation of Disability Inventory: Development, standardization, and administration manual.* Boston: New England Medical Center Hospital/Trustees of Boston University.

Hammer, D. (1997). Discovery learning and discovery teaching. *Cognition and Instruction, 15*(4), 485–529.

Harris, K., & Pressley, M. (1991). The nature of cognitive strategy instruction: Interactive strategy instruction. *Exceptional Child, 57*, 392–404.

Hart, T., Buchhofer, R., & Vaccaro, M. (2004). Portable electronic devices as memory and organizational aids after traumatic brain injury: A consumer survey study. *Journal of Head Trauma Rehabilitation, 18*, 725–734.

Hart, T., Hawkey, K., & Whyte, J. (2002). Use of a portable Voice Organizer to remember therapy goals in traumatic brain injury rehabilitation: A within-subjects trial. *Journal of Head Trauma Rehabilitation, 17*, 556–570.

Hartley, L. L. (1995). *Cognitive-communicative abilities following brain injury: A functional approach.* San Diego: Singular Publishing.

Haslam, C., Gilroy, D., Black, S., & Beesley, T. (2006). How successful is errorless learning in supporting memory for high and low-level knowledge in dementia. *Neuropsychological Rehabilitation, 16*(5), 505–536.

Haslam, C., Moss, Z., & Hodder, K. (2010, May). Are two methods better than one?: Evaluating the effectiveness of combining errorless learning with vanishing cues. *Journal of Clinical and Experimental Neuropsychology*, 1–13. [Epub ahead of print]

Hawley, K., Cherry, K., Boudreaux, E., & Jackson, M. (2008). A comparison of adjusted spaced retrieval versus a uniform expanded retrieval schedule for learning a name–face association in older adults with probable Alzheimer's disease. *Journal of Clinical and Experimental Neuropsychology, 30*(6), 639–649.

Haynes, R. B., Ackloo, E., Sahota, N., McDonald, H. P., & Yao, X. (2008). Interventions for enhancing medication adherence. *Cochrane Database of Systematic Reviews (Online), 2*(2), CD000011.

Henry, J. D., Phillips, L. H., Crawford, J. R., Ietswaart, M., & Summers, F. (2006). Theory of mind following traumatic brain injury: The role of emotion recognition and executive dysfunction. *Neuropsychologia*, , xx–xx.

Henry, K. D., Rosemond, C., & Eckert, L. B. (1998). Effect of number of home exercises on compliance and performance in adults over 65 years of age. *Physical Therapy, 78*, 270–277.

Hettema, J., Steele, J., & Miller, W. R. (2005). Motivational interviewing. *Annual Review of Clinical Psychology, 1*, 91–111.

Hillary, F. G., Schultheis, M. T., Challis, B. H., Millis, S. R., Carnevale, G. J., Glashi, T., et al. (2003). Spacing of repetitions improves learning and memory after moderate and severe TBI. *Journal of Clinical and Experimental Neuropsychology, 25*(1), 49–58.

Hitchcock, C. H., Dowrick, P. W., & Prater, M. A. (2003). Video self-modeling intervention in school-based settings: A review. *Remedial and Special Education, 24*(1), 36–46.

Hoepner, J., & Turkstra, L. S. (2010). Video-based administration of the LaTrobe Communication Questionnaire for Adults with Traumatic Brain Injury and Their Communication Partners. (Unpublished).

Holland, A. L. (2007). *Counseling in communication disorders: A wellness perspective.* San Diego: Plural Publishing.

Holland, A. L., & Fridriksson, J. (2001). Aphasia management during the early phases of recovery following stroke. *American Journal of Speech–Language Pathology, 10*(1), 19–28.

Holmes, C. F., Fletcher, J. P., Blaschak, M. J., & Schenck, R. C. (1997). Management of shoulder dysfunction with an alternative model of orthopaedic physical therapy intervention: A case report. *Journal of Orthopaedic and Sports Physical Therapy, 26*, 347–354.

Hopper, T., Drefs, S. J., Bayles, K. A., Tomoeda, C. K., & Dinu, I. (2008). The effects of modified spaced-retrieval training on learning and retention of face–name associations by individuals with dementia. *Neuropsychological Rehabilitation, 20*(1), 81–102.

Hopper, T., Mahendra, N., Kim, E., Azuma, T., Bayles, K. A., Cleary, S. J., et al. (2005). Evidence-based practice recommendations for working with individuals with dementia: Spaced-retrieval training. *Journal of Medical Speech–Language Pathology, 13*(4), 27–34.

Horvath, A. O., & Luborsky, L. (1993). The role of the therapeutic alliance in psychotherapy. *Journal of Consulting and Clinical Psychology, 61*(4), 561–573.

Horvath, A. O., & Symonds, B. D. (1991). Relation between working alliance and outcome in psychotherapy: A meta-analysis. *Journal of Counseling Psychology, 38,* 139–149.

Huckans, M., Pavawalla, S., Demadura, T., Kolessar, M., Seeve, A., Roost, N., et al. (2010). A pilot study examining effects of group-based cognitive strategy training on self-reported cognitive problems, psychiatric symptoms, functioning and compensatory strategy use in OIF/OEF veterans with persistent mild cognitive disorder and history of trauma and brain injury. *Journal of Rehabilitation Research and Development, 47*(1), 43–60.

Hughes, C. A., Ruhl, K. L., Schumaker, J. B., & Deshler, D. D. (2002). Effects of instruction in an assignment completion strategy on the homework performance of students with learning disabilities in general education classes. *Learning Disabilities: Research and Practice, 17*(1), 1–18.

Hunkin, N. A., & Parkin, A. J. (1995). The method of vanishing cues: An evaluation of its effectiveness in teaching memory impaired individuals. *Neuropsychologia, 33*(10), 1255–1279.

Hunkin, N. M., Squires, E. J., Parkin, A. J., & Tidy, J. A. (1998a). Are the benefits of errorless learning dependent on implicit memory? *Neuropsychologia, 36*(1), 25–36.

Hunkin, N. M., Squires, E. J., Aldrich, F. L., & Parkin, A. J. (1998b). Errorless learning and the acquisition of word processing skills. *Neuropsychological Rehabilitation, 8*(4), 433–449.

Jan, M., Hung, J., Lin, J. C., Wang, S., Liu, T., & Tang, P. (2004). Effects of a home program on strength, walking speed, and function after total hip replacement. *Archives of Physical Medicine and Rehabilitation, 85,* 1943–1951.

Jette, A. M., Rooks, D., Lachman, M., Lin, T. H., Levenson, C., Heislein, D., et al. (1998). Home-based resistance training: Predictors of participation and adherence. *The Gerontologist, 38,* 412–421.

Judge, K. S., Menne, H. L., & Whitlatch, C. J. (2009). Stress process model for individuals with dementia. *The Gerontologist, 50*(3), 294–302.

Kagan, A., Black, S., Duchan, J., Mackie, N., & Square, P. (2001). Training volunteers as conversation partners using "Supported Conversation for Adults With Aphasia" (SCA): A controlled trial. *Journal of Speech, Language, and Hearing Research, 44,* 624–638.

Kalla, T., Downes, J. J., & van den Broeck, M. (2001). The pre-exposure technique: Enhancing effects of errorless learning in the acquisition of face–name associations. *Neuropsychological Rehabilitation, 11*(1), 1–16.

Kaschel, R., Sala, S., Cantagallo, A., Fahlbck, A., Laaksonen, R., & Kazen, M. (2002). Imagery mnemonics for the rehabilitation of memory: A randomised group controlled trial. *Neuropsychological Rehabilitation, 12*(2), 127–153.

Katz, M. M., & Lyerly, S. B. (1963). Methods for measuring adjustment and social behavior in the community: I. Rationale, description, discriminative validity and scale development. *Psychological Reports, 13*(2 Mono. Suppl. No. 4-V13), 503–535.

Kavale, K. A., & Forness, S. R. (2000). What definitions of learning disability say and don't say: A critical analysis. *Journal of Learning Disabilities, 33,* 239–256.

Kennedy, M. R., Krause, M. O., & Turkstra, L. S. (2008). An electronic survey about college experiences after traumatic brain injury. *NeuroRehabilitation, 23*(6), 511–520.

Kennedy, M. R. T., & Coelho, C. (2005). Self-regulation after traumatic brain injury: A framework for intervention of memory and problem solving. *Seminars in Speech and Language, 26,* 242–255.

Kennedy, M. R. T., Coelho, C., Turkstra, L., Ylvisaker, M., Sohlberg, M. M., Yorkston, K., et al. (2008). Intervention for executive functions after traumatic brain injury: A systematic review, meta-analysis and clinical recommendations. *Neuropsychological Rehabilitation*, 18(3), 257–299.

Kennedy, M. R. T., Linhart, S., & Brady, B. (2006). Metamemory for narratives after traumatic brain injury: Does timing matter?

Kennedy, M. R. T., & Tursktra, L. (2006). Group intervention studies in the cognitive rehabilitation of individuals with traumatic brain injury: Challenges faced by researchers. *Neuropsychology Review*, 16(4), 151–159.

Kern, R. S., Green, M. F., Mintz, J., & Liberman, R. P. (2003). Does 'errorless learning' compensate for neurocognitive impairments in the work rehabilitation for persons with schizophrenia? *Psychological Medicine*, 33, 432–433.

Kern, R. S., Green, M. F., Mitchell, S., Kopelowicz, A., Mintz, J., & Liberman, R. P. (2005). Extensions of errorless learning for social problem-solving deficits in schizophrenia. *American Journal of Psychiatry*, 162(3), 513–519.

Kern, R. S., Liberman, R. P., Kopelowicz, A., Mintz, J., & Green, M. F. (2002). Applications of errorless learning for improving work performance in persons with schizophrenia. *American Journal of Psychiatry*, 159, 1921–1926.

Kern, R. S., Wallace, C. J., Hellman, S. G., Womack, L. M., & Green, M. F. (1996). A training procedure for remediating WCST deficits in chronic psychotic patients: An adaptation of errorless learning principles. *Journal of Psychiatric Research*, 30(4), 283–294.

Kerns, K. A., & Thomson, J. (1998). Implementation of a compensatory memory system in a school age child with severe memory impairment. *Pediatric Rehabilitation*, 2, 77–87.

Kilgard, M. P., & Merzenich, M. M. (1998). Cortical map reorganization enabled by nucleus basalis activity. *Science*, 279, 1714–1718.

Kim, A., Vaughn, S., Wanzek, J., & Wei, S. (2004). Graphic organizers and their effects on the reading comprehension of students with LD: A synthesis of research. *Journal of Learning Disabilities*, 37(2), 105–119.

Kim, H. J., Burke, D. T., Dowds, M. M., Boone, K., & Park, G. J. (2000). Electronic memory aids for outpatient brain injury: Follow-up findings. *Brain Injury*, 14, 187–196.

Kim, H. J., Burke, D. T., Dowds, M. M., & George, J. (1999). Utility of a microcomputer as an external memory aid for a memory-impaired head injury patient during inpatient rehabilitation. *Brain Injury*, 13, 147–150.

King, A. C. (1994). Community and public health approaches to the promotion of physical activity. *Medicine and Science in Sports and Exercise*, 26, 1405–1412.

Kinsella, G. J., Mullaly, E., Rand, E., Ong, B., Burton, C., Price, S., et al. (2009). Early intervention for mild cognitive impairment: A randomised controlled trial. *Journal of Neurology, Neurosurgery, and Psychiatry*, 80(7), 730–736.

Kinsella, G. J., Ong, B., Storey, E., Wallace, J., & Hester, R. (2007). Elaborated spaced-retrieval and prospective memory in mild Alzheimer's disease. *Neuropsychological Rehabilitation*, 17(6), 688–706.

Kirsch, N. L., Levine, S. P., Fallon-Krueger, M., & Jaros, L. A. (1987). Focus on clinical research: The microcomputer as an "orthotic" device for patients with cognitive deficits. *The Journal of Head Trauma Rehabilitation*, 2(4), 77–86.

Kirsch, N. L., Levine, S. P., Lajiness-O'Neill, R., & Schnyder, M. (1992). Computer-assisted interactive task guidance: Facilitating the performance of a simulated vocational task. *Journal of Head Trauma Rehabilitation*, 7(3), 13–25.

Kirsch, N. L., Shenton, M., & Rowan, J. (2004a). A generic 'in-house' alphanumeric paging system for prospective activity impairments after traumatic brain injury. *Brain Injury*, 18, 725–734.

Kirsch, N. L., Shenton, M., Spril, E., Rowan, J., Simpson, R., Schreckenghost, D., et al. (2004b).

Web-based assistive technology interventions for cognitive impairments after traumatic brain injury: A selective review and two case studies. *Rehabilitation Psychology, 49,* 200–212.

Kirwan, T., Tooth, L., & Harkin, C. (2002). Compliance with hand therapy programs: Therapists' and patients' perceptions. *Journal of Hand Therapy, 15,* 31–40.

Kleim, J. A., & Jones, T. A. (2008). Principles of experience-dependent neural plasticity: Implications for rehabilitation after brain damage. *Journal of Speech, Language, and Hearing Research, 51*(1), S225–S239.

Komatsu, S., Mimura, M., Kato, M., Wakamatsu, N., & Kashima, H. (2000). Errorless and effortful processes involved in the learning of face–name associations by patients with alcoholic Korsakoff's syndrome. *Neuropsychological Rehabilitation, 10*(2), 113–132.

Kosma, M., Cardinal, B. J., & McCubbin, J. A. (2005). A pilot study of a web-based physical activity motivational program for adults with physical disabilities. *Disability and Rehabilitation, 27,* 1435–1442.

Krause, M., Wendt, J., Dressel, A., Berneiser, J., Kessler, C., Hamm, A. O., et al. (2009). Prefrontal function associated with impaired emotion recognition in patients with multiple sclerosis. *Behavioural Brain Research, 205*(1), 280–285.

Landis, J., Hanten, G., Levin, H. S., Li, X., Ewing-Cobbs, L., Duron, J., et al. (2006). Evaluation of the errorless learning technique in children with traumatic brain injury. *Archives of Physical Medicine and Rehabilitation, 87*(6), 799–805.

Larkins, B. M., Worrall, L. E., & Hickson, L. M. (2004). Stakeholder opinion of functional communication activities following traumatic brain injury. *Brain Injury, 18*(7), 691–706.

Lauer, A. (2004). Measuring positive and negative factors of device discontinuance. Unpublished Masters Thesis, University of Wisconsin, Milwaukee.

Law, B., & Ste-Marie, D. M. (2005). Effects of self-modeling on figure skating jump performance and psychological variables. *European Journal of Sport Science, 5*(3), 143–152.

Lawson, M. J., & Rice, D. N. (1989). Effects of training use of executive strategies on a verbal memory problem resulting from closed head injury. *Journal of Clinical and Experimental Neuropsychology, 6,* 8420–8854.

Lekeu, F., Wojtasik, V., Van Der Linden, M., & Salmon, E. (2002). Training early Alzheimer patients to use a mobile phone. *Acta Neurologica Belgica, 102,* 114–121.

Lemoncello, R. R. (2008). A within-subjects experimental evaluation of the television assisted prompting (TAP) system to maximize completion of home-delivered swallow strengthening exercises among individuals with co-occurring acquired swallowing and cognitive impairments (doctoral dissertation, University of Oregon, 2008). *Dissertation Abstracts International: Section B, 69*(8-B), 4714.

Lemoncello, R. R., & Sohlberg, M. M. (2005). *Practicing what the instructional research preaches: How do SLPs rate?* Paper presented at the American Speech–Language–Hearing Association Convention, San Diego, CA.

Leng, N. R. C., Copello, A. G., & Sayegh, A. (1991). Learning after brain injury by the method of vanishing cues: A case study. *Behavioral Psychotherapy, 19,* 173–181.

Lenker, J., & Paquet, V. L. (2004). A new conceptual model for assistive technology outcomes research and practice. *Assistive Technology, 16,* 1–10.

Lesgold, A. M. (2001). The nature and methods of learning by doing. *American Psychologist, 56,* 964–973.

Levine, B., Robertson, I. H., Clare, L., Carter, G., Hong, J., Wilson, B. A., et al. (2000). Rehabilitation of executive functioning: An experimental-clinical validation of goal management training. *Journal of the International Neuropsychological Society, 6,* 299–312.

Levinson, R. (1997). The planning and execution assistant and trainer (PEAT). *The Journal of Head Trauma Rehabilitation, 12*(2), 85–91.

Linscott, R. J., Knight, R. G., & Godfrey, H. P. (1996). The Profile of Functional Impairment in Communication (PFIC): A measure of communication impairment for clinical use. *Brain Injury, 10*(6), 397–412.

Lloyd, J., Riley, G., & Powell, T. (2009). Errorless learning of novel routes through a virtual town in people with acquired brain injury. *Neuropsychological Rehabilitation, 19*(1), 98–109.

Logemann, J. A. (2005). The role of exercise programs for dysphagia patients. *Dysphagia, 20,* 139–140.

Logsdon, R. G., McCurry, S. M., Pike, K. C., & Teri, L. (2009). Making physical activity accessible to older adults with memory loss: A feasibility study. *Gerontologist, 4,* S94–S99.

LoPresti, E. F., Mihailidis, A., & Kirsch, N. L. (2004). Assistive technology for cognitive rehabilitation: State of the art. *Neuropsychological Rehabilitation, 14,* 5–39.

LoPresti, E. F., Simpson, R. C., & Kirsch, N., Schreckenghost, D., & Hayashi, S. (2008). Distributed cognitive aid with scheduling and interactive task guidance. *Journal of Rehabilitation Research and Development, 45*(4), 505–522.

Lough, S., Kipps, C. M., Treise, C., Watson, P., Blair, J. R., & Hodges, J. R. (2006). Social reasoning, emotion and empathy in frontotemporal dementia. *NeuroPsychologia, 44*(6), 950–958.

Lowe, M. R., & Cautela, J. R. (1978). A self-report measure of social skill. *Behavioral Therapy, 9,* 535–544.

Lubinsky, T., Rich, J., & Anderson, N. (2009). Errorless learning and elaborative self-generation in healthy older adults and individuals with amnestic mild cognitive impairment: Mnemonic benefits and mechanisms. *Journal of International Neuropsychological Society, 15,* 704–716.

Lysack, C., Dama, M., Neufeld, S., & Andreassi, E. (2005). Compliance and satisfaction with home exercise: A comparison of computer-assisted video instruction and routine rehabilitation practice. *Journal of Allied Health, 34*(2), 76–82.

Maas, E., Robin, D. A., Austermann-Hula, S. N., Freedman, S. E., Wulf, G., Ballard, J. J., et al. (2008). Principles of motor learning in treatment of motor speech disorders. *American Journal of Speech–Language Pathology, 17,* 277–298.

Malec, J. F., Smigielski, J. S., & DePompolo, R. W. (1991). Goal attainment scaling and outcome measurement in postacute brain injury rehabilitation. *Archives of Physical Medicine and Rehabilitation, 72*(2), 138–143.

Manasse, N. J., Hux, K., & Snell, J. (2005). Teaching face–name associations to survivors of traumatic brain injury: A sequential treatment approach. *Brain Injury, 19*(8), 633–641.

Manheim, L. M., Halper, A. S., & Cherney, L. (2009). Patient-reported changes in communication after computer-based script training for aphasia. *Archives of Physical Medicine and Rehabilitation, 90*(4), 623–627.

Manley, K., Collins, B. C., Stenhoff, D. M., & Kleinert, H. (2008). Using a system of least prompts procedure to teach telephone skills to elementary students with cognitive disabilities. *Journal of Behavioral Education, 17,* 221–236.

Marchand-Martella, N. E., Slocum, T. A., & Martella, R. C. (2004). *Introduction to direct instruction.* Upper Saddle River, NJ: Pearson Education, Inc.

Markowitsch, H. (1998). Cognitive neuroscience of memory. *Neurocase, 4,* 429–435.

Martins, S., Guillery-Girard, B., Jambaque, I., Dulac, O., & Eustache, F. (2006). How do children suffering severe amnesic syndrome acquire new concepts? *NeuroPsychologia, 44*(14), 2792–2805.

Mastos, M., Miller, K., Eliasson, A. C., & Imms, C. (2007). Goal-directed training: Linking theories of treatment to clinical practice for improved functional activities of daily life. *Clinical Rehabilitation, 21*, 47–55.

Mastropieri, M. A., Scruggs, T. E., Bakken, J. P., & Whedon, C. (1996). Reading comprehension: A synthesis of research in learning disabilities. In T. E. Scruggs & M. A. Mastropieri (Eds.), *Advances in learning and behavioral disabilities* (Vol. 10, pp. 277–303). Greenwich, CT: JAI.

McCarty, D. L. (1980). Investigations of a visual imagery mnemonic device for acquiring face–name associations. *Journal of Experimental Psychology: Human Learning and Memory, 6*(2), 145–155.

McDonald, H. P., Garg, A. X., & Haynes, R. B. (2002). Interventions to enhance patient adherence to medication prescriptions: Scientific review. *Journal of the American Medical Association, 288*(22), 2868–2879.

McDonald, S., Flanagan, S., & Rollins, J. (2002). The Awareness of Social Inference Test (TASIT). Austin, TX: Harcourt Assessment.

McDonald, S., Tate, R., Togher, L., Bornhofen, C., Long, E., Gertler, P., et al. (2008). Social skills treatment for people with severe, chronic acquired brain injuries: A multicenter trial. *Archives of Physical Medicine and Rehabilitation, 89*(9), 1648–1659.

McGann, W., Werven, G., & Douglas, M. M. (1997). Social competence and head injury: A practical approach. *Brain Injury, 11*(9), 621–628.

McGraw-Hunter, M., Faw, G. D., & Davis, P. K. (2006). The use of video self-modelling and feedback to teach cooking skills to individuals with traumatic brain injury: A pilot study. *Brain Injury, 20*(10), 1061–1068.

McKenna, P., Clare, L., & Baddeley, A. D. (1995). Schizophrenia. In A. D. Baddeley, B. Wilson, & F. N. Watts (Eds.), *Handbook of memory disorders*. West Sussex, UK: Wiley.

McKitrick, L. A., Camp, C. J., & Black, W. (1992). Prospective memory intervention in Alzheimer's disease. *Journal of Gerontology: Psychological Sciences, 47*, P337–P343.

McWreath, M. (2005). Picturing aphasia. Available online at *www.aphasia.tv*.

Meichenbaum, D., & Turk, D. C. (1987). *Facilitating treatment adherence: A practitioner's guidebook*. New York: Plenum Press.

Melton, A. K., & Bourgeois, M. S. (2005). Training compensatory memory strategies via telephone for persons with TBI. *Aphasiology, 19*(3–5), 353–364.

Merriam-Webster's Collegiate Dictionary. (1986). Springfield, MA: Merriam-Webster, Inc.

Metzler-Baddeley, C., & Snowden, J. S. (2005). Brief report: Errorless versus errorful learning as a memory rehabilitation approach in Alzheimer's disease. *Journal of Clinical and Experimental Neuropsychology, 27*, 1070–1079.

Miller, R. G., Rosenberg, J. A., Gelinas, D. F., Mitsumoto, H., Newman, D., Sufit, R., et al. (1999). Practice parameter: The care of the patient with amyotrophic lateral sclerosis (an evidence-based review): Report of the Quality Standards Subcommittee of the American Academy of Neurology. *Neurology, 52*, 1311–1325.

Miller, W. R., & Rollnick, S. P. (2002). *Motivational interviewing: Preparing people for change* (2nd ed.). New York: Guilford Press.

Moffat, N. (1984). Strategies of memory therapy. In B. A. Wilson & N. Moffat (Eds.), *Clinical management of memory problems*. Beckenham, UK: Croom Helm.

Montessori, M., & George, A. (1912). *Scientific pedagogy as applied child education in "The Children's Houses."* New York: Stokes.

Mooney, P., Ryan, J., Uhing, B., Reid, R., & Epstein, M. (2005). A review of self-management interventions targeting academic outcomes for students with emotional and behavioral disorders. *Journal of Behavioral Education, 14*, 203–221.

Morris, D. M., Taub, E., & Mark, V. W. (2006). Constraint-induced movement therapy: Characterizing the intervention protocol. *Europa Medicophysica, 42*, 257–268.

Morris, L. S., & Schulz, R. M. (1992). Patient compliance–an overview. *Journal of Clinical Pharmacy and Therapeutics, 17*, 283–295.

Muller, F., Simion, A., Reviriego, E., Galera, C., Mazaux, J. M., Barat, M., et al. (2009). Exploring theory of mind after severe traumatic brain injury. *Cortex, 46*(9), 1088/1099.

Newbigging, E. D., & Laskey, J. W. (1995). Riding the bus: Teaching an adult with a brain injury to use a transit system to travel independently to and from work. *Brain Injury, 10*, 543–550.

Norman, G. J., Zabinski, M. F., Adams, M. A., Rosenberg, D. E., Yaroch, A. L., & Atienza, A. A. (2007). A review of eHealth interventions for physical activity and dietary behavior change. *American Journal of Preventive Medicine, 33*(4), 336–345.

Oberg, L., & Turkstra, L. S. (1998). Use of elaborative encoding to facilitate verbal learning after adolescent traumatic brain injury. *Journal of Head Trauma Rehabilitation, 13*(3), 44–62.

O'Carroll, R. E., Russell, H. H., Lawrie, S. M., & Johnstone, E. C. (1999). Errorless learning and the cognitive rehabilitation of memory-impaired schizophrenic patients. *Psychological Medicine, 29*, 105–112.

Olney, S. J., Nymark, J., Brouwer, B., Culham, E., Day, A., Heard, J., et al. (2006). A randomized controlled trial of supervised versus unsupervised exercise programs for ambulatory stroke survivors. *Stroke, 37*, 476–481.

Olswang, L., & Bain, B. (1994). Data collection: Monitoring children's treatment progress. *American Journal of Speech–Language Pathology, 3*, 55–66.

O'Neil-Pirozzi, T. M., Strangman, G. E., Goldstein, R., Katz, D. I., Savage, C. R., Kelkar, K., et al. (2010). A controlled treatment study of internal memory strategies (I-MEMS) following traumatic brain injury. *Journal of Head Trauma Rehabilitation, 25*(1), 43–51.

Ownsworth, T. L., & McFarland, K. (1999). Memory remediation in long-term acquired brain injury: Two approaches in diary training. *Brain Injury, 13*(8), 605–626.

Ownsworth, T. L., Quinn, H., Fleming, J., Kendall, M., & Shum, D. (2010). Error self regulation following traumatic brain injury: A single case study evaluation of metacognitive skills training and behavioral practice interventions. *Neuropsychological Rehabilitation, 20*(1), 59–80.

Page, M., Wilson, B., Shiel, A., Carter, G., & Norris, D. (2006). What is the locus of the errorless-learning advantage? *Neuropsychologia, 44*, 90–100.

Palincsar, A. S., & Brown, A. L. (1984). Reciprocal teaching of comprehension-fostering and monitoring activities. *Cognition and Instruction, 1*, 117–175.

Parkin, A. J., Hunkin, N. M., & Squires, E. J. (1998). Unlearning John Major: The use of errorless learning in the reacquisition of proper names follow herpes simplex encephalitis. *Cognitive Neuropsychology, 15*(4), 361–375.

Paul, D. R., Frattali, C. M., Holland, A. L., Thompson, C. K., Caperton, C. J., & Slater, S. C. (2004). *The American Speech–Language–Hearing Association Quality of Communication Life Scale (QCL): Manual*. Rockville, MD: American Speech–Language–Hearing Association.

Philippi, C. L., Mehta, S., Grabowski, T., Adolphs, R., & Rudrauf, D. (2009). Damage to association fiber tracts impairs recognition of the facial expression of emotion. *Journal of Neuroscience, 29*(48), 15089–15099.

Pitel, A. L., Perruchet, P., Vabret, F., Desgranges, B., Eustache, F., & Beaunieux, H. (2010). The advantage of errorless learning for the acquisition of new concepts' labels in alcoholics. *Psychological Medicine, 40*(3), 497–502.

Pope, J. W., & Kern, R. S. (2006). An "errorful" learning deficit in schizophrenia? *Journal of Clinical and Experimental Neuropsychology, 28*, 101–110.

Premack, D., & Woodruff, G. (1978). Does the chimpanzee have a theory of mind? *Behavioral and Brain Sciences, 1*(4), 515–526.

Quemada, J. I., Cespedes, J. M., Ezkerra, J., Ballesteros, J., Ibarra, N., & Urruticoechea, I. (2003). Outcome of memory rehabilitation in traumatic brain injury assessed by neuropsychological tests and questionnaires. *Journal of Head Trauma Rehabilitation, 18,* 532–540.

Ram, N., & McCullagh, P. (2003). Self-modeling: Influence on psychological responses and physical performance. *Sport Psychologist, 17*(2), 220–241.

Randolph, C. (2001). *Repeatable battery for the assessment of neuropsychological status* (1st ed.). San Antonio, TX: Psychological Corporation.

Rath, J., Simon, D., Langenbahn, D. M., Sherr, R. L., & Diller, L. (2003). Group treatment of problem solving deficits in outpatients with traumatic brain injury: A randomized outcome study. *Neuropsychological Rehabilitation, 13,* 461–488.

Raymer, A. M., Beeson, P., Holland, A., Kendall, D., Maher, L. M., Martin, N., et al. (2008). Translational research in aphasia: From neuroscience to neurorehabilitation. *Journal of Speech, Language, and Hearing Research, 51*(1), S259–S275.

Reid, R., Trout, A., & Schartz, M. (2005). Self-regulation interventions for children with attention deficit/hyperactivity disorder. *Exceptional Children, 71*(4), 361–377.

Resnicow, K., Davis, R. E., Zhang, G., Konkel, J., Strecher, V. J., Shaikh, A. R., et al. (2008). Tailoring a fruit and vegetable intervention on novel motivational constructs: Results of a randomized study. *Annals of Behavioral Medicine, 35*(2), 159–169.

Rickards-Schlichting, K. A., Kehle, T. J., & Bray, M. A. (2004). A self-modeling intervention for high school students with public speaking anxiety. *Journal of Applied School Psychology, 20*(2), 47–60.

Riley, G., & Heaton, S. (2000). Guidelines for the selection of a method of fading cues. *Neuropsychological Rehabilitation, 10*(2), 133–149.

Riley, G. A., Sotirious, D., & Jaspal, S. (2004). Which is more effective in promoting implicit and explicit memory: The method of vanishing cues or errorless learning without fading? *Neuropsychological Rehabilitation, 14*(3), 257–283.

Robison, J., Curry, L., Gruman, C., Porter, M., Henderson, C. R., Jr., & Pillemer, K. (2007). Partners in caregiving in a special care environment: Cooperative communication between staff and families on dementia units. *Gerontologist, 47*(4), 504–515.

Robison, J. I., & Rogers, M. A. (1994). Adherence to exercise programmes: Recommendations. *Sports Medicine, 17,* 39–52.

Rollnick, S., Mason, P., & Butler, C. (1999). *Health behavior change: A guide for practitioners.* Edinburgh, NY: Churchill Livingstone.

Rosenshine, B., & Meister, C. (1994). Reciprocal teaching: A review of the research. *Review of Educational Research, 64*(4), 479–530.

Roth, R. M., Isquith, P. K., & Gioia, G. A. (2005). Behavior Rating Inventory of Executive Function (Adult ed.). Lutz, FL: Par.

Ruis, C., & Kessels, R. P. C. (2005). Effects of errorless learning and errorful face–name associative learning in moderate–severe dementia. *Aging Clinical and Experimental Research, 17*(6), 514–517.

Rust, K., & Smith, R. O. (2006). Perspectives of outcome data from assistive technology developers. *Assistive Technology Outcomes and Benefits, 3*(1), 34–52.

Sackett, D. L., Straus, S. E., Richardson, W. S., Rosenberg, W., & Haynes, R. B. (2001). *Evidence-based medicine: How to practice and teach EBM.* London: Churchill-Livingstone.

Sander, A. M., Clark, A., Atchison, T., & Rueda, M. (2009). A web-based videoconferencing approach to training caregivers in rural areas to compensate for problems related to traumatic brain injury. *Journal of Head Trauma Rehabilitation, 24*(4), 248–261.

Scherer, M., Jutai, J., Fuhrer, M., Demers, L., & DeRuyter, F. (2007). A framework for modelling the selection of assistive technology devices (ATDs). *Disability and Rehabilitation: Assistive Technology, 2*(1), 1–8.

Scherer, M. J., Hart, T., Kirsch, N., & Schulthesis, M. (2005). Assistive technologies for cognitive disabilities. *Critical Reviews in Physical and Rehabilitation Medicine, 17,* 195–215.

Schmitter-Edgecombe, M., Fahy, J. F., Whelan, J. P., & Long, C. (1995). Memory remediation after severe closed head injury: Notebook training vs. supportive therapy. *Journal of Consulting and Clinical Psychology, 63*(3), 484–489.

Selznick, L., & Savage, R. C. (2000). Using self-monitoring procedures to increase on-task behavior with three adolescent boys with brain injury. *Behavioral Interventions, 15*(3), 243–260.

Simard, J. M., Wiederkehr, S., Bergeron, M. E., Turgeon, Y., Hudon, C., & Tremblay, I. (2010). Efficacy of a cognitive training programme for mild cognitive impairment: results of a randomised controlled study. *Neuropsychology Rehabilitation,* 2010 Jun; *20*(3), 377–405. Epub 2009 Dec 1.

Sirtori, V., Corbetta, D., Moja, L., & Gatti, R. (2009). Constraint-induced movement therapy for upper extremities in patients with stroke. *Stroke,* , xx–xx.

Sluijs, E. M. (1991). A checklist to assess patient education in physical therapy practice: Development and reliability. *Physical Therapy, 71,* 561–569.

Sluijs, E. M., & Knibbe, J. J. (1991). Patient compliance with exercises: Different theoretical approaches to short and long-term compliance. *Patient Education and Counseling, 17,* 191–204.

Sluijs, E. M., Kok, G. J., & van der Zee, J. (1993). Correlates of exercise compliance in physical therapy. *Physical Therapy, 73,* 771–786.

Smidt, N., de Vet, H. C. W., Bouter, L. M., & Dekker, J. (2005). Effectiveness of exercise therapy: A best-evidence summary of systematic reviews. *Australian Journal of Physiotherapy, 51,* 71–85.

Sohl, S. J., & Moyer, A. (2007). Tailored interventions to promote mammography screening: A meta-analytic review. *Preventive Medicine, 45*(4), 252–261.

Sohlberg, M. M. (2006). Evidence-based instructional techniques for training procedures and knowledge in persons with severe memory impairment. *Revista de Neuropsicologia, 1*(1), 14–19.

Sohlberg, M. M., Avery, J., Kennedy, M. R. T., Coelho, C., Ylvisaker, M., Turkstra, L., et al. (2003). Practice guidelines for direct attention training. *Journal of Medical Speech–Language Pathology, 11*(3), 19–39.

Sohlberg, M. M., Ehlhardt, L., & Kennedy, M. (2005). Instructional techniques in cognitive rehabilitation: A preliminary report. *Seminars in Speech and Language, 26*(4), 268–279.

Sohlberg, M. M., Kennedy, M. R. T., Avery, J., Coelho, C., Turkstra, L., Ylvisaker, M., et al. (2007). Evidence based practice for the use of external aids as a memory rehabilitation technique. *Journal of Medical Speech Pathology, 15*(1), xv–li.

Sohlberg, M. M., & Mateer, C. (2001a). *Attention Process Training Test.* Lash & Associates.

Sohlberg, M. M., & Mateer, C. A. (2001b). *Cognitive rehabilitation: An integrated neuropsychological approach.* New York: Guilford Press.

Sohlberg, M. M., Mateer, C. A., Penkman, L., Glang, A., & Todis, B. (1998). Awareness intervention: Who needs it? *Journal of Head Trauma Rehabilitation, 13*(5), 27–43.

Sohlberg, M. M., McLaughlin, K., Pavese, A., Heidrich, A., & Posner, M. (2000). Evaluation of attention process training in persons with acquired brain injury. *Journal of Clinical and Experimental Neuropsychology, 22*(5), 656–676.

Sohlberg, M. M., Sprunk, H., & Metzelaar, K. (1988). Efficacy of an external cueing system of an individual with severe frontal lobe damage. *Cognitive Rehabilitation, 6*(4), 36–41.

Souvignier, E., & Mokhlesgerami, J. (2006). Using self-regulation as a framework for implementing strategy-instruction to foster reading comprehension. *Learning and Instruction, 16,* 57–71.

Spikman, J. M., Boelen, D. H. E., Lamberts, K. F., Brouwer, W. H., & Fasottie, L. (2010). Effects of a multifaceted treatment program for executive dysfunction after acquired brain injury on indications of executive functioning in daily life. *Journal of the International Neuropsychological Society, 16,* 118–129.

Squire, L. R. (1992). Declarative and nondeclarative memory: Multiple brain systems supporting learning and memory. *Journal of Cognitive Neuroscience, 4,* 232–243.

Squires, E. J., Hunkin, N. M., & Parkin, A. J. (1996). Memory notebook training in a case of severe amnesia: Generalizing from paired associate learning to real life. *Neuropsychological Rehabilitation, 6*(1), 55–65.

Squires, E. J., Hunkin, N. M., & Parkin, A. J. (1997). Errorless learning of novel associations in amnesia. *Neuropsychologia, 35*(8), 1103–1111.

Stapleton, S., Adams, M., & Atterton, L. (2007). A mobile phone as a memory aid for individuals with traumatic brain injury: A preliminary investigation. *Brain Injury, 21*(4), 401–411.

Stark, C., Stark, S., & Gordon, B. (2005). New semantic learning and generalization in a patient with amnesia. *Neuropsychology, 19*(2), 139–151.

Stein, M., Carnine, D., & Dixon, R. (1998). Direct instruction: Integrating curriculum design and effective teaching practice. *Intervention in School and Clinic, 33,* 227–233.

Strangman, G., O'Neil-Pirozzi, T. M., Burke, D., Cristina, D., Goldstein, R., Rauch, S. L., et al. (2005). Functional neuroimaging and cognitive rehabilitation for people with traumatic brain injury. *American Journal of Physical Medicine and Rehabilitation, 84*(1), 62–75.

Surian, L., & Siegal, M. (2001). Sources of performance on theory of mind tasks in right hemisphere-damaged patients. *Brain and Language, 78,* 224–232.

Suzman, K. B., Morris, R. D., Morris, M. K., & Milan, M. A. (1997). Cognitive-behavioral remediation of problem solving deficits in children with acquired brain injury. *Journal of Behavioral Therapy and Experimental Psychiatry, 28,* 203–212.

Svoboda, E., Richards, B., Polsinelli, A., & Guger, S. (2009). A theory-driven training programme in the use of emerging commercial technology: Application to an adolescent with severe memory impairment. *Neuropsychological Rehabilitation, 20*(4), 562–586.

Swanson, H. L. (1999). Instructional components that predict treatment outcomes for students with learning disabilities: Support for the combined strategy and direct instruction model. *Learning Disabilities Research and Practice, 14*(3), 129–140.

Swanson, H. L. (2001). Searching for the best model for instructing students with learning disabilities. *Focus on Exceptional Children, 34*(2), 2–15.

Swanson, H. L., Carson, C., & Sachse-Lee, C. M. (1996). A selective synthesis of intervention research for students with learning disabilities. *School Psychology Review, 25,* 370–391.

Swanson, H. L., & Hoskyn, M. (1998). A synthesis of experimental intervention literature for students with learning disabilities: A meta-analysis of treatment outcomes. *Review of Educational Research, 68*(277–322).

Taber, T. A., Alberto, P. A., Seltzer, A., & Hughes, M. (2003). Obtaining assistance when lost in the community using cell phones. *Research and Practice for Persons with Severe Disabilities, 28,* 105–116.

Tailby, R., & Haslam, C. (2003). An investigation of errorless learning in memory-impaired patients: Improve the technique and clarifying the theory. *Neuropsychologia, 41,* 1230–1240.

Tate, R., Hodgkinson, A., Veerabangsa, A., & Maggiotto, S. (1999). Measuring psychosocial recovery after traumatic brain injury: Psychometric properties of a new scale. *Journal of Head Trauma Rehabilitation, 14*(6), 543–557.

Thoene, A. I. T., & Glisky, E. (1995). Learning name–face associations in memory impaired patients: A comparison of procedures. *Journal of the International Neuropsychological Society, 1*(1), 29–38.

Todd, M., & Barrow, C. (2008). Touch type: The acquisition of a useful complex perceptual–motor skill. *Neuropsychological Rehabilitation, 18*(4), 486–506.

Togher, L., Hand, L., & Code, C. (1996). A new perspective on the relationship between communication impairment and disempowerment following head injury in information exchanges. *Disability and Rehabilitation, 18*(11), 559–566.

Togher, L., McDonald, S., Code, C., & Grant, S. (2004). Training communication partners of people with traumatic brain injury: A randomised controlled trial. *Aphasiology, 18*(4), 313–335.

Tompkins, C. A., Scharp, V. L., Fassbinder, W., Meigh, K. M., & Armstrong, E. M. (2008). A different story on "theory of mind" deficit in adults with right hemisphere brain damage. *Aphasiology, 22*(1), 42–61.

Tonks, J., Williams, W. H., Frampton, I., Yates, P., & Slater, A. (2007). Reading emotions after child brain injury: A comparison between children with brain injury and non-injured controls. *Brain Injury, 21*(7), 731–739.

Trappe, S., Williamson, D., & Godard, M. (2002). Maintenance of whole muscle strength and size following resistance training in older men. *Journals of Gerontology Series A: Biological Sciences and Medical Sciences, 57,* B138–B143.

Troyer, A., Murphy, K., Anderson, N., Moscovitch, M., & Craik, F. (2008). Changing everyday memory behaviour in amnestic mild cognitive impairment: A randomized controlled trial. *Neuropsychological Rehabilitation, 18*(1), 65–88.

Tulving, E., & Markowitsch, H. J. (1998). Episodic and declarative memory: Role of the hippocampus. *Hippocampus, 8*(3), 198–204.

Turkstra, L. S. (2001). Partner effects in adolescent conversations. *Journal of Communication Disorders, 34*(1–2), 151–162.

Turkstra, L. S. (2008). Conversation-based assessment of social cognition in adults with traumatic brain injury. *Brain Injury, 22*(5), 397–409.

Turkstra, L. S., & Bourgeois, M. S. (2005). Intervention for a modern day HM: Errorless learning of practical goals. *Journal of Medical Speech Language Pathology, 13*(3), 205–212.

Turkstra, L. S., Dixon, T. M., & Baker, K. K. (2004). Theory of mind and social beliefs in adolescents with traumatic brain injury. *NeuroRehabilitation, 19*(3), 245–256.

Turkstra, L. S., Holland, A. L., & Bays, G. A. (2003). The neuroscience of recovery and rehabilitation: What have we learned from animal research? *Archives of Physical Medicine and Rehabilitation, 84*(4), 604–612.

Turkstra, L. S., McDonald, S., & DePompei, R. (2001). Social information processing in adolescents: Data from normally developing adolescents and preliminary data from their peers with traumatic brain injury. *Journal of Head Trauma Rehabilitation, 16*(5), 469–483.

van den Broek, M. D., Downes, J., Johnson, Z., Dayus, B., & Hilton, Z. (2000). Evaluation of an electronic memory aid in the neuropsychological rehabilitation of prospective memory deficits. *Brain Injury, 14,* 455–462.

Van der Linden, M., Meulemans, T., & Lorrain, D. (1994). Acquisition of new concepts by two amnesic patients. *Cortex, 30,* 305–317.

van Hout, M. S., Wekking, E. M., Berg, I. J., & Deelman, B. G. (2008). Psychosocial and cognitive rehabilitation of patients with solvent-induced chronic toxic encephalopathy: A randomised controlled study. *Psychotherapy and Psychosomatics, 77*(5), 289–297.

Vargha-Khadem, F., Gadian, D. G., Watkins, K. E., Connelly, A., Van Paesschen, W., & Mishkin, M. (1997). Differential effects of early hippocampal pathology on episodic and semantic memory. *Science, 277*(5324), 376–380.

Varni, J. W., Seid, M., & Rode, C. A. (1999). The PedsQL: Measurement model for the Pediatric Quality of Life inventory. *Medical Care, 37*(2), 126–139.

Velicer, W. F., Prochaska, J. O., & Redding, C. A. (2006). Tailored communications for smoking cessation: Past successes and future directions. *Drug and Alcohol Review, 25*(1), 49–57.

Verhaeghe, S., Defloor, T., & Grypdonck, M. (2005). Stress and coping among families of patients with traumatic brain injury: A review of the literature. *Journal of Clinical Nursing, 14*(8), 1004–1012.

von Cramon, D. Y., & Matthes-von Cramon, G. (1994). Back to work with a chronic dysexecutive syndrome? (A case report). *Neurpsychological Rehabilitation, 4,* 399–417.

von Cramon, D. Y., Matthes-von Cramon, G., & Mai, N. (1991). Problem solving deficits in brain injured patients: A therapeutic approach. *Neuropsychological Rehabilitation, 1,* 45–64.

Wade, S. L., Carey, J., & Wolfe, C. R. (2006). An online family intervention to reduce parental distress following pediatric brain injury. *Journal of Consulting and Clinical Psychology, 74*(3), 445–454.

Wade, T. K., & Troy, J. C. (2001). Mobile phones as a new memory aid: A preliminary investigation using case studies. *Brain Injury, 15,* 305–320.

Walz, N. C., Yeates, K. O., Taylor, H. G., Stancin, T., & Wade, S. L. (in press). Theory of mind skills 1 year after traumatic brain injury in 6- to 8-year-old children. *Journal of Neuropsychology.*

Warren, S. F., Fey, M. E., & Yoder, P. J. (2007). Differential treatment intensity research: A missing link to creating optimally effective communication interventions. *Mental Retardation and Developmental Disabilities, 13,* 70–77.

Webb, P. M., & Gluecauf, R. L. (1994). The effects of direct involvement in goal setting on rehabilitation outcome for persons with traumatic brain injuries. *Rehabilitation Psychology, 39,* 179–188.

Weeks, D. L., Brubaker, J., Byrt, J., Davis, M., Hamann, L., & Reagan, J. (2002). Videotape instruction versus illustrations for influencing quality of performance, motivation, and confidence to perform simple and complex exercises in health subjects. *Physiotherapy Theory and Practice, 18,* 65–73.

West, R. (1995). Compensatory strategies for age-associated memory impairment. In A. D. Baddeley, B. A. Wilson, & F. N. Watts (Eds.), *Handbook of memory disorders* (pp. 481–500). New York: Wiley.

Whiteneck, G. G., Charlifue, S. W., Gerhart, K. A., Overholser, J. D., & Richardson, G. N. (1992). Quantifying handicap: A new measure of long-term rehabilitation outcomes. *Archives of Physical Medicine and Rehabilitation, 73*(6), 519–526.

Whitman, T. L., Spence, B. H., & Maxwell, S. (1987). A comparison of external and self-instructional teaching formats with mentally retarded adults in a vocational training setting. *Research in Developmental Disabilities, 8,* 371–388.

Willer, B., Rosenthal, M., Kreutzer, J. S., & Gordon, W. A. (1993). Assessment of community integration following rehabilitation for traumatic brain injury. *Journal of Head Trauma Rehabilitation, 8*(2), 75–87.

Wilson, B. A. (1991). Long-term prognosis of patients with severe memory disorders. *Neuropsychological Rehabilitation, 1,* 117–134.

Wilson, B. A. (1992). Memory therapy in practice. In W. B. A. & N. Moffat (Eds.), *Clinical management of memory problems* (2nd ed., pp. 120–153). London: Chapman & Hall.

Wilson, B. A. (1995). Management and remediation of memory problems in brain-injured adults. In A. D. Baddeley, B. A. Wilson, & F. N. Watts (Eds.), *Handbook of memory disorders* (pp. 451–479). New York: Wiley.

Wilson, B. A. (2009). *Memory rehabilitation: Integrating theory and practice*. New York: Guilford Press.

Wilson, B. A., Baddeley, A., Evans, J., & Shiel, A. (1994). Errorless learning in the rehabilitation of memory impaired people. *Neuropsychological Rehabilitation, 4*(3), 307–326.

Wilson, B. A., Emslie, H. C., Quirk, K., & Evans, J. J. (2001). Reducing everyday memory and planning problems by means of a paging system: A randomized control crossover study. *Journal of Neurology, Neurosurgery and Psychiatry, 70*, 477–482.

Wilson, B. A., Evans, J. J., Emslie, H., & Malinek, V. (1997). Evaluation of NeuroPage: A new memory aid. *Journal of Neurology, Neurosurgery, and Psychiatry, 63*, 113–115.

Winter, J., & Hunkin, N. M. (1999). Relearning in Alzheimer's disease. *International Journal of Geriatric Psychiatry, 14*, 983–990.

World Health Organization. (2001). *International classification of functioning, disability and health* (Report). Geneva: Switzerland. Available at *www.who.int/icihd/index.htm*.

Wright, P., Rogers, N., Hall, C., Wilson, B., Evans, J., Emslie, H., et al. (2001). Comparison of pocket-computer memory aids for people with brain injury. *Brain Injury, 15*, 787–800.

Yancy, W. S., & Boan, J. (2006). Adherence to diet recommendations. In H. B. Bosworth, E. Z. Oddone, & M. Weinberger (Eds.), *Patient treatment adherence: Concepts, interventions, and management* (1 ed., pp. 95–123). Mahwah, NJ: Erlbaum.

Yasuda, K., Misu, T., Beckman, B., Watanabe, O., Ozawa, Y., & Nakamura, T. (2002). Use of an IC Recorder as a voice output memory aid for patients with prospective memory impairment. *Neuropsychological Rehabilitation, 12*, 155–166.

Yesavage, J. A. (1984). Relaxation and memory training in 39 elderly patients. *American Journal of Psychiatry, 141*, 778–781.

Ylvisaker, M., Coehlo, C., Kennedy, M., Sohlberg, M., Turkstra, L., Avery, J., et al. (2002). Reflections on evidence-based practice and rational clinical decision making. *Journal of Medical Speech–Language Pathology, 10*(3), 25–33.

Ylvisaker, M., & Feeney, T. J. (1998). *Collaborative brain injury intervention: Positive everyday routines*. San Diego, CA: Singular.

Ylvisaker, M., & Feeney, T. (2000). Reconstruction of identity after brain injury. *Brain Impairment, 1*(1), 12–28.

Ylvisaker, M., Feeney, T., & Capo, M. (2007). Long-term community supports for individuals with co-occurring disabilities after traumatic brain injury: Cost effectiveness and project-based intervention. *Brain Impairment, 8*(3), 276–292.

Ylvisaker, M., Turkstra, L. S., & Coelho, C. (2005). Behavioral and social interventions for individuals with traumatic brain injury: A summary of the research with clinical implications. *Seminars in Speech and Language, 26*(4), 256–267.

Young, A., Newcombe, F., de Haan, E., Small, M., & Hay, D. (1993). Face perception after brain injury. *Brain, 116*, 941–959.

Young, D. A., Zakzanis, K. K., Campbell, Z., Freyslinger, M. G., & Meichenbaum, D. H. (2002). Scaffolded instruction remediates Wisconsin Card Sorting Test deficits in schizophrenia: A comparison to other techniques. *Neuropsychological Rehabilitation, 12*(3), 257–287.

Zencius, A., Wesolowski, M. D., & Burke, W. H. (1990). A comparison of four memory strategies with traumatically brain-injured clients. *Brain Injury, 4*, 33–38.

Zlotowitz, S., Fallow, K., Illingworth, V., Liu, C., Geenwood, R., & Papps, B. (2010). Teaching action sequences after a comparison of modeling and moulding techniques. *Clinical Rehabilitation, 24*(7), 632–638.

Index